Statistics for Biology and Health

For other titles published in this series, go to
http://www.springer.com/series/2848

M. Elizabeth Halloran • Ira M. Longini, Jr.
Claudio J. Struchiner

Design and Analysis of Vaccine Studies

Springer

M. Elizabeth Halloran
Center for Statistics and Quantitative Infectious Diseases
University of Washington, and Fred Hutchinson Cancer Research Center
1100 Fairview Avenue N.
Seattle WA 98109-1024, USA
betz@u.washington.edu

Ira M. Longini, Jr.
Center for Statistics and Quantitative Infectious Diseases
University of Washington, and Fred Hutchinson Cancer Research Center
1100 Fairview Avenue N.
Seattle WA 98109-1024, USA
longini@scharp.org

Claudio J. Struchiner
Escola Nacional de Saúde Pública
Fundação Oswaldo Cruz
Rio de Janeiro RJ 21041-210, Brazil
stru@fiocruz.br

ISSN 1431-8776
ISBN 978-1-4614-2488-8 e-ISBN 978-0-387-68636-3
DOI 10.1007/978-0-387-68636-3
Springer New York Dordrecht Heidelberg London

Printed on acid-free paper

Springer is part of Springer Science+Business Media (www.springer.com)

Dedicated to those lives saved by vaccination

Preface

Immunization is one of the great advances in public health. Figure 0.1 shows a camel with a solar-powered refrigerator on his back carrying vaccines across a hot desert to the far reaches of civilization. Many vaccines contain live viruses that need to be kept cold, or the vaccine viruses will die, and the vaccines will lose their ability to produce an immune response. Thus a continuous chain of refrigeration, the cold chain, from the origin to delivery of some vaccines needs to be maintained. The inspiration of the camel image is that it represents the dedication of the world to bring vaccines to everyone.

The first major success, and the origin of the word vaccination (*vacca* for cow), was Jenner's introducing cowpox-based vaccine against smallpox in the late 18th century. After nearly a century hiatus, at the end of the 19th century, inoculations against cholera, typhoid, plague (caused by bacteria) and rabies (caused by a virus) were developed. By the early 20th century, statisticians of the stature of Karl Pearson, Major Greenwood, and Udny Yule were heartily involved in discussions of evaluating these vaccines in the field. In the 1920s, new vaccines included pertussis, diptheria, tetanus, and bacille Calmette-Guérin against tuberculosis. The 1930s saw development of yellow fever, influenza, and rickettsia vaccines. After World War II, the advent of cell cultures in which viruses could grow enabled production of polio vaccine and vaccines against measles, mumps, rubella, varicella, and adenovirus, among others (Plotkin et al 2008). Further new technologies allowed new generations of vaccines to replace old ones against particular pathogens. Research is ongoing on vaccines against malaria, HIV, and many others where the infectious agent outwits not only the researchers but also our natural immune response. Some vaccines are highly efficacious, and protective effects are recognizable even without subtle statistics. Others are less efficacious, so that study design and statistical analysis are more challenging.

Statistical inference made great advances in the 20th century and is continuing into the 21st (Efron 1998). The development of statistics, clinical trial design, and epidemiological methods in the 20th century had their counterparts in advances in vaccine studies as well. The focus has historically been on evaluating the direct protective effects of immunization in the individuals who are immunized. Due to the

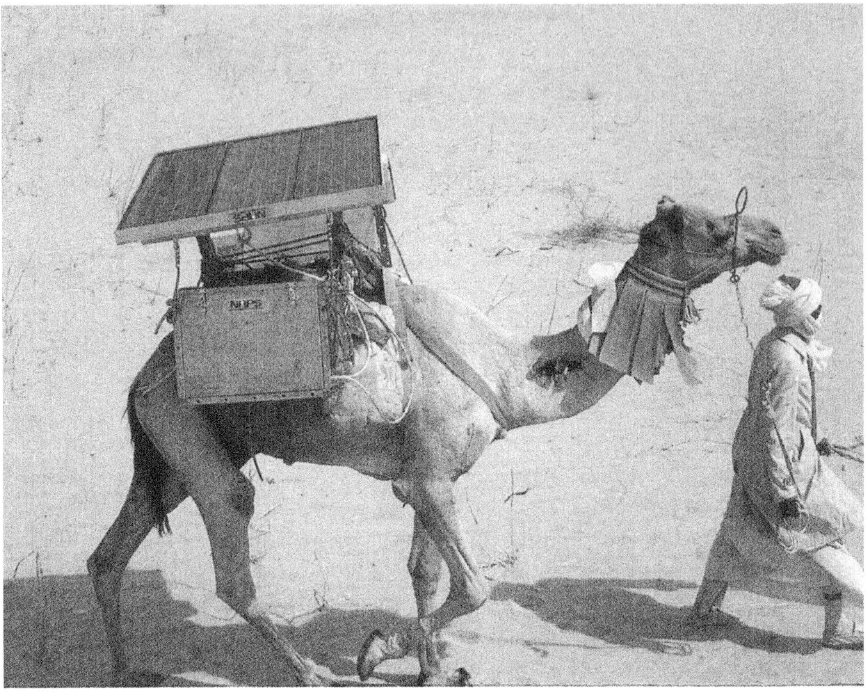

Fig. 0.1 Camel with a refrigerator powered by solar electricity with vaccines being kept in the cold chain. Image courtesy of Naps Systems Oy, Finland.

dependent happening nature of infectious diseases (Ross 1916), widespread immunization can have many different kinds of effects in populations, including in the unvaccinated individuals. Increasing interest is being given to the indirect effects of vaccination in addition to the direct protective effects. The same dependent happening structure results in what seems at first glance to be a single vaccine effect breaking into several that have an intrinsic relation to one another through the transmission system. And as we look closer, even the effects of vaccines at the individual level differentiate into a multidimensional palette. Because the effects of vaccination generally need to be evaluated in the field, studies take place in the wild, in a manner of speaking, where the dynamic population of the infectious agent of interest is circulating with the humans as hosts.

Our aim with this book is to present a unified view of vaccine effects and vaccine field studies, showing their relation to one another. We present a systematic framework of different effects of vaccination at the individual and at the population level. Different approaches to vaccine studies have been developed by researchers working on particular infectious diseases and particular vaccines. Our focus is on general principles that can be applied to many infectious diseases and many vaccines. As an analogy, people who specialize in particular musical instruments are pianists, clarinetists, or violinists. But then there are musicians who can play just about any instrument. Our view here is more from the point of view of the musician than of the violinist. The field is growing and changing rapidly. We hope the general framework provided here will prove useful in organizing, deepening, and refining your view about the effects of vaccination as it has ours.

This book is intended to serve three audiences: researchers specializing in vaccine and infectious disease studies; scientists interested in understanding vaccine and infectious disease studies; and students in statistics, biostatistics, epidemiology or infectious diseases. The prerequisites for understanding much of the material in the book are minimal. Our goal has been to explain most essential concepts in simple language. It is not necessary to understand statistical inference to understand the key ideas and overarching framework of the book. However, the models and analytic methods require comfort with equations and statistical inference, which we do not explain here. We do not assume knowledge of infectious disease epidemiology or immunology. We have included material on concepts of infectious disease epidemiology and dynamic models because they are integral to our approach. We also include a brief chapter on vaccines and the immune response to infection and vaccination for those readers not familiar with the somewhat daunting terminology of immunology.

Many colleagues have collaborated with us over the years on aspects of evaluating vaccine efficacy under dependent happenings. Jim Koopman, Eduardo Massad, and Marie-Pierre Préziosi have been particularly close and instrumental in our thinking. Many former graduate students contributed our research, including Cheryl Addy, Haitao Chu, Greg Golm, and Phil Rhodes. We particularly appreciate the ongoing research with Michael Hudgens and Yang Yang, former students, now our colleagues. Current students who contributed to this volume include Nicole Basta, Laura Matrajt, and Jonathan Sugimoto. We thank our colleague Wasima Rida for her dedication and thoughtful comments in reviewing most of the chapters on the long path to completion of this book. Finally, we appreciate our editor John Kimmel, whose (nearly infinite) patience and support saw us through.

Much of our research presented in this book was supported by the National Institute of Allergy and Infectious Disease grants R01-AI32042, R29-AI31057, and R01-40846, and by the Brazilian Reseach Council (CNPq), for which we are truly grateful.

Seattle, Rio de Janeiro,
August 2009

M. Elizabeth Halloran
Ira M. Longini, Jr.
Claudio J. Struchiner

Contents

Chapter 1
Introduction and Examples

1.1 The Need of Vaccine Studies Framework

Vaccine efficacy and vaccine effectiveness, VE, are generally estimated as one minus some measure of relative risk, *RR*, in the vaccinated group compared to the unvaccinated group:

$$VE = 1 - RR \,. \tag{1.1}$$

The groups being compared could be composed of individuals or of populations or communities.

Historically, interest focused on evaluating protective effects of vaccination. Study designs and statistical analysis played a role even with early immunizations. In the November 5, 1904, issue of the *British Medical Journal*, Karl Pearson published a criticism of the Antityphoid Committee's report on the anti-typhoid inoculation statistics from the South African War and from India. The Committee's report had recommended continued use of anti-typhoid inoculation. Armed with the correlation coefficient and the Theory of Correlation, Pearson reanalyzed the data and claimed that the correlations between protection against disease and inoculation ranged from 0.021 and 0.445, mostly around 0.1, with the correlations against mortality in a similar range. He compared these values with his analysis of the relation of recovery from smallpox with smallpox vaccination, which were in the range 0.576 and 0.769. Although he demurred somewhat due to his lack of knowledge about typhoid, he wrote that the results were such as "would justify suspension of [anti-typhoid inoculation] as a routine method" (p. 1244). He suggested "that a more effective serum or effective method of administration must be found before inoculation ought to become a routine practice in the army" (p. 1245). The immunologist A. E. Wright countered the following week, writing that although he did not understand the correlation coefficient, the mortality was reduced four- to sixfold, so that Pearson's conclusion must be wrong and that the Medical Advisory Board, who had heeded the criticism, could not "hide behind Professor Pearson's petticoats" (p. 1345). In addition to low correlation, Pearson was also arguing about the variability

M.E. Halloran et al., *Design and Analysis of Vaccine Studies*, Statistics for Biology and Health, DOI 10.1007/978-0-387-68636-3_1,

of the data. The argument continued in the *British Medical Journal* weekly for a full nine weeks until December 31, 1904, when Pearson finally gave up continuing the controversy after Wright refused to deal with what he had called "statistical minutiae" (p. 1614) and the "mathematical expression" (p. 1727).

In 1915, the statisticians Major Greenwood and Udny Yule published a treatise on "The Statistics of Anti-typhoid and Anti-cholera Inoculations, and the Interpretation of such Statistics in general" in the *Proceedings of the Royal Society of Medicine*. The 85-page paper begins, "Hardly any subjects within the range of preventive medicine is of more immediate importance than the methods of prophylaxis which ought to be adopted with respect to typhoid fever and cholera" (p. 113). In addition to presenting much of the data available at that time from field studies of anti-typhoid and anti-cholera inoculations, the paper develops a general approach to analyzing and interpreting such data. They lay out the conditions for valid inference and use the Pearson chi-square to calculate significance of the effect of inoculation against disease and mortality. They discuss heterogeneity in susceptibility and protection, and the role of a possible threshold immune level for protection.

Person-time analysis was not invented yet, so they discussed the problem of people being inoculated during the course of the epidemic, thus changing their status. Figure 1.1 shows two tables with data on anti-typhoid inoculation from the original Greenwood and Yule (1915) paper. The problem was whether to "class as inoculated those who were so at the date of the last return made or only those actually inoculated at the time of arrival on the foreign station" (p. 120). In the former case, shown in Table I of Figure 1.1, there may be an exaggeration of the "number of men who were inoculated during the whole exposure to infection," and in the latter case, shown in Table II, one would underestimate it "because many inoculations were done shortly after arrival"(p. 120).

In 1939, Kendrick and Eldering reported on a large pertussis vaccine field trial in Michigan. Figure 1.2 shows data from the Kendrick and Eldering (1939) paper on number of cases and person-time at risk in the pertussis trials. Figure 1.3 shows data from the Kendrick and Eldering (1939) paper on number of cases and number of exposures to pertussis in the trial. Vaccine efficacy can be computed using both kinds of data. It is not unusual for a vaccine study to present two such analyses, one that takes exposure to infection into account and one that does not. In this book, we present a framework that shows how the two approaches are related through assumptions about the underlying transmission. Both the Greenwood and Yule (1915) and the Kendrick and Eldering (1939) papers pre-date formal randomized studies and discuss in detail potential sources of bias and conditions for valid inference.

In 1954, an enormous field study of the Salk killed poliomyelitis vaccine was undertaken with great publicity in the United States. A total of 1,829,916 children participated in the nationwide study. The Summary Report of the trial by Thomas Francis, Jr. of the University of Michigan and colleagues was published early in 1955 in the *American Journal of Public Health*. In December 1955, K. A. Brownlee, a statistician at the University of Chicago, wrote an invited, highly critical review article for the *Journal of the American Statistical Association* on the statistics of the 1954 polio vaccine trials. The original design plan, called the Observed Control

TABLE I.—ANTI-TYPHOID COMMITTEE'S DATA.

First arrangement.

	Not attacked	Attacked	Total
Inoculated	10,322 ...	56 ...	10,378
Not inoculated	8,664 ...	272 ...	8,936
Total	18,986 ...	328 ...	19,314

$\chi^2 = 180{\cdot}38$. P = less than 0·0001.

TABLE II.—ANTI-TYPHOID COMMITTEE'S DATA.

Second arrangement.

	Not attacked	Attacked	Total
Inoculated	6,759 ...	56 ...	6,815
Not inoculated	11,396 ...	272 ...	11,668
Total	18,155 ...	328 ...	18,483

$\chi^2 = 56{\cdot}23$. P = less than 0·0001.

Fig. 1.1 Two tables from the original Greenwood and Yule (Proc R Soc Med, 8(part 2):113–194, 1915) paper containing data on anti-typhoid inoculations and attack rates in the military. The two tables represent two differing arrangements of the data. Reprinted with permission of the Royal Society of Medicine.

Study, was "to administer vaccine to children in the second grade of school; the corresponding first and third graders would not be inoculated, but would be kept under observation for the occurrence of poliomyelitis in comparison with the inoculated second graders" (Francis et al 1955, p. 1). This procedure was followed in 127 areas, mostly counties, in 33 states with a population of first, second, and third graders of 1,080,680.

During implementation of the trial, someone noticed this was not a blinded study and that other factors such as differences in age might lead to bias. So, to "have data which could provide an accurate gauge of the effect, free of possible bias in diagnosis and reporting" (Francis et al 1955, p. 1), the plan was changed in mid-stream. In the second plan, called the Placebo Control Study, "children of the first, second, and third grades would be combined. One half would receive vaccine; the other matching half, serving as strict controls, would receive a solution of similar appearance" (Francis et al 1955, p. 1). This procedure was followed in 84 areas in 11 states with a population of first, second, and third graders of 749,239. Fewer than half of the children were in the second part of the study. Brownlee's colorful judgment was that "It is a pity that explicit credit is not given to whomever was responsible for this change. However, only 41 percent of the trial was rescued and the remaining 59 percent blundered along its stupid and futile path" (Brownlee 1955, p. 1007). Despite possible design flaws, the vaccine was determined to have a 72% efficacy

TABLE 9

Incidence of pertussis in test and control groups based on period at risk

Time at risk and subsequent attack	Groups in study		
	Both groups	In-jected	Con-trol
Number of children	4212	1815	2397
Person-years	4575	2268	2307
Number of attacks	400	52	348
Annual pertussis attack rate per 100	8.7	2.3	15.1

PEARL KENDRICK AND GRACE ELDERING

Fig. 1.2 Results of a pertussis vaccine trial in Michigan, USA, in the 1930s (from Kendrick and Eldering, Am J Hyg, Sect B, 38:133, 1939, reprinted with permission of the American Journal of Epidemiology).

(lower 5% confidence limit 61) against paralytic polio in the Placebo Study Areas and 62% efficacy (lower 5% confidence limit 51) in the Observed Study Areas. The Salk killed injected polio vaccine and Sabin live oral polio vaccines transformed the epidemiology of the disease. Transmission of the three polio virus strains has been eliminated in most countries of the world.

In 1916, Sir Ronald Ross published his treatise on The Theory of Happenings in the *Proceedings of the Royal Society of London*. Ross had already been awarded the second Nobel prize in medicine for elucidating that malaria was transmitted by mosquitoes. He was also an amateur mathematician who developed the early mathematical models of malaria and interventions (Ross 1911; Ross 1915). In his quite general 1916 treatise, Ross wrote,

> Different kinds of happenings may be separated into two classes, namely (a) those in which the frequency of the happening is *independent* of the number of individuals already affected; and (b) those in which the frequency of the happening *depends on this quantity*...to class (b) belong infectious diseases, membership of societies and sects with propagandas, trade-unions, political parties, etc., due to propagation from within, that is, individual to individual. (p. 211)

TABLE 12

Persons in the study series exposed to pertussis according to "type" of exposure and proportions of those exposed who were attacked

	Classification according to history of exposure				No history of exposure
	Definite in own household	Definite in other household	Indefinite	Total	
Both groups					
No. of exposures...	243	161	166	570	3642
Attacks...	172	39	14	225	175
Per cent...	70.8	24.2	8.4	39.5	4.8
Vaccine group					
No. of exposures...	83	100	114	297	1518
Attacks...	29	5	4	38	14
Per cent...	34.9	5.0	3.5	12.8	0.9
Control group					
No. of exposures...	160	61	52	273	2124
Attacks...	143	34	10	187	161
Per cent...	89.4	55.7	19.2	68.5	7.6

PEARL KENDRICK AND GRACE ELDERING

Fig. 1.3 Results of a pertussis vaccine trial in Michigan, USA, in the 1930s (from Kendrick and Eldering, Am J Hyg, Sect B, 38:133,1939, reprinted with permission of the American Journal of Epidemiology).

The happenings are more commonly called events or occurrences today. In infectious diseases, most infection events are dependent happenings, depending on how many people or vectors are already infected.

Due to the dependent happenings in infectious diseases, vaccination can produce several different kinds of effects at both the individual and the population level. In an individual, vaccination can induce a biologically protective response against infection and/or disease, and/or reduce the degree or duration of infectiousness for other individuals. Widespread vaccination in a population can reduce transmission and produce indirect effects, even in individuals who were not vaccinated.

An early description of indirect and overall effects of immunization was given in 1792 by William Buchan, a Scottish physician in Edinburgh. Variolization, inoculation against smallpox using live smallpox virus, had been introduced from Turkey a half century earlier as a means to prevent severe smallpox and scarring.

> We have been the more full upon this subject [of the importance of smallpox inoculation] because the benefits of inoculation cannot be extended to society by an other means than making the practice general. While it is confined to a few, it must prove hurtful to the whole. By means of it the contagion is spread, and is communicated to many who otherwise never would have had the disease. Accordingly it is found that more die of the smallpox now than before inoculation was introduced; and this important discovery, by which alone more lives might be saved than by all the endeavors of the Faculty [of Medicine], is in a great measure lost by its benefits not being extended to the whole community. (p. 218)

This is an example illustrating that not all indirect and overall effects of immunization programs are necessarily beneficial.

During the 20th century, two for the most part distinct mathematical areas developed. One was in the fields of statistics and inference, including the development of the randomized trial, and further developments of clinical trials and epidemiological study design. The primary focus of vaccine studies was on evaluating direct protection in vaccinated compared with unvaccinated people. Most of these methods assumed an independent happening structure in the data. The underlying dynamics of transmission of the infectious agent did not play an important role. Epidemic theory made great advances in the 20th century as well. Both deterministic and stochastic models of infectious disease dynamics and interventions were developed. Especially with the advent of computers, models could become more complex. Epidemic theory and computer models could be used to study potential indirect effects of widespread vaccination or other interventions. However, the relation of the field studies, prospective data collection, statistical analysis and the underlying transmission dynamics remained largely unexplored.

In the latter decades of the 20th century, interest began to grow in evaluating more than just the direct protective effects of vaccination (Fine 1993; Clemens et al 1996). During the 1980's, hope flourished that effective malaria vaccines were imminent. The malaria parasite has three main stages of its life cycle in humans, one for infection, one for disease, and one for transmission to the mosquitoes. Vaccines were being developed to protect against each of the separate stages. The problem of designing studies to evaluate a vaccine that blocked transmission from humans to mosquitoes but did not confer direct protection to the immunized individual led naturally to the idea of using community-randomized designs to evaluate the reduction in overall incidence due to use of such a vaccine.

In the early 1990s the *Hemophilus influenzae b* (Hib) conjugate vaccines were introduced. Young children were vaccinated with the result that incidence of invasive disease in young infants nearly disappeared. This effect was apparently due to a large reduction in carriage of the infectious agent in the nasal passages (Adegbola et al 2005). More recently, similar phenomena are being observed with meningococcal conjugate vaccines (Ramsay et al 2003) and pneumococcal conjugate vaccines (Hennessy et al 2005). Thus, interest has grown in accurate evaluation of the changes in transmission and incidence of invasive disease by reducing carriage in contrast to just direct protection against invasive disease.

During a primary pneumococcal vaccine trial conducted in the 1990's, some concern developed about whether the number of events being observed in the study would be sufficient to support licensure of the vaccine. A community-randomized study was designed and implemented to evaluate the reduction in incidence of widespread vaccination, especially the reduction in the vaccinated children in the communities where vaccination was offered compared to the unvaccinated in the control communities (Moulton et al 2001). The idea of the study was that it would lend support to the primary study. However, the vaccine was licensed before completion of the community-randomized study, so that the latter trial was interrupted.

In general, interest in evaluating possible indirect effects of widespread vaccination either before or after licensure is growing. Currently it is generally believed that HIV vaccines will not prevent infection, but could limit growth of the virus in the blood and reduce infectiousness for others. Such vaccine could have potentially important public health benefits which would be good to evaluate prospectively. Influenza researchers have believed for decades that children are responsible for most of the transmission of influenza in the community (Monto et al 1969). Vaccination of children has been promoted as a public health measure to reduce transmission in adults and high-risk groups who might themselves not respond well to immunization. A community-based study in Texas to evaluate the effects of vaccinating schoolchildren against influenza on adults has been ongoing in Texas, USA, since 1998 (Piedra et al 2007).

Pertussis vaccines have been in widespread use since the 1930s. Considerable controversy raged over whether pertussis vaccination had any effect on the circulation of the bacteria on the population (Fine and Clarkson 1982). Indirect evidence based on population-dynamic arguments suggested that the circulation of the bacteria was not reduced, just serious disease. A study in Niakhar, Senegal, was conducted in the early 1990s of pertussis vaccination, in which the primary interest was in the protective effects of vaccination. The data had information on exposure to infection, thus also allowed estimation of the effect of the vaccine on reducing transmission from vaccinated breakthrough cases compared with transmission from unvaccinated cases (Préziosi and Halloran 2003a) as well as the effect of vaccination on the severity of disease in those who did develop pertussis (Préziosi and Halloran 2003b).

These are only a few recent examples of growing interest in evaluating more complex effects of vaccination in populations. Our goal in this book is to provide a systematic framework for understanding the different effects of vaccination and how they relate to one another through the underlying transmission dynamics and dependent happenings. We consider principles of study design and statistical analysis in this context.

1.2 Scope and Outline of the Book

Different types of studies are required for different phases of vaccine development. The statistical problems in vaccine studies range from small sample exact analysis for sample sizes of two to eight animals or people, to randomized field trials with hundreds to several thousands of people, to community trials with hundreds of thousands of participants, and finally to surveillance in populations with hundreds of millions of inhabitants. The early phase of vaccine development involves searching for candidate vaccine antigens. These include in vitro studies as well as testing in animals. More recently, designer approaches to vaccine discovery using computer models of various parts of the infectious agent and the immune system have been developed. Once a candidate antigen is found, then a vaccine is formulated. If appropriate animals are available for that particular infectious agent, then the vaccine candidate will be tested for safety, immunogenicity, and possibly efficacy against experimental challenge with the infectious agent.

Then the vaccine goes into humans for various phases of clinical testing. Phase I is primarily safety and possibly immunogenicity. Phase II studies are further safety and immunogenicity testing in humans. Phase III studies are generally field evaluations of direct protective efficacy, with further accumulation of safety data. Recently, there has been some discussion of integrating evaluation of indirect effects for some vaccines into Phase III studies. The Phase III studies are the field studies that are generally used to apply for licensure of a vaccine. Once a vaccine is licensed, then the efficacy and safety of the vaccine in regular usage is often monitored and evaluated using a variety of studies. The post-licensure studies are somewhat generically referred to as Phase IV studies. Phase II studies are generally not designed to be large enough to evaluate the protective efficacy of the vaccine. Phase IIb studies have been proposed that are something like proof-of-concept studies (Fleming 1996). They are powered possibly to estimate an effect with moderate significance. The idea is that the trial might be expanded to be larger if there is some evidence of an effect.

The Phases III and IV studies are the main focus of our book, in that we focus on field studies. In defining the various effects of vaccination and their relation to one another, we implicitly assume a randomized study, with observational studies being departures from the randomized study (Rosenbaum 1995). Departures from the randomized study can result in confounding and types of biases. Our general paradigm is that of causal inference. Aspects of our book are largely conceptual, showing the interface among study design, statistical analysis, and epidemic theory, and implications for interpretation. After giving an overview of the book, in the remainder of Chapter 1, we introduce some key definitions in infectious disease research and causal inference.

Chapter 2 presents a systematic framework for thinking about many of the different types of vaccination effects and the study designs and estimators used to evaluate them. This chapter is based on a paper by Halloran et al (1997) we call the Table Paper because it lays out a two-dimensional table (Table 2.2) showing several of the main vaccine efficacy and effectiveness estimators. Struchiner et al (1990) and Halloran and Struchiner (1991) introduced four basic study designs for dependent happenings for differentiating and evaluating direct effects and indirect, total, and overall population-level effects of vaccination. Motivated by the malaria vaccine discussions of the 1980s, Struchiner, Halloran and colleagues differentiated the efficacies of vaccines against infection, disease, and transmission (Struchiner et al 1989; Halloran et al 1989). Longini and Koopman (1982) proposed methods to analyze household studies in which information on contacts between infectives and susceptibles allow the estimation of the effect of covariates on the transmission probabilities and the probability of infection from the community. Rhodes et al (1996) showed formally the relation among the various estimators of protective effects of vaccination using counting process models to formulate the dependent happening relation. The framework in Chapter 2 is a unification of these various ideas. Much of the book expands those aspects presented within this framework. At the conceptual level, our emphasis is on the many different measures of vaccine efficacy and how they relate to each other.

Chapter 3 provides a brief introduction to the immune response to infection, the basis for the idea of prophylatic immunization, and a brief chronicle of the development of vaccines. This is intended to help the reader who does not know immunology and vaccines to be able to read the rest of the book. Vaccine safety is of key importance in vaccine studies. Preclinical animal studies and Phase I and II clinical trials are designed to evaluate immunogenicity and safety, thus are also included in Chapter 3. The idea of herd immunity, the level of immunity to an infectious agent in a population, in contrast to the immune response within an individual, is presented.

Chapter 4 introduces dynamic models and assumptions about mixing patterns in a population. The chapter focuses on the Reed–Frost model and stochastic, discrete-time methods. The chapter demonstrates randomness and the use of stochastic models to investigate direct, indirect, total, and overall effects of vaccination programs. The Reed–Frost model is the basis of estimation procedures in later chapters. Chapter 5 focuses on the basic reproductive number R_0 and the role of vaccination. A simple deterministic differential equation is presented, but such models do not play a large role in this book. These two chapters can be read on their own as an introduction to dynamic infectious disease models.

Chapters 6 through 9 focus on studies for evaluating the direct protective effects of vaccination. Chapter 6 presents the estimands and estimators for the measures of protective efficacy that do not condition on exposure to infection. Specifically, these include the most common estimators of vaccine efficacy based on the incidence rate, hazard rate, and cumulative incidence. Cumulative incidence is often called the attack rate in infectious diseases. Several examples of field studies are presented. The chapter covers general considerations of designing a study, including choice of populations and comparison populations, choice of outcomes, sample size determination, and randomized versus observational studies. Chapter 7 discusses different distributions of protection in a population and the implications for study design. The problems of estimating vaccine efficacy in the presence of heterogeneity in protection or exposure to infection or if efficacy wanes are considered. Chapter 8 considers case-control studies in vaccine evaluation. The choice of outcome measures and the use of validation sets for nonspecific outcomes are presented. Chapter 9 presents the evaluation of the effects of vaccination on post-infection outcomes, such as whether vaccination reduces the probability of clinical illness if a person becomes infected.

Chapters 10 through 12 present studies in households and other small transmission units and methods for their analysis. In particular, the chapters present methods for estimating vaccine efficacy for infectiousness and direct protective effects of vaccination when exposure to infection information is available. Chapter 10 presents several examples of studies in households and other small transmission units and discusses considerations of study design. Chapter 11 presents statistical analyses that assume the households or other transmission units are nested within a community. Chapter 12 presents methods of analysis assuming the households or transmission units are independent of each other, including the conventional secondary attack rate analysis.

Chapter 13 focuses on estimation of the indirect, total, and overall effects of widespread vaccination. The framework is the study designs for dependent happenings. The first part presents approaches comparing incidence before and after implementing a vaccination strategy in a population. The second part presents cluster-randomized designs in which several communities are compared.

Chapter 14 discusses issues related to the limitations of randomization to control for confounding and interpretation of estimates when baseline transmission, pre-existing immunity, and vaccine-induced protection interact to produce apparently different efficacy of vaccination in different populations. Chapter 15 focuses on evaluating immunological correlates and surrogates of protection.

Many new developments in vaccine trial design have been made possible by advances in biological specimen collection, immunology, and genome scans and sequencing of infectious agents. However, a future book on vaccine studies will be the one to cover these in more detail.

1.3 Concepts in Infectious Disease Research

Each infectious agent has its own life cycle, modes of transmission, population dynamics, evolutionary pressures, and molecular and immunological interaction with its host. The transmission cycle may involve a particular insect or other vector, and consequently its ecology. Studies and interventions need to take the particular transmission, dynamics, and natural history of each infectious agent into account.

However, some underlying principles of transmission and dynamics are common to many infectious diseases. These principles are captured in a wide variety of mathematical and statistical models. Because for the infectious agent, the human host population is its ecological niche, some of the principles come from general theories of populations, evolution, and ecology. (see Burnet and White 1972; McNeill 1976). Some of the principles have their origins in infectious disease epidemiology. In this section we present some general concepts of infectious disease epidemiology.

1.3.1 Transmission

Transmission from one host to another is fundamental to the survival strategy of most infectious agents. One measure of the success of an infectious agent is how effectively it is transmitted. The *transmission probability* p is the probability that, given a contact between an infective source and a susceptible host, successful transfer of the infectious agent will occur so that the susceptible host becomes infected. The transmission probability depends on the type and definition of a contact, the

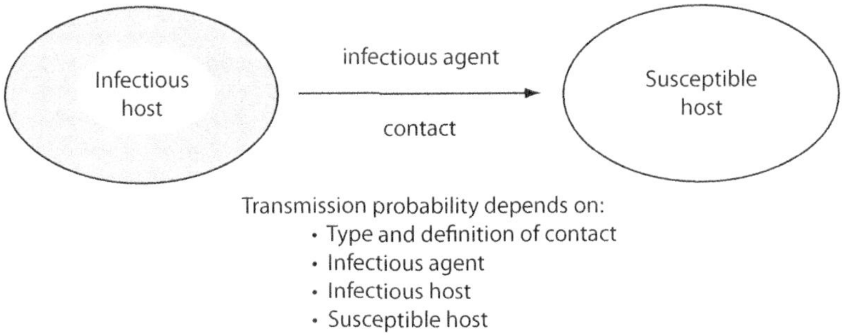

Fig. 1.4 Transmission from an infectious host to a susceptible host.

infectious agent of interest, characteristics of the infectious host, and characteristics of the susceptible host (Figure 1.4).

1.3.2 Time line of infection

Once a host is infected, the natural history of infection within a host can be described with reference to either infectiousness or disease (Figure 1.5). Both time lines begin with the successful infection of the susceptible host by the infectious agent. The natural history of infectiousness includes the *latent period*, the time interval from infection to becoming infectious, and the *infectious period*, during which time the host could infect another host or vector. Eventually the host becomes noninfectious, either by clearing the infection, possibly developing immunity, or by death. The host can also become noninfectious while still harboring the infectious agent. The host may also become an infectious *carrier* if he recovers from disease (ie, asymptomatic), but continues to carry the infection, often remaining infectious.

The natural history of disease in the infected host includes the *incubation period*, the time from infection to symptomatic disease, and the *symptomatic period*. The probability of developing symptomatic disease after becoming infected is the *pathogenicity* of the interaction of the infectious agent with the host. Eventually the host leaves the symptomatic state, either by recovering from the symptoms or by death. If the infectious agent has provoked an autoimmune response in the host, symptoms can continue even after the infectious agent is cleared. An *inapparent case* or *silent infection* is a successful infection that does not produce symptoms in the host. Inapparent cases can be infectious.

Although the disease process and its associated time line are important to the infected person and to a physician, the dynamics of infectiousness are important for propagation of the infectious agent and for public health. The relation of the two time lines to each other is specific to each infectious agent and can have important implications for study design, modeling, and public health.

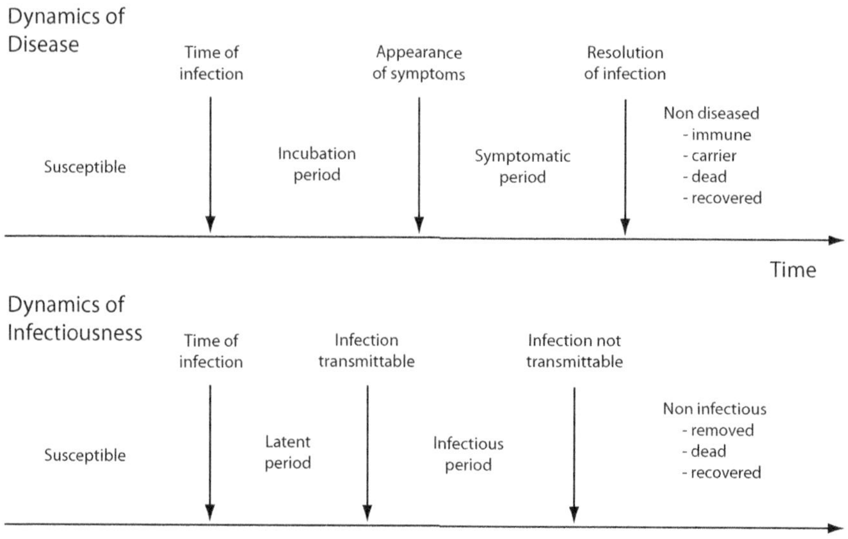

Fig. 1.5 General time lines of infection and disease.

HIV poses a particular problem for public health because the virus has a short latent period and a long incubation period. A person infected with HIV could infect many people before symptoms develop. *Plasmodium falciparum*, one of the parasites that causes human malaria, has an incubation period of about 14 days, but the infective stages of the parasite do not appear until about 10 days after the first symptoms. Thus, early treatment of symptoms with a drug that also kills or prevents infective stages could have an important effect on transmission.

The role of changes in behavior relative to the development of infectiousness and symptoms is also important. It is possible to add a third time line related to behavioral aspects, such as withdrawal to the home with symptoms, going to the hospital, or other aspects that influence how infectives expose other susceptibles, or how susceptibles alter their exposure. Figure 1.6 shows the consensus time line of infection, disease, and behavior of smallpox infection and disease for an unmodified smallpox, that is, the course in an infected individual who was not previously vaccinated (Longini et al 2007a). Once again the relation between the onset of infectiousness and symptoms is key because the symptoms influence the behavior.

Figure 1.7 shows a time line for influenza symptoms and the time course of viral shedding of six people infected with influenza. There is considerable uncertainty about how much of the infectiousness occurs before symptoms develop. This is important for choosing among public health interventions and for dynamic modeling.

Elveback et al (1976) developed an influenza model that distinguished between illness and infection attack rates. The infected people become infectious, but only a fraction of them develop overt disease. In many studies of infectious agents, it is easier to use overt disease as the outcome, rather than infection, because infection

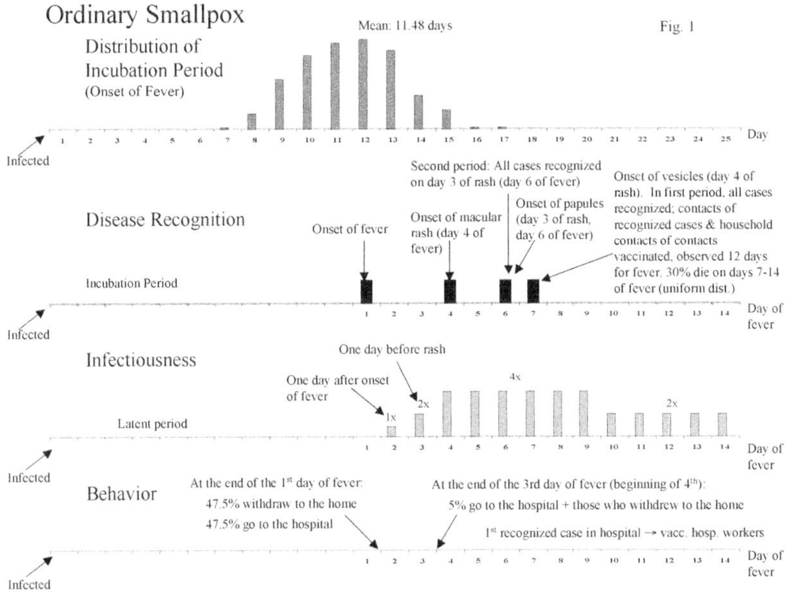

Fig. 1.6 Smallpox time lines of infection, disease, and behavior (Longini et al 2007a).

may be difficult to ascertain. If many infections are inapparent, however, using overt disease would result in underestimation of the level of exposure to infection in the population. Estimation of the incubation and latent periods can be difficult because the time of infection as well as the onset and end of infectiousness are often difficult to observe. Bayesian estimation methods can be used.

1.3.3 Basic reproductive number, R_0 and generation interval, T_g

Another key quantity in infectious disease epidemiology is the basic reproductive number, R_0, pronounced "are-zero" or "are-naught". R_0 is defined as the expected number of new infectious hosts that one typical infectious host will produce during his or her infectious period in a large population that is completely susceptible. This definition applies for small infectious agents, such as viruses and bacteria, also called *microparasites* (Anderson and May 1991) Understanding R_0 is important for public health applications and for describing the population biology of a parasite in a population of hosts. R_0 does not include the new cases produced by the secondary cases, or cases farther down the chain. It also does not include secondary cases who do not become infectious. R_0 is a measure of the transmissibility of the strain in

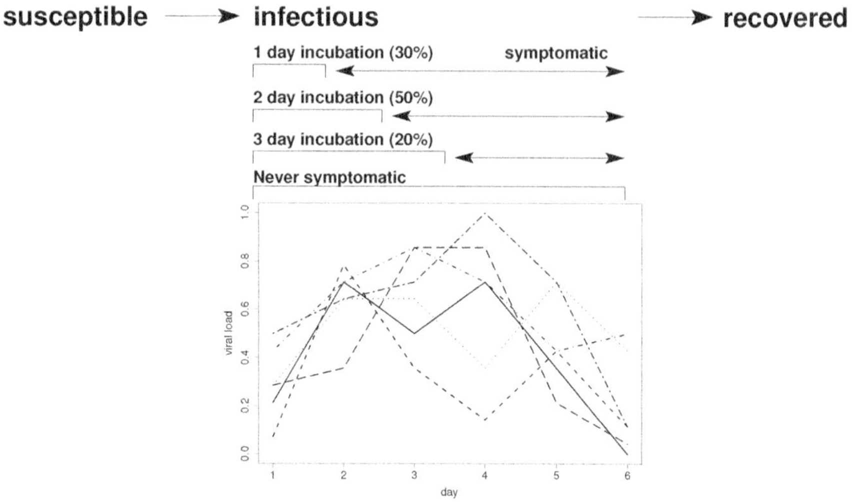

Fig. 1.7 Influenza time course of symptoms and viral shedding. The incubation period can be one, two, or three days. Some of the people remain asymptomatic. The graph shows the level of viral shedding of six people challenged with influenza virus (data from Baccam et al 2006).

the population and largely determines the proportion of the population that will be infected in an epidemic.

The generation time, or generation interval, T_g, is the average time between infection of an index case and infection of the secondary cases produced. Serial times, or serial intervals, are defined as the times between occurrence of observable events, such as the onset of clinical symptoms (Svensson 2006). If the generation interval is estimated based on the average time between the onset of symptoms or ascertainment of an index case and the onset of symptoms or ascertainment of the secondary cases produced, additional variability must be taken into account. The rate of growth of an epidemic is determined approximately by the ratio R_0/T_g (Fraser et al 2004). Because the generation time of influenza is on the order of 2 to 3 days, and that of smallpox is on the order of 10 to 14 days, influenza epidemics are much more explosive than a smallpox outbreak would be. The goal of intervention is to reduce R_0 so that $R_0 < 1$, which for simple assumptions about population mixing requires transmission rates to be reduced by a fraction $1 - 1/R_0$.

The concept of R_0 comes from general population theory and refers to the expected number of reproducing offspring that one reproducing member of the population will produce in the absence of overcrowding. With larger parasites such as worms, called *macroparasites*, R_0 is the expected number of mature female offspring that one female will produce in her lifetime. In macroparasitic diseases, the parasites are often distributed in a skewed fashion among their hosts which influences the design of intervention programs. We do not consider macroparasitic diseases in this book. Chapters 4 and 5 have more discussion of R_0.

1.4 Causal Inference and Vaccine Effects

In many parts of this book our approach draws on the potential outcomes approach to causal inference (Rubin 1980, Holland 1986, Robins 1986). Causal inference is a framework for carefully defining causal estimands, that is, the quantities that one wants to estimate, and then articulating the conditions and assumptions under which they can be estimated from the observed data. A potential outcome is the outcome that a person would have if a person received a particular treatment. Receiving the treatment does not necessarily occur. Suppose that infection, yes or no, is the outcome of interest. One can imagine that a person would have one potential outcome (not infected) if vaccinated and a possibly, but not necessarily, different (infected) potential outcome if that person were not vaccinated. Generally, in this framework, the potential outcomes are assumed to be determined before a person receives either treatment. That is, the potential outcomes are assumed fixed before any assignment to either vaccine or control. One can define the causal effect at the individual level. The individual causal effect of treatment A compared to treatment B is defined as the difference (or ratio) in the potential outcome under treatment A and the potential outcome under treatment B.

The Fundamental Problem of Causal Inference (Holland 1986) is that generally only one of the potential outcomes of an individual can be observed. That is, generally, if we assign a person to receive either vaccine or control, then we will observe the outcome under that assignment, but not observe the outcome under the other assignment. So, to define an effect that we can observe, we use a population of individuals. The population average causal effect (ACE) is the difference of the expectation of the potential outcomes if everyone received treatment A and the expectation of the potential outcomes if everyone received treatment B. It is still not possible to observe this. However, under two assumptions, we can estimate the population average causal effect from the observed data.

The first assumption generally made is that the treatment assignment in one person does not affect the potential outcome in another person. This was called the assumption of no interference by Cox (1958). Rubin (1980) called it the Stable Unit Treatment Assumption (SUTVA). Technically, SUTVA includes as well the assumption that all treatments and their potential outcomes are represented in the model, which we assume is true throughout. Then, if there are only two treatments, say, vaccine and control, then the representation with just two potential outcomes is adequate.

The second assumption required is the specification of the mechanism of assignment of the treatments to the individuals. A very useful assignment mechanism is randomization. Under the assumption of no interference between the individuals in the study, and the assumption that treatments A and B were assigned randomly, then the observed difference in the average outcome in individuals assigned A and the individuals assigned B is equal to the population average causal effect.

To formalize the above ideas, we need at least three elements in the model, a population of units, at least two treatments (the causes), and the response variables, or potential outcomes of interest. Suppose we have a population of individual people,

Table 1.1 Four kinds of people and the individual causal effects based on potential outcomes

Stratum	$Y(Z=1)$	$Y(Z=0)$	Causal Effect
Immune	0	0	0
Harmed	1	0	−1
Protected	0	1	1
Doomed	1	1	0

$i = 1,\ldots,n$. For simplicity, assume here just two levels of treatment Z, say, vaccine and control, denoted by $Z = 1$ for vaccine and $Z = 0$ for control. The two potential outcomes Y could be infected and not infected, represented by $Y = 1$ if infected and $Y = 0$ if not infected. Let $Y_i(Z = 1)$ and $Y_i(Z = 0)$ represent the potential outcomes for person i under vaccine and control. Then the *individual causal effect* in person i of vaccine compared with control is $Y_i(0) - Y_i(1)$. For example, if person i would be infected if he received control ($Y_i(0) = 1$) and he would not be infected if he received vaccine ($Y_i(1) = 0$), then the individual causal effect in person i is

$$Y_i(0) - Y_i(1) = 1 - 0 = 1. \tag{1.2}$$

Because the individual causal effects are not observable, we proceed to the population average causal effect. Assume that we randomly assign $n_0 = n/2$ of the population to vaccine and to control. Under the assumptions of SUTVA and randomization (and compliance), the population average causal effect is

$$\begin{aligned} E\{Y(0) - Y(1)\} &= E\{Y(0)\} - E\{Y(1)\} \\ &= E\{Y(0)|Z = 0\} - E\{Y(1)|Z = 1\} \\ &= \frac{\Sigma_{i=0}^{n_0} Y_i(0)|Z = 0}{n_0} - \frac{\Sigma_{i=0}^{n_0} Y_i(1)|Z = 1}{n_0}, \end{aligned} \tag{1.3}$$

which is identifiable from the observed data.

Four types of individuals are possible in the population defined by their pairs of potential outcomes under vaccine and control (Table 1.1). First, they could be uninfected whether they receive vaccine or control. These people are called immune (even outside the vaccine literature). They could be infected if they receive vaccine, but remain uninfected if they receive control. These people are considered harmed by the vaccine. They could remain uninfected if they receive vaccine, but become infected if they receive control, called protected by the vaccine. They could become infected under both vaccine and control. These people are called doomed. The causal inference framework based on potential outcomes induces an inherent heterogeneity in the population. In some infectious disease papers, the four types of people are called never infected, harmed, protected, and always infected.

The four different types of people are latent groups that cannot be identified without further assumptions. For example, if a vaccinated person becomes infected, that person could be either a person harmed by vaccination or a person doomed to become infected. If we make the assumption that the vaccine does not harm people, that is, there are no individuals in the harmed stratum, then we know that the infected vaccinated person must be in the doomed stratum. Also, under this assumption, we know that an unvaccinated person who does not get infected must be in the immune stratum. A vaccinated person who does not get infected, however, could belong to either the immune or the protected stratum.

The assumption of randomization to specify estimators of the estimands of interest in equation (1.3) demonstrates how randomization can serve as the point of departure for estimating effects of interest. Observational studies in which the vaccine assignment is not randomized are subject to biases, but can be viewed as departures from the randomized experiment. By making our assumptions about how an observational study departs from a randomized study explicit, we can understand how our estimates of the estimand of interest differ from what we might have observed in a randomized study.

The flavor of causal inference courses through various aspects of this book. Causal inference methods help in understanding vaccine effects on post-infection outcomes in Chapter 9. Causal inference underlies new approaches to evaluating immunological surrogates of protection in Chapter 15. Clearly, the assumption of no interference contradicts the situation in dependent happenings in infectious diseases (Halloran and Struchiner 1995). If the potential outcomes depend on the treatments that other people receive then people have more than just two potential outcomes (Rubin 1978). In Chapter 13, we consider relaxing the assumption of no interference to evaluate indirect, total, and overall effects within the causal inference framework. The potential outcome approach to causal inference is not everyone's cup of tea. Our goal in this book is to present many ideas related to evaluating vaccines within populations and make them accessible to a wide audience, so only parts of the book are expressly formulated in terms of causal inference. The simple statement of comparing what the outcome would be with vaccine compared to what it would have been with control, the basis of most vaccine studies, has an implicit reference to the framework of causal inference.

Problems

1.1. Consider the data from the pertussis vaccine trial in Figures 1.2 and 1.3.
(a) How do the attack rates in the children with definite exposure compare to the attack rates in children with no history of exposure in Figure 1.3?
(b) How do the attack rates in children with definite exposure in Figure 1.3 compare with the attack rates in Figure 1.2 where exposure is not taken into account?
(c) Compare the size of the denominators in different categories in the two figures.
(d) What could be possible sources of differences in estimates of vaccine efficacy based on data from the two figures?

1.2. Give one explanation for how widespread pertussis vaccination might substantially reduce the number of clinical cases in a population but not change the circulation of the bacteria.

1.3. Suppose in a population that $R_0 = 4$ for both mumps and HIV. What else do you need to know to be able to say something about the relative speed of the epidemics of the two infections?

1.4. From a public health perspective, would you say that it is better the latent period be shorter than the incubation period or vice versa? Why?

1.5. To which two strata in Table 1.1 could an unvaccinated person who becomes infected belong?

Chapter 2
Overview of Vaccine Effects and Study Designs

2.1 Introduction

In this chapter, we present a systematic framework showing the relation among many of the different vaccination effects and the parameters and study designs to estimate them. This framework provides a structure for thinking about the different vaccine effects of interest and how they are related to one another. We present different versions of vaccine efficacy and effectiveness as one minus some measure of relative risk, *RR*:

$$VE = 1 - RR .$$

We focus on the relation between the vaccine effects of interest and the choice of comparison groups, the unit of observation, the choice of parameter, and the amount of information about the transmission system required for estimation. The framework draws on the dependent happening relation in infectious diseases. Although the framework is not exhaustive, many designs not considered explicitly in this overview are special cases of these general designs. Our primary concern in this chapter is conceptual. Details of study design and methods of estimation and inference are left to following chapters.

2.2 Vaccine Effects of Interest

Table 2.1 lists several different vaccine effects. Historically, the primary focus has been how well vaccination protects the vaccinated individual. VE_S, the vaccine efficacy for susceptibility, is a measure of how protective vaccination is against infection. With most infectious agents, the major interest is in preventing clinical illness. In evaluating vaccines against such infectious agents, such as measles, influenza, or pertussis, ascertainment is often by observing individuals clinically, who then might have a biological test done to confirm the infectious agent under study. In this case,

M.E. Halloran et al., *Design and Analysis of Vaccine Studies*, Statistics for Biology and Health, DOI 10.1007/978-0-387-68636-3_2,

Table 2.1 Vaccine effects of interest

Symbol	Definition
VE_S	Vaccine efficacy for susceptibility
VE_{SP}	Vaccine efficacy for susceptibility to disease
VE_{col}	Vaccine efficacy for colonization
VE_P	Vaccine efficacy for progression, pathogenicity
VE_I	Vaccine efficacy for infectiousness
VE_T	Total vaccine efficacy
VE_{IIa}	Indirect effects of vaccination in those not vaccinated
VE_{IIb}	Total effects of vaccination in those vaccinated
VE_{III}	Overall population-level effects

asymptomatic infections would not be ascertained. VE_{SP} denotes vaccine efficacy against disease. However, many times, both in this book and the literature in general, the distinction between the two is made clear simply by the case definition used in the study and the ascertainment method. Unless required for clarity or because the discussion is about the distinction of the two, we use VE_S to represent both VE_S and VE_{SP} in many places.

VE_{col} measures the efficacy against colonization (Auranen et al 2000, Käyhty et al 2006). Many infectious agents, such as pneumococcal, meningococcal, and *Hemophilus influenzae b* bacteria, colonize the nose and throat passages without causing overt disease. Colonized individuals generally are asymptomatic, but they play a central role in transmission. They can transmit to other susceptible individuals who in their turn develop severe disease. Recent interest is growing in evaluating the effect of vaccination on colonization. It is an aim of one of the Gates' Grand Challenge Grants. (See www.pneumocarr.org in Finland.) Pneumococcal and meningococcal carriage acquisition rates can be estimated conditional on exposure to infection or unconditionally. The rate of acquisition of pneumococcal carriage can also be used as the outcome measure to estimate vaccine efficacy, VE_{acq} (Rinta-Kokko et al 2009).

VE_P, vaccine efficacy for progression or pathogenicity, measures the efficacy of vaccination in preventing a post-infection outcome (Halloran et al 1994c). Depending on the situation, the measure of interest can be the effect of prophylactic vaccination on the rate or probability of progressing to disease, conditional on being infected. If ascertainment is on disease, VE_P could be a measure of the effect of vaccination on the probability of severe disease. VE_P could also measure the reduction in duration of being infected, such as in pneumococcal colonization. Although VE_S, VE_{SP}, and VE_P are all measures of the direct protective effects of vaccination, there is an important difference. The main distinction between VE_S or VE_{SP} and in contrast to VE_P is that studies to estimate VE_S and VE_{SP} evaluate an outcome in participants who are susceptible to infection, whereas studies to estimate VE_P evaluate an outcome in participants who are already infected. The denominators in the two different types of studies are different. In randomized studies, as long as the outcome is the first outcome of interest after randomization, whether infection,

VE_S, or disease, VE_{SP}, the validity of the comparison is preserved. However, the exposure to infection needs to be taken into account.

A vaccinated person who becomes infected may be less infectious to other susceptibles or be infectious for a shorter period of time. The vaccine efficacy for infectiousness, VE_I, measures the reduction in the ability of a vaccinated infected person compared to an unvaccinated infected person to transmit the infectious agent to others. The combined effect of having both individuals in a contact being vaccinated compared to neither being vaccinated is denoted by VE_T. Both VE_I and VE_T are of interest because a vaccine that reduces infectiousness could have important public health consequences (Halloran et al 1994c; Farrington 2003).

Widespread vaccination can have indirect effects for unvaccinated people as well as for vaccinated people. The indirect effects are due to the change in collective level of immunity in the population, the herd immunity, due to vaccination. Differentiation of the population-level effects in the unvaccinated and vaccinated groups is important because they might not be the same. The former is called indirect vaccination effectiveness, VE_{IIa}, the latter total vaccination effectiveness, VE_{IIb}. The overall effectiveness of a vaccination strategy or allocation within a particular population, VE_{III}, is the weighted average of the outcomes in the vaccinated and the unvaccinated people

To evaluate direct protective effects of vaccination, VE_S, VE_{SP}, and VE_P, usually the individual is the unit of observation. To evaluate VE_I, generally small transmission units, such as households or partnerships in which contacts can be defined, are needed (Fine et al 1988; Préziosi and Halloran 2003b; Halloran et al 2003b). This type of study in small transmission units can also be used to evaluate VE_S or VE_{SP}. To evaluate the population level effects, the unit of observation becomes the population, so that generally several populations need to be included in the study. Table 2.2 provides an overview of several different types of effects and the parameters used to estimate the effects.

2.3 Vaccine Efficacy for Susceptibility, VE_S (VE_{SP})

We first consider study designs for estimating the protective effects of vaccination, VE_S (VE_{SP}). In Table 2.2, these are represented in the column labeled "susceptibility". The estimates of VE_S are obtained from the relative risk of infection or disease in the vaccinated individuals compared with the unvaccinated individuals:

$$VE_S = 1 - \frac{\text{R(vaccinated people)}}{\text{R(unvaccinated people)}},$$

where R denotes one of the measures of risk. The measure of risk can be a form of the transmission probability, which conditions on exposure to infection, or the incidence rate, hazard rate, or cumulative incidence (attack rate), which do not condition on exposure to infection. In Table 2.2, the amount of information about the transmission system required for the efficacy estimates decreases from Level I in the top row to Level IV in the bottom row.

2.3.1 VE_S conditional on knowledge of exposure to infection

The top row of Table 2.2 contains measures of VE that rely on information about exposure to infection and contacts between infectious individuals and susceptible individuals. The first is a measure of VE_S based on the transmission probability, $VE_{S,p}$. Let the *transmission probability*, denoted p_{ij}, be the probability that, conditional upon a contact between an infective source with covariate status i and a susceptible host with covariate status j, successful transfer and establishment of the infectious agent will occur. A related concept is the *secondary attack rate* (SAR_{ij}), defined as the proportion of susceptibles with covariate status j making contact with an infectious person of covariate status i who becomes infected. The SAR is a special case of the transmission probability.

Let 0 and 1 denote being unvaccinated and vaccinated. Then, for example, p_{01} denotes the transmission probability per contact from an unvaccinated infective person to a vaccinated uninfected person. Let $p_{.0}$ and $p_{.1}$ denote the transmission probability to unvaccinated and vaccinated susceptibles, where the dot in the subscript can denote any vaccine status or an average across the population.

Then $VE_{S,p}$ based on the transmission probability or secondary attack rate (Table 2.2, top row) is estimated from

$$VE_{S,p} = 1 - \frac{p_{.1}}{p_{.0}} = 1 - \frac{\frac{\text{vaccinated infections}}{\text{vaccinated contacts}}}{\frac{\text{unvaccinated infections}}{\text{unvaccinated contacts}}}$$

or

$$VE_{S,SAR} = 1 - \frac{SAR_{.1}}{SAR_{.0}} = 1 - \frac{\frac{\text{vaccinated infections}}{\text{vaccinated contacts}}}{\frac{\text{unvaccinated infections}}{\text{unvaccinated contacts}}}.$$

Estimating vaccine efficacy from the transmission probability ratios requires information on who is infectious and when, and whom they contact and how. The concept of a *contact* is very broad and must be defined in each particular study. Often it is defined for individuals within a small transmission unit such as a household or sexual partnership.

Table 2.2 Parameters used for measuring various effects of vaccination. The levels form a hierarchy, with higher levels requiring less information about the transmission system, with only level I requiring actual contact information*.

Level	Parameter Choice	Comparison Groups and Effect			
		Susceptibility	Infectiousness	Combined Change in Susceptibility and Infectiousness	
	Conditional on exposure to infection:				
I	Transmission probability, p Secondary attack rate, SAR	$VE_{S.p}\dagger = 1 - \frac{p_{\cdot 0}}{p_{\cdot 1}}$	$VE_{I.p} = 1 - \frac{p_{1\cdot}}{p_{0\cdot}}$	$VE_{T.p} = 1 - \frac{p_{11}}{p_{00}}$	
		Study Design			
		I Direct	IIa Indirect	IIb Total	III Overall
	Unconditional:				
II	Incidence rate, IR	$VE_{S.IR} = 1 - \frac{IR_{A1}}{IR_{A0}}$	$VE_{IIa.IR} = 1 - \frac{IR_{A0}}{IR_{B0}}$	$VE_{IIb.IR} = 1 - \frac{IR_{A1}}{IR_{B0}}$	$VE_{III.IR} = 1 - \frac{IR_{A\cdot}}{IR_{B\cdot}}$
	Hazard rate, λ	$VE_{S.\lambda} = 1 - \frac{\lambda_{A1}}{\lambda_{A0}}$	$VE_{IIa.\lambda} = 1 - \frac{\lambda_{A0}}{\lambda_{B0}}$	$VE_{IIb.\lambda} = 1 - \frac{\lambda_{A1}}{\lambda_{B0}}$	$VE_{III.\lambda} = 1 - \frac{\lambda_{A\cdot}}{\lambda_{B\cdot}}$
III	Proportional hazards, PH	$VE_{S.PH} = 1 - e^{\beta_1}$	NA	NA	NA
IV	Cumulative incidence, CI Attack rates, AR	$VE_{S.CI} = 1 - \frac{CI_{A1}}{CI_{A0}}$	$VE_{IIa.CI} = 1 - \frac{CI_{A0}}{CI_{B0}}$	$VE_{IIb.CI} = 1 - \frac{CI_{A1}}{CI_{B0}}$	$VE_{III.CI} = 1 - \frac{CI_{A\cdot}}{CI_{B\cdot}}$

* From Halloran et al 1997. The subscripts 0 and 1 denote unvaccinated and vaccinated people, respectively. Population A contains both vaccinated and unvaccinated people. All people in population B are unvaccinated (see Figure 2.3). The subscripts S, I, and T denote susceptibility, infectiousness, and combined effects. The Cox proportional hazards estimator is denoted by e^{β_1}. Time has been omitted from the table for notational clarity.

† Vaccine efficacy/effectiveness; NA, not applicable

There are two main ways to design a study to estimate the relative transmission probabilities. The first method, called the secondary attack rate (Fox et al 1970; Fine et al 1988), or case-contact rate method, has been used since the pertussis vaccine trials in the 1930s (Kendrick and Eldering 1939) to estimate vaccine efficacy. Another method of estimating the transmission probability is based on the Bernoulli model. In this case, we observe susceptible people, count the number of contacts they make with infectives, count the number of these susceptible people who become infected, and use a transmission model to estimate the transmission probability and related covariate effects. These approaches are presented in more detail in Chapters 4 and 10 through 12.

2.3.2 *VE_S not conditional on knowledge of exposure to infection*

Information on exposure to infection is often difficult or impossible to collect. More commonly, studies are designed to estimate VE_S from events per person-time of potential rather than actual exposure or simply from the proportion of people who become infected in the vaccinated compared to the unvaccinated groups. Standard parameters for estimating VE_S that do not require exposure to infection information are incidence rates, hazard rates, or cumulative incidence (attack rate).

In estimating direct protective effects of vaccination, Greenwood and Yule (1915) gave three conditions necessary for valid inference:

1. The persons must be, *in all material respects,* alike.
2. The effective exposure to the disease must be identical in the case of inoculated and uninoculated persons.
3. The criteria of the fact of inoculation and of the fact of the disease having occurred must be independent.

Double-masked randomized trials are designed to ensure that these criteria are met. If the criteria are met, and the vaccinated and unvaccinated groups are equally exposed to infection, any differences in the risk in the two groups is likely due to the biological effects of the vaccine.

Primary vaccine efficacy studies often report $VE_{S,IR}$ based on relative events per person-time,

$$VE_{S,IR} = 1 - \frac{\text{vaccinated events/person-time}}{\text{unvaccinated events/person-time}}. \tag{2.1}$$

The usual assumption is that the numbers of events follow a Poisson distribution. Similarly, investigators may estimate the hazard rates in the vaccinated and unvaccinated, $\lambda_1(t)$ and $\lambda_0(t)$, using survival analysis methods. Then the VE_S is based on the hazard rate ratio

$$VE_{S,\lambda}(t) = 1 - \frac{\lambda_1(t)}{\lambda_0(t)}. \tag{2.2}$$

When covariates such as age and gender are added, the analyses are stratified by the covariates or Poisson regression can be used. Under the assumption that the effect of the vaccine is multiplicative, constant, and homogeneous, the Cox proportional hazards model can be used to estimate $\text{VE}_{S,PH}$. In this case, it is not necessary to estimate the hazard rate in the unvaccinated group, but only the relative hazard rate. This requires only the ordering of the infection times. Covariates, including time-dependent covariates, can easily be incorporated using standard software.

In an early example of estimating $\text{VE}_{S,IR}$, the study by Kendrick and Eldering (1939) of pertussis vaccine reported the number of cases per person-time (Figure 1.2). The study is described in Section 10.2.2. The vaccinated and control groups had 1815 and 2397 children, respectively, who contributed 2268 and 2307 person-years at risk. There were 52 cases in the vaccinated and 348 cases in the control group, so

$$\widehat{\text{VE}}_{S,IR} = 1 - \frac{\frac{52 \text{ cases}}{2268 \text{ person-years}}}{\frac{348 \text{ cases}}{2307 \text{ person-years}}} = 0.85 \tag{2.3}$$

More recently, Urdaneta et al. (1998) presented estimates of $\text{VE}_{S,IR}$ as the result of a randomized, placebo-controlled field trial of SPf66 malaria vaccine in Costa Marques, Rondonia, Brazil. A total of 572 participants completed the three-dose vaccine schedule and were followed for 18 months. The 287 vaccinated individuals contributed a total of 12,178 person-weeks at risk, and 76 first *P. falciparum* malaria episodes were observed among them. In the placebo group, 285 individuals contributed 11,698 person-weeks at risk and 85 cases leading to an estimate of $\widehat{\text{VE}}_{S,IR} = 0.14$.

In some studies, it is possible to compute both a conditional and an unconditional estimate of vaccine efficacy from a single study. The Kendrick and Eldering (1939) study on pertussis vaccine also had information on children who had been exposed to pertussis within their own households (Figure 1.3). In the vaccinated group, 29 of 83 exposed children developed pertussis, and 143 of 160 exposed children in the unvaccinated group developed pertussis. Thus, the estimate of $\text{VE}_{S,p}$ is

$$\widehat{\text{VE}}_{S,p} = 1 - \frac{29 \text{ cases}/83 \text{ vac exposed}}{143 \text{ cases}/160 \text{ unvac exposed}} = 0.61\ . \tag{2.4}$$

Although everyone is included in the estimate of $\text{VE}_{S,IR}$, only the children with presumed exposure to infection are included in the $\text{VE}_{S,p}$ estimate. The interpretations of the two estimates are also different, because one measures the protection conferred as measured by infections per person time and the other by the probability of an infection per potentially infectious contact.

Estimation of $\text{VE}_{S,CI}(T)$ based on the cumulative incidence requires only information about whether persons are infected by the end of the study at time T, that is, final value data:

$$VE_{S,CI}(T) = 1 - \frac{\text{vaccinated infection events/persons–at–risk}}{\text{unvaccinated infection events/persons–at–risk}}$$
$$= 1 - \frac{CI_1(T)}{CI_0(T)} . \quad (2.5)$$

As an example, Greenwood and Yule (1915) used the cumulative incidence in studying the efficacy of anti-typhoid inoculation in the troops in the early part of the twentieth century (Figure 1.1). In one analysis, Greenwood and Yule assumed that the denominators were based on the vaccinated and unvaccinated groups at the beginning of the study. They had 56 cases of typhoid in 10,378 vaccinated soldiers, and 272 cases in 8936 unvaccinated soldiers. The estimated efficacy based on these numbers is

$$\widehat{\mathrm{VE}}_{S,CI}(T) = 1 - \frac{56 \text{ cases}/10,378 \text{ at-risk}}{272 \text{ cases}/8936 \text{ at-risk}} = 0.82 . \quad (2.6)$$

A more recent example is from a double-blinded randomized trial of live attenuated influenza vaccine compared with inactivated influenza vaccine in children (Belshe et al 2007). In this trial, of the 3936 children who received inactivated vaccine, 338 developed culture-confirmed cases of influenza. Of the 3912 children who received live-attenuated vaccine, 153 cases developed. Based on these numbers,

$$\widehat{\mathrm{VE}}_{S,CI}(T) = 1 - \frac{153 \text{ cases}/3912 \text{ at-risk}}{338 \text{ cases}/3936 \text{ at-risk}} = 0.54 .$$

This is called the relative efficacy of two vaccines, rather than the absolute efficacy, because there is no control or placebo group.

Which method is used to estimate VE_S (VE_{SP}) in a particular study depends on the type and duration of the study, the infectious agent and its transmission mode, the resources available, and the assumptions of the distribution of protection within the vaccinated group. Chapters 6 through 8 consider estimation of VE_S from the unconditional parameters in detail.

2.4 Hierarchy of VE_S Measures

The different VE_S parameters require differing levels of information and make different demands on study design and data collection (Rhodes et al 1996). The levels I through IV in Table 2.2 form a hierarchy, with higher levels requiring less information about the transmission system, and only Level I requiring actual contact information. Because $\mathrm{VE}_{S,p}$ based on the transmission probability is defined conditional on exposure to infection, it is called a conditional parameter, and the other measures are called unconditional parameters. Incidence rates or hazard rates require the time to event and the period of potential exposure of each person under study. The hazard rate in infectious diseases is often called the *force of infection*. A

Cox proportional hazards model requires only the ordering of the event times. An estimate of cumulative incidence requires only final value data, that is, whether an infection occurred by the end of the study. Correspondingly, in Table 2.2, $VE_{S,IR}$ based on incidence rates and $VE_{S,\lambda}$ are Level II parameters, $VE_{S,PH}$ based on Cox proportional hazards is Level III, and $VE_{S,CI}$ based on cumulative incidence or final value data is Level IV.

Because of the dependent happening structure of events in infectious diseases, there is an intrinsic relation among the different parameters on which the VE_S estimators are based. Understanding this relation helps to see the relation of the different estimators of VE_S to one another. Figure 2.1 illustrates the dependent happening relation of the hierarchy of parameters to one another. Section 2.9 develops the relation formally.

Let p_{ij} be the transmission probability as defined above. Let c denote the contact rate in a population assuming that people are randomly mixing, and let $P(t)$ denote the prevalence of infectives at time t. Then the hazard rate $\lambda(t)$ (or incidence rate or force of infection) at time t can be expressed as the product of the contact rate, the transmission probability, and the probability that a contact is infectious:

$$\lambda(t) = cp_{ij}P(t). \tag{2.7}$$

So even if the different components of the hazard rate are not measured, we can consider the underlying process that is producing the infections we observe. Similarly, the cumulative incidence, $CI(T)$, at some time T is a function of the hazard rate during the follow-up period, and thus also a function of the transmission probability, contact rate, and prevalence of infection in the contacts. Even though the cumulative incidence estimate is a sort of black-box estimator, it is useful in vaccine studies to think about the underlying transmission system that would produce the observed final values.

Expression (2.7) represents the fundamental dependent happening relation of Ross (1916). The frequency of happenings in the susceptible individuals depends on the number already affected, in this case, the prevalence of infective individuals in the people making contact with the susceptible individuals. The different estimators do not require information about the contacts or the prevalence of infectious people necessarily. However, interpretation of the estimates can vary depending on the assumptions about the underlying transmission system.

2.5 Vaccine Efficacy for Infectiousness, VE_I

The efficacy of a vaccine in reducing infectiousness, VE_I, can be estimated epidemiologically by comparing the per-contact transmission probability from vaccinated people who become infected with the transmission probability from unvaccinated people who become infected. The relative risk comparison groups are defined according to the vaccination status of the infectious person contacting the susceptible

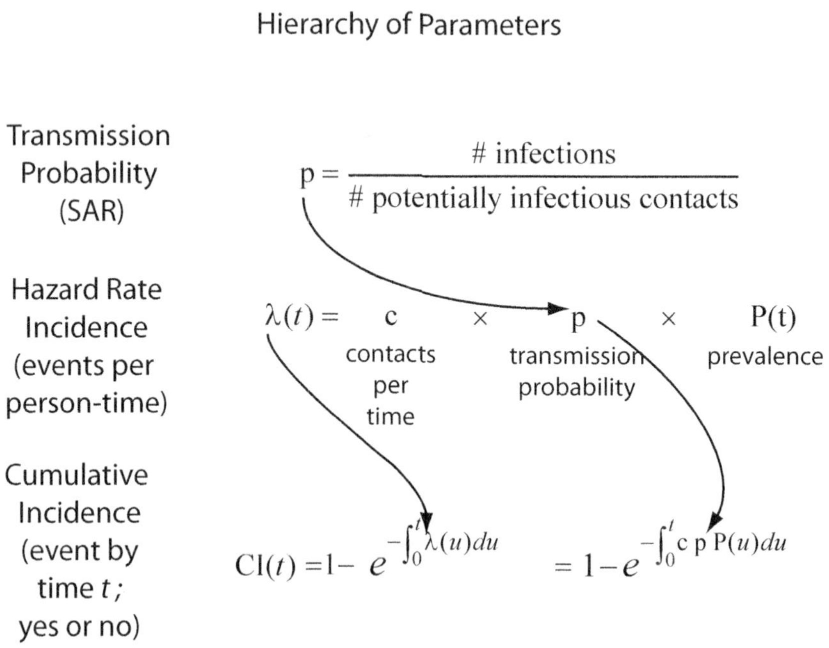

Fig. 2.1 Hierarchy of VE_S parameters showing the dependent happening relation among them.

person (Halloran and Struchiner 1995). In Table 2.2, the VE_I estimator is shown in the second column of the top row of conditional parameters. The third column contains the estimate of combined effect of the vaccine in reducing the transmission probability if both the infectious person and the susceptible person in the contact are vaccinated (VE_T). In contrast to VE_S, which can be estimated using either conditional or unconditional parameters, the VE_I and VE_T can generally be estimated using only conditional measures such as the transmission probability or secondary attack rate (Koopman and Little 1995; Longini et al 1996; Préziosi and Halloran 2003b; Halloran et al 2003b).

Studies for estimating VE_I can be incorporated into those for estimating $VE_{S,p}$ based on the transmission probability, if the vaccination status of the infectious person in a contact is known. The analysis can then simply stratify on the vaccination status of both the infectious and susceptible persons in the contact to get estimates of VE_S, VE_I, and VE_T. In the case of the binomial model, the likelihood can be constructed from the different contributions of each contact, where the parameters for relative susceptibility and for relative infectiousness are built directly into the likelihood (Longini et al 1996; Hudgens et al 2001).

In general, there are at least seven measures potentially of interest. Considering the estimates of VE based on the relative secondary attack rates, there are three main unstratified vaccine effects:

$$VE_{S.1/.0} = 1 - \frac{SAR_{.1}}{SAR_{.0}}, \quad VE_{I1./0.} = 1 - \frac{SAR_{1.}}{SAR_{0.}},$$
$$VE_T = 1 - \frac{SAR_{11}}{SAR_{00}}. \tag{2.8}$$

If one stratifies on the vaccine status of both the infective person and the susceptible person, then there are four further stratified measures of VE_S and VE_I:

$$VE_{S01/00} = 1 - \frac{SAR_{01}}{SAR_{00}}, \quad VE_{S11/10} = 1 - \frac{SAR_{11}}{SAR_{10}},$$
$$VE_{I10/00} = 1 - \frac{SAR_{10}}{SAR_{00}}, \quad VE_{I11/01} = 1 - \frac{SAR_{11}}{SAR_{01}}. \tag{2.9}$$

Chapters 10 through 12 consider estimation of the conditional parameters based on transmission probabilities and SARs from studies in households and other small transmission units in detail.

2.5.1 Estimating multiple levels of parameters

Statistical models have been developed to express both the within household transmission probability and the unconditional probability of being infected from the community at large (Longini and Koopman1982; Hudgens et al 2001; O'Neill et al 2000; Becker et al 2003). In some vaccine studies, information on contacts within transmission units such as households or sexual partnerships may be available, but the individuals may also be exposed to infection outside the transmission unit. Some individuals in a study might not be members of clearly defined transmission units. These models are considered in detail in Chapters 10 through 12.

2.6 Vaccine Efficacy for Progression or Pathogenesis, VE_P

VE_P measures the effect of vaccination on some outcome that occurs only in people who get infected. It requires comparison of the post-infection outcome, for example, morbidity or mortality, in infected vaccinated people with that in infected unvaccinated people. The interest could be the vaccine effect on the probability of developing disease if infected, that is, the effect on pathogenicity. The interest could be on effect on the time from infection to development of disease, that is, the rate of progression from infection to disease. The interest could be on the effect of vaccination on reducing the severity of disease or probability of death in symptomatic cases. For binary outcomes, such as becoming symptomatic or not, developing severe disease or not, or death or not, VE_P would be estimated by one minus the ratio in the vaccinated compared to the unvaccinated, including in the calculation only those people who had become infected:

Table XLIII.

Degree of effective vaccination	Strength to resist small-pox when incurred		
	Deaths	Recoveries	Total
Cicatrix absent	94	383	477
Cicatrix present	42	1,562	1,604
Total	136	1,945	2,081

Fig. 2.2 VE_P: Death versus recovery in smallpox: Greenwood and Yule (Proc R Soc Med, 8(part 2):113–194, 1915). Cicatrix present indicates effective vaccination; cicatrix absent indicates no effective vaccination. Reprinted with permission of the Royal Society of Medicine.

$$VE_P = 1 - \frac{\frac{\text{no. severe vaccinated cases}}{\text{all vaccinated cases}}}{\frac{\text{no. severe unvaccinated cases}}{\text{all unvaccinated cases}}} . \tag{2.10}$$

Based on data in Greenwood and Yule (1915) on the effect of smallpox vaccination to prevent death by comparing the number of cases recovering to those dying of smallpox (Figure 2.2), the estimate of VE_P of smallpox vaccination to prevent death is

$$\widehat{VE}_P = 1 - \frac{\frac{\text{no. deaths in vaccinated cases}}{\text{all vaccinated cases}}}{\frac{\text{no. deaths in unvaccinated cases}}{\text{all unvaccinated cases}}} \tag{2.11}$$

$$= 1 - \frac{42/1604}{94/477} = 0.87 .$$

For such binary outcomes, a simple relation among VE_{SP}, VE_S, and VE_P is

$$VE_{SP} = 1 - (1 - VE_S)(1 - VE_P). \tag{2.12}$$

That is, the vaccine efficacy against the severe outcome is a function of the vaccine efficacy against infection and the vaccine efficacy against the severe post-infection outcome in those people who become infected, illustrated further in Section 5.2.3. The relation (2.12) assumes that there is no selection bias due to vaccination in those who become infected. Considerable recent research has been devoted to estimating the effects of vaccination on post-infection outcomes (Préziosi and Halloran 2003a), particularly on understanding potential selection bias (Gilbert et al 2003a; Hudgens et al 2003; Hudgens and Halloran 2006; Jemiai et al 2007). VE_P is discussed in detail in Chapter 9.

2.7 Contact Rates and Exposure Efficacy

Vaccinated people may alter their contact and exposure to infection patterns if they believe the vaccine is protective. *Exposure* or *behavior efficacy* is the relative increase or decrease in the relative risk of infection or disease due to the change in exposure to the infectious agent (Halloran et al 1994b). For example, if we consider the components of the hazard rate as discussed above, changes in exposure to the infectious agent can occur in the rate of contacts, in the prevalence of infection in the contact groups, or in the transmission probability through changing the type of contact. In nonrandomized or observational studies, the vaccinated and unvaccinated groups often differ in their exposure to infection, resulting in biased estimates of VE_S. Although VE_S estimates based on the transmission probability require more information than those based on the unconditional parameters, they are less sensitive to bias from unequal exposure to infection in the two groups. The overall effect of biological protection and change in exposure to infection might be of interest for understanding the public health consequences of vaccination. Study designs need to be explicit about differentiating factors related to susceptibility, such as vaccination status, and factors related to exposure to infection.

2.8 Indirect, Total, and Overall Effectiveness

Struchiner et al (1990) and Halloran and Struchiner (1991) define study designs for dependent happenings that allow evaluation of the indirect, total, and overall effects of vaccination (Figure 2.3). The population-level effects of vaccination are defined within the context of a particular intervention program, or allocation of vaccination, thus the unit of inference is the population. Several populations or communities need to be included in the study to take potential variability into account. Exactly what the intervention program of interest is will depend on the vaccine and the target population for vaccination. The comparisons may be made between different levels of vaccination coverage, between allocation within different age groups, or otherwise defined subgroups (Monto et al 1969; Moulton et al 2001).

In Table 2.2 and Figure 2.3, the different type of population-level effects are considered on the simple example that no vaccination has taken place in population *B*, and a proportion of people are vaccinated in population *A*. The control population may be the same population that receives the vaccination, but before the vaccination program started. The direct effects of vaccination can be evaluated within the population that receives the vaccination program, and are forms of VE_S, VE_{SP}, and VE_P.. The indirect effects of the vaccine given a particular allocation of vaccination is then the comparison of the incidence or other outcome of interest in the unvaccinated people in community *A* compared to the unvaccinated people in the unvaccinated community *B*. These comparisons are called designs type IIa. The indirect effectiveness measures are denoted VE_{IIa}. The total effects of the combination of being vaccinated and the allocation is the outcome in the vaccinated people in the

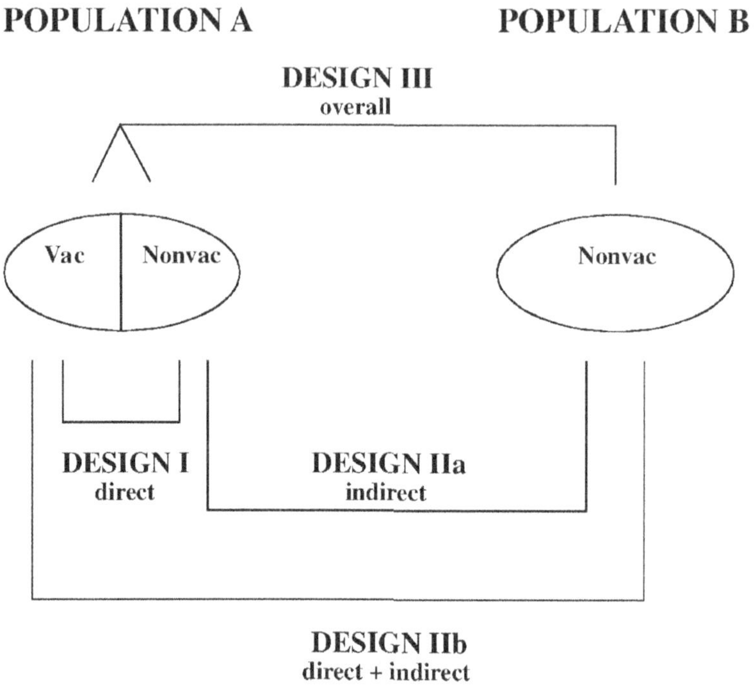

Fig. 2.3 Study designs for dependent happenings. Types of effects of vaccination programs and different study designs based on comparison populations for their evaluation (Halloran and Struchiner 1991, Epidemiology, 2:331–338. Reprinted with permission).

communities *A* compared to that of the unvaccinated people in the unvaccinated communities *B*. These comparisons are called designs type IIb, and the total effectiveness measures are denoted VE_{IIb}. The overall effectiveness of the vaccine and allocation compare the average outcomes in the vaccinated communities with those of the unvaccinated communities. These comparisons are called designs type III, and the overall effectiveness measures are denoted VE_{III}. Table 2.2 contains examples of the VE_{IIa}, VE_{IIb}, and VE_{III} based on the usual unconditional measures incidence rate, hazard rate, and cumulative incidence. The proportional hazards model is not included because the baseline hazard would presumably differ across populations. Many other measures could be used as the outcome measure, including average age of infection or the basic reproductive number, R_0, and the reproductive number, R.

In choosing the communities or populations, it is important to ensure that they are separated as much as possible in every way that is relevant for transmission. Transmission patterns can differ greatly among communities. It is necessary to give some thought to the likely transmission patterns and sources of exposure to infection in a population. These transmission patterns will greatly influence the magnitude of the indirect effects. Variability could swamp out the estimates of the effects of vaccination. Matching by transmission characteristics might be desirable (Hayes et al 1995). Interpretability and general applicability of quantitative results to other settings may be limited, although qualitative trends might hold (Halloran and Struchiner 1995).

Comparisons across communities would also allow study of other biological questions. For example, vaccines might contain only particular serotypes or strains of an organism. Widespread vaccination could allow the expansion of non-vaccine serotypes that had been less important before vaccination (Lipsitch 2000; Singleton et al 2007; Peters and Poehling 2007) or put evolutionary pressure on the existing strains.

Conducting a trial to evaluate effectiveness across several different populations or communities does not preclude evaluating VE_S or VE_I of vaccination within the populations. A Phase III vaccine trial can be designed to answer several questions at the same time. Generally, one scientific question will be designated the primary goal of the study, and others secondary or ancillary goals. The primary analysis will be planned to evaluate the primary scientific question. Randomization within a population can be used to answer efficacy questions, and comparison across populations can be used to evaluate the indirect and overall effects of vaccination. There is a trade-off in designing studies to measure both direct and indirect effects of vaccination between vaccinating high numbers of people so that indirect effects are high, and vaccinating too many people so that the number of events in the vaccinated populations is too low to estimate VE_S or VE_I well.

Randomized community trials fall into the category of cluster- or group-randomized trials where whole social units, rather than independent individuals are randomly assigned to treatment groups (Hayes et al 1995; Koepsell et al 1992; Donner et al 1998; Prentice 1995; Klar et al 1995; Murray 1998, Hayes and Moulton 2009). Because vaccines are administered to individuals, randomization can occur at two stages, namely the group level and the individual level within groups (Hudgens and Halloran 2008).In general, assignment mechanisms other than randomization could be in place at the two levels. That is, either allocation of the vaccination strategy to populations might not be randomized or allocation of the individual vaccination within populations or both might not be randomized. The analysis and sample size calculations need to take the clustering and possible group-randomization into account. Methods for estimating indirect, total, and or overall effects are discussed in more detail in Chapter 13.

2.8.1 Hypothetical example

Figure 2.4 shows a simple example of estimating the direct, indirect, total, and overall effects using just two populations, each with a population $N = 1000$. We assume that the populations are identical. We base our estimates on the number of cases at the end of an epidemic, the attack rate or cumulative incidence, say, at the end of an influenza season. In population A, 700 people are randomly vaccinated and the other 300 are unvaccinated. In population B, we consider separately the 700 people

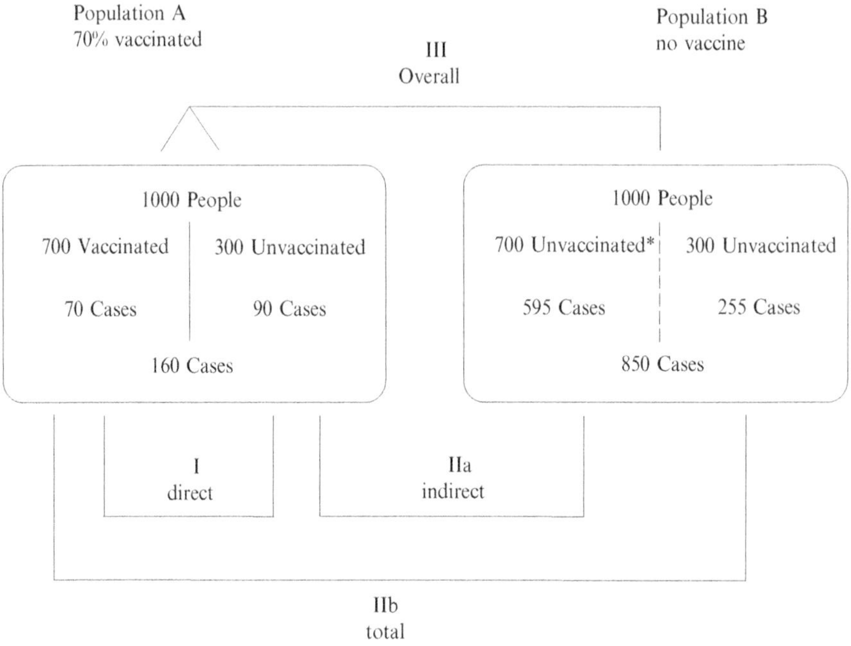

Fig. 2.4 An example of estimating direct, indirect, total, and overall effects of vaccination. The * represents the people who would have been vaccinated if Population B had had the vaccination strategy.

who would have been vaccinated and the 300 who would not have been vaccinated, if population B had received vaccine. In population B, we observe 850 cases, so the attack rate is $AR_B = 0.85$. Due to randomization, the attack rate is the same in those who would have received vaccine as those who would not have received vaccine, so 595 of the 850 cases are in the 700 people who would have received vaccine, and 255 of the cases are in the 300 people who would not have received vaccine. In population A, there are 70 cases in the 700 vaccinated people and 90 cases in the 300 unvaccinated people, for a total of 160 cases, and an attack $AR_A = 0.16$. The $AR_{A1} = 0.10$ in the vaccinated and $AR_{A0} = 0.30$ in the unvaccinated. The VE estimates of interest are

$$VE_{\text{direct}} = 1 - \frac{0.10}{0.30} = 0.66, \quad VE_{IIa} = 1 - \frac{0.30}{0.85} = 0.65,$$

$$VE_{IIb} = 1 - \frac{0.10}{0.85} = 0.88, \quad VE_{III} = 1 - \frac{0.16}{0.85} = 0.81.$$

The direct vaccine efficacy is a measure similar to the prevented fraction in the exposed, where the exposure is vaccination (Greenland and Robins 1988; Robins and Greenland 1989). The prevented number of cases in the vaccinated group can be computed from the prevented fraction times the number of people vaccinated. However, the situation is different with dependent happenings than with the usual prevented fraction in the exposed when events are independent of one another. If we used the usual prevented fraction in the exposed, we would compute the number of cases we would have expected in the vaccinated individuals in population A by assuming the attack rate if they had not been vaccinated would have been the same as that observed in the unvaccinated individuals in population A. Under this assumption, we would have expected $(90/300) \times 700 = 210$ cases in the vaccinated individuals if they had not been vaccinated. The number of cases prevented by vaccination would be calculated to be $210 - 70 = 140$. However, this does not take into account that the number of cases in the unvaccinated group in population A is also decreased by indirect effects. To compute the total number of cases prevented in the vaccinated by vaccination and the vaccination program, we need to use the 595 cases in the 700 people in population B who would have been vaccinated. Then the total number of actually prevented cases in the vaccinated people is $595 - 70 = 525$. Using the usual prevented fraction in the exposed underestimates the actual number of cases prevented because it does not take the indirect effects into account. The overall cases prevented by vaccination is $850 - 160 = 690$.

2.8.2 Influenza example

Monto et al (1969) estimated both the protective efficacy, VE_S, and the overall effect, VE_{III}, of an influenza vaccination program. They vaccinated 85% of the school-age children in Tecumseh, Michigan, against Hong Kong influenza just before the epidemic in 1968. The 10-week epidemic period was from November 17, 1968, to January 26, 1969. The weekly mean influenza illness rates in vaccinated and unvaccinated children were 0.072 and 0.090, respectively. This yields an approximate estimate of $VE_{S,IR} \approx 1 - 0.072/0.090 = 0.20$, which is rather low. The overall influenza illness cumulative incidence in Tecumseh for the epidemic period was 0.14, and the adjusted overall influenza cumulative incidence in unvaccinated, neighboring Adrian, Michigan, was 0.42 for the same period. Using the methods of study design III, the overall effectiveness of vaccinating 85% of Tecumseh's school children is estimated to be $VE_{III,CI} \approx 1 - 0.14/0.42 = 0.67$.

2.9 Counting Process Models for Hierarchy of Parameters

In this section, we present a part of the formal development of the hierarchy of parameters based on counting process models found in Rhodes et al (1996). Before that, there had been little effort to relate the different measures of vaccine efficacy to one another formally, or their interpretation in terms of the underlying contact and infection processes. (This section is very technical and may be skipped.)

2.9.1 *Contact, infection, susceptibility, and infectiousness processes*

2.9.1.1 Overview

Rhodes et al (1996) extended counting process models for infection rates (Becker 1982, 1985, 1989) to incorporate contact rates between individuals, infectiousness of the infectives, and variables affecting susceptibility to infection, such as vaccination, given that such a contact had occurred. Using these counting process models, they demonstrate that the commonly used relative risk parameters form a hierarchy requiring different amounts of information about the contact and infection processes. The emphasis is on the distinction between exposure opportunity and actual exposure, and the amount of information that we have about these. Separation of the contact and the infection processes allows quantification of the different contributions of the contact process, infectiousness, and susceptibility in the estimated relative risk of infection in the comparison groups.

Table 2.3 contains an overview of the hierarchy levels of information that could be known about a population of interacting hosts with an infectious agent circulating in it. The hierarchy presented in Table 2.2 is a simplified version of the formal hierarchy, with the major difference in the interpretation of Level II. At a minimum, we need to know those covariates that are relevant to susceptibility as well as who is actually susceptible. The hierarchy goes from Level I to IV, or from (a) to (f), as information is either lost or ignored. In (a), we know all contacts between individuals, whereas in (b), we only know when infective individuals contact susceptibles. Level (b) is analogous to a vaccine efficacy study using the household secondary attack rate, studies in tuberculosis using contact tracing to estimate transmission probabilities, or discordant partner studies to estimate the transmission probability of HIV. Levels IIA and IIB, or (c) and (d), have information only on contacts that lead to infection, or the times at which individuals are infectious, respectively. These levels have important differences, but share enough similarities that they are developed in tandem. The analysis of the former has the form of a Poisson regression. At Level III, we know just the infection times, which under certain conditions leads to a stratified Cox regression analysis. Finally, at Level IV, we only know that a person becomes infected sometime during the study period. This provides information for an analysis based on the cumulative incidence or distribution function, such as vaccine efficacy based on the attack rates.

2.9.1.2 Notation and definitions

All processes defined below occur in continuous time and are orderly, ie, multiple points do not occur at any time t. Also, there are no tied jumps for pairs of processes of the same type involving different individuals, eg, no two infections can occur at the same time. Some pairs of processes of different types may jump at the same time

Table 2.3 Level and amount of information for each history (Rhodes et al 1996)

Level		Type of Information for Each History
I	(a)	All contacts between individuals and outcomes of those contacts (whether an infection is transmitted)
	(b)	Only those contacts between infective and susceptible individuals and infection outcome of those contacts
IIA	(c)	Only contacts leading to infections (who infects whom)
IIB	(d)	Infectious periods, ie, the times at which individuals become and cease to be infectious
III	(e)	The times at which individuals become infected
IV	(f)	Whether an infection occurs to each individual in some time period $(0,T]$

(eg, see C_{ij} and N_{ij} below). Consider a closed population of n individuals. Let $C_{ij}(t)$ be the counting process for person j contacting person i $(j \rightarrow i)$, $i, j = 1, \ldots, n, i \neq j$. (Notation of the subscripts for the infectives and susceptibles is reversed in this section from the other sections in the book.) We set $C_{ij}(0) = 0$ for all i, j, ie, we disregard all contacts that occur before the start of the study. For a study of length T, let t_{ijk} represent times in $(0,T]$ at which $j \rightarrow i$, $k = 1, \ldots, C_{ij}(T) = c_{ij}$. For an epidemic, T refers either to the end of the epidemic or to some preset ending time. For an endemic situation, T is some selected time at which an analysis is to be performed.

Let $N_{ij}(t)$ be the counting process for the process j infects i, ie, $dN_{ij}(t) = 1$ if person j infects person i at time t. Let δ_{ijk} be an indicator variable for whether the contact at t_{ijk} results in an infection (ie, $\delta_{ijk} = dN_{ij}(t_{ijk})$). Let $N_{i.}(t) = \sum_j N_{ij}(t)$. Let $\delta_i = N_{i.}(T) - N_{i.}(0)$, ie, $\delta_i = 1$ if person i becomes infected in $(0,T]$ and 0 if not. It is possible that $N_{i.}(0) = 1$ which indicates that person i was infected before the start of the current study. However, here we are interested only in counting infections that occur after time 0. We assume that the infection can occur at most once, ie, $N_{i.}(t) \leq 1$.

Let $I_j(t) = 1$ if person j is infectious at time t and $I_j(t) = 0$ otherwise. A person is infectious immediately after becoming infected (no latent period). Let $S_i(t) = 1$ if person i is susceptible at time t and $S_i(t) = 0$ otherwise. We define both sets of these processes to be left continuous. Thus, I_j and S_i are predictable processes (Bremaud 1981).

2.9.1.3 Intensities for contact processes

Let the intensity of the contact process C_{ij} be denoted by $\lambda_{ij}(t)$ $(\lambda_{ii}(t) = 0)$, ie,

$$\lambda_{ij}(t) = \lim_{\Delta \rightarrow 0} \frac{\Pr((C_{ij}(t+\Delta) - C_{ij}(t)) = 1 | \mathscr{H}_t)}{\Delta}, \tag{2.13}$$

where $\mathscr{H}_t$ is some history (Bremaud 1981). Informally, by a history we mean some observed information arising from various processes on the time interval

$(0,t]$. Technically, $\mathscr{H}_t$ is a σ-algebra generated by these processes on $(0,t]$. Several such histories may be of interest. We assume that the λ_{ij} are constants that can be parametrized using covariates $\mathbf{G}_i$ and $\mathbf{G}_j$ and a set of parameters $\theta = (\theta_1, \ldots, \theta_R)$, where $R << n(n-1)$, the number of pairs of individuals.

More generally, the contact rates could vary over time, such as cyclically, or be history-dependent. For example, the occurrence of an infection could cause a person j to reduce his or her activity and thus lower the intensities λ_{ij} for all i. We do not consider this aspect further, and drop the notation for $\mathbf{G}_j$.

2.9.1.4 Intensities for infection processes

Consider any C_{ij} contact process discussed earlier. The contact process plus the infection outcomes, δ_{ijk}, constitute a marked counting process (Bremaud 1981; Arjas 1989). Consider the multivariate infection process $\mathbf{N}(t) = \{N_{1.}(t), \ldots, N_{n.}(t)\}$. The process $N_{..}(t) = \sum_{i=1}^{n} N_{i.}(t)$ plus the identity and covariate values of the person infected at each jump is also a marked counting process. Let the function $\rho(t)$ denote the probability that an event occurring at time t in the original process will be retained by a thinned process. If $\lambda(t)$ is an intensity for the original process and $\rho(t)$ is predictable, the intensity for the thinned process is $\rho(t)\lambda(t)$ (Bremaud 1981).

Each infection process N_{ij} is a thinned version of the corresponding contact process C_{ij}. Let $p(t;\mathbf{z}_i,\mathbf{z}_j,\beta)$ represent the probability that a contact $j \to i$ at time t results in an infection if person j is infectious and person i is susceptible. This is also called the transmission probability. The $\mathbf{z}_i$ are covariates associated with susceptible i, $\mathbf{z}_j$ are covariates associated with infective j, and β is a vector of unknown parameters. If either $I_j(t)$ or $S_i(t)$ is 0, a point from C_{ij} has probability 0 of being accepted. If both $I_j(t)$ and $S_i(t)$ are 1, the point is accepted with probability $p(t;\mathbf{z}_i,\mathbf{z}_j,\beta)S_i(t)I_j(t)$. The time- and history-dependent probability $\rho_{ij}(t)$ that a point from C_{ij} will be accepted for N_{ij} is $p(t;\mathbf{z}_i,\mathbf{z}_j,\beta)$. A dependence on $\mathbf{z}_j$ implies that persons are differentially infectious. For simplicity, here we assume that all infectives are equally infectious, and drop the dependence on $\mathbf{z}_j$. An intensity for $N_{ij}(t)$ may then be written as

$$\alpha_{ij}(t) = \lambda_{ij}(t)p(t;z_i,\beta)S_i(t)I_j(t)\ , \tag{2.14}$$

where the infection process is a thinned version of the contact process.

2.9.2 *Information levels and types of statistical analyses*

In most of the development here, the covariates associated with the contact parameters are assumed to be the same for all individuals. $\mathbf{Z}_i$ and $\mathbf{G}_i$ denote covariates associated with the susceptibility and contact parameters.

2.9.2.1 Level I

In the first level of information, either all contacts between individuals and outcomes of those contacts are known, or contacts between infectives and the susceptibles whom they contact during their infectious period:

$$\mathscr{H}_t^I = \sigma\{C_{ij}(s),\ N_{ij}(t),\ I_j(s),\ S_i(s),\ \mathbf{Z}_i(s),\ \mathbf{G}_i(s),\ 0 \le s \le t\}.$$

The analysis remains the same for evaluating covariates related to susceptibility because only contacts between infectives and susceptibles enter into the analysis. Estimation of the contact process will differ, however. The log-likelihood of observing contacts at the set of points $\{t_{ijk} : i, j = 1, \dots, n, k = 1, \dots, C_{ij}(T)\}$ (Fleming and Harrington 1991) is given below in terms of stochastic integrals:

$$\log L(C) = \sum_{i=1}^{n}\sum_{j=1}^{n}\int_0^T \log(\lambda_{ij}(t))dC_{ij}(t) - \sum_{i=1}^{n}\sum_{j=1}^{n}\int_0^T \lambda_{ij}(t)dt. \qquad (2.15)$$

The conditional likelihood for the infection outcome marks (the N_{ij} processes) given the C_{ij}, $\mathbf{Z}_i$, S_i, and I_j processes is

$$\prod_{i=1}^{n}\prod_{j=1}^{n}\prod_{k=1}^{c_{ij}}\{I_j(t_{ijk})S_i(t_{ijk})p(t_{ijk};\mathbf{z}_i,\beta)\}^{\delta_{ijk}} \times \{1 - I_j(t_{ijk})S_i(t_{ijk})p(t_{ijk};\mathbf{z}_i,\beta)\}^{(1-\delta_{ijk})}.$$

We assume that the λ_{ij} are parametrized by $\theta = (\theta_1, \dots, \theta_R)$ and that $p(t_{ijk};\mathbf{z}_i,\beta) = \exp(\beta\mathbf{z}_i)$, where β has length H. 0^0 is defined as 1. Because p lies in the interval [0,1], in general we would want $\hat{\beta} \le 0$. Let $\gamma_{ijk} = I_j(t_{ijk})S_i(t_{ijk})$. Then

$$IC_{i.} = \sum_{j=1}^{n}\sum_{k=1}^{c_{ij}} \gamma_{ijk},$$

that is, the total contacts made on person i by infectives while person i was susceptible. Assuming sufficient regularity such that the interchange of the various integrals and derivatives is justified, and making appropriate substitutions, the $R + H$ score equations for Level I can be written as

$$\frac{\partial \log L(C,N)}{\partial \theta_r} = \sum_{i=1}^{n}\sum_{j=1}^{n}\int_0^T \frac{1}{\lambda_{ij}(t)}\frac{\partial \lambda_{ij}(t)}{\partial \theta_r}dC_{ij}(t) - \sum_{i=1}^{n}\sum_{j=1}^{n}\int_0^T \frac{\partial \lambda_{ij}(t)}{\partial \theta_r}dt,$$

$$\frac{\partial \log L(C,N)}{\partial \beta_h} = \sum_{i=1}^{n}\delta_i z_{hi} - \sum_{i=1}^{n}(IC_{i.} - \delta_i)\frac{z_{hi}\exp(\beta\mathbf{z}_i)}{1 - \exp(\beta\mathbf{z}_i)}. \qquad (2.16)$$

These equations are formally equivalent to a log-linear binomial regression where each person i with covariate $\mathbf{z}_i$ contributes $IC_{i.}$ trials with outcome δ_i. The score equations for β and θ can be solved separately. The information equations for this level and the score and information equations for all other levels are given in Rhodes et al (1994).

2.9.2.2 Level II

In Level IIA the source of each infection is known, that is, who infects whom, as well as how long each person is infectious. Level IIA is the last level with any direct contact information at all. On Level IIB, it is known who is infectious and how long, but not who infects whom. The time that a person remains infectious plus contact rates with other individuals gives a measure of the exposure opportunity that this person provides to other individuals, after taking into account when each was susceptible: Level IIA,

$$\mathscr{H}_t^{IIA} = \sigma\{N_{ij}(s), I_j(s), S_i(s), \mathbf{Z}_i(s), \mathbf{G}_i(s),\ 0 \le s \le t\};$$

Level IIB,

$$\mathscr{H}_t^{IIB} = \sigma\{N_{i.}(s), I_j(s), S_i(s), \mathbf{Z}_i(s), \mathbf{G}_i(s),\ 0 \le s \le t\}.$$

In most cases, information for pattern IIA will be difficult to obtain because of the necessity of observing who infects whom. When the C_{ij} processes are not directly observed, we treat the N_{ij} processes as thinned versions of the C_{ij}. Using expression (2.14) for the intensity of N_{ij}, Rhodes et al (1996) give the log-likelihood for level IIA.

Without knowledge of the contact process, we cannot estimate both the set of parameters λ_{ij} (or the θ) and the parameter β_0 corresponding to a constant term in $\mathbf{z}_i$. We must incorporate the value $\exp(\beta_0)$ into the λ_{ij} functions and deal with a new set of parameters $\lambda_{ij}^* = \lambda_{ij}\exp(\beta_0)$. We also refer to the new set of parameters θ_1^* (note: $\theta_1^* \neq \theta_1 \exp(\beta_0)$ except in special cases). In this instance, the β and θ^* equations cannot be solved separately. However, the score equations for β have the form of a Poisson regression if the terms involving one portion of the log-likelihood,

$$\sum_{j=1}^{n} \lambda_{ij}^* \int_0^T I_j(t) S_i(t) dt, \tag{2.17}$$

are known. Thus, estimation proceeds by alternating between solving the θ^* equations and the β equations. Certain choices of the parametrization for the λ_{ij}^* lead to both sets of equations conforming to a Poisson regression model.

The intensities for the $N_{i.}$ processes are obtained by summing the intensities of the corresponding N_{ij} processes (Bremaud 1981). Level IIB has the same limitation in terms of not being able to estimate β_0 and λ_{ij} separately. The log-likelihood is given in Rhodes et al (1996).

2.9.2.3 Level III

We know the times at which infections occur and which individuals were susceptible as well as the values of all covariate processes. We do not observe how long each person remains infectious. Thus, for Level III,

$$\mathscr{H}_t^{III} = \sigma\{N_{i.}(s),\ S_i(s),\ \mathbf{Z}_i(s),\ \mathbf{G}_i(s),\quad 0 \le s \le t\}.$$

We proceed by writing a complete likelihood for the marked counting process $N_{..}(t) = \sum_{i=1}^n N_{i.}(t)$ and then decomposing it into components. The mark corresponds to the identity of the person infected when the combined process jumps. The contribution to the likelihood for the interval (t_{d-1}, t_d) where t_d is the time of the dth event in the process $N_{..}$ is broken into two parts:

(a) L(no event for $N_{..}$ in (t_{d-1}, t_d), event for $N_{..}$ at $t_d | \mathscr{H}_t^{III}$, $t_{d-1} \le t \le t_d$),
(b) L(identity of person infected at t_d|event at t_d, set of individuals susceptible at time t_d, $\mathscr{H}_t^{III}$, $0 \le t < t_d$).

The first term is obtained by treating $N_{..}$ as the sum of thinned point processes and the second by considering the conditional probability of the identity of the infected individual given the set of individuals susceptible at time t_d. Level III has the same limitation in terms of not being able to estimate β_0 and λ_{ij} separately. The expressions for the log-likelihoods are in Rhodes et al (1996).

The conditional probabilities may depend on the contact parameters and on the I_j processes. In some instances, depending on the form of the $\mathbf{G_i}$ covariates, strata can be formed in which the conditional probability does not involve either the contact parameters or the I_j processes. For example, if the $\lambda_{ij}(t)$ are all equal to a constant value λ, the conditional probability is free of both the above quantities. Also, consider the case where each individual belongs to one of K mixing groups. In that circumstance we can work with $N_{k..}$, $k = 1, \ldots, K$, the total infection processes in each of the K groups. Part b is then the conditional distribution of the mark given the actual set of individuals who were susceptible at time t_d in the group in which the infection occurred.

The Cox regression model has an advantage over analyses IIA and IIB in that no modification needs to be made for the situation where the study population constitutes only a portion of the entire population. For example, if one conducts a vaccine trial in a limited age group of the population and collects infection data only for that age group, the Poisson-based methods could not be formulated correctly because one would not know the total exposure potential of the children in the trial.

2.9.2.4 Level IV

For Level IV we know whether each individual has been infected in $(0, T]$ but not when the infection occurred:

$$\mathscr{H}_t^{IV} = \sigma\{N_{i.}(T), \mathbf{Z}_i(0), \mathbf{G}_i(0)\}.$$

Table 2.4 Estimates of β_1 and estimated variances for β_1 assuming homogeneous mixing† (Rhodes et al 1996)

Level	Estimator	Variance Estimator
I	$\log\left(\frac{n_1 IC_0}{n_0 IC_1}\right)$	$\frac{1-\hat{p}_0}{n_0}+\frac{1-\hat{p}_1}{n_1}$
II	$\log\left(\frac{n_1 L_0}{n_0 L_1}\right)$	$\frac{1}{n_0}+\frac{1}{n_1}$
III	No closed form	No closed form
IV	$\log\left[\frac{\log\{-\log(1-\hat{p}_1)\}}{\log\{-\log(1-\hat{p}_0)\}}\right]$	$\sum_{i=0}^{1}\frac{\hat{p}_1}{m_i(1-\hat{p}_i)\{(1-\hat{p}_i)\}^2}$

†IC_i is the number of contacts made on individuals in group i by infectives while those individuals in group i were susceptible. n_i is the number of infections in each group during the study. L_i is the total time that susceptibles in group i were exposed to infectives. m_j is the initial number of susceptibles in group i, $\hat{p}_i = n_i/m_i$.

The analysis has the form of a binary regression, although the link is the complementary log–log link (ie, $\log(-\log(p))$). Censoring or late entry is not permitted, nor is it possible to incorporate time-dependent covariates. Thus, we restrict attention to the values of covariates at the start of study.

Consider the probability that an individual i with covariates $\mathbf{z}$ would escape uninfected over the time period $(0,T]$ if we were given the full history of the infectiousness processes for all other individuals.

$$\Pr(N_{i.}(T)=0|I_j,\mathbf{Z}_i) = 1-p_i(T) = \exp\left[-\exp(\beta\mathbf{z}_i)\int_0^T\sum_{j=1}^{n}\lambda_{ij}(t)I_j(t)dt\right],$$

or

$$\log(-\log(1-p_i(T))) = \beta\mathbf{z}_i + \log\int_0^T\sum_{j=1}^{n}\lambda_{ij}(t)I_j(t)dt = \beta\mathbf{z}_i+\gamma_i\,. \quad (2.18)$$

If the terms γ_i are unique to each individual, estimation of the parameters of interest, β, is not possible, because each individual adds a new parameter to the analysis. However, if among the n individuals there are a limited number of γ parameters, estimation is possible. Thus, although the I_j processes are not observable, under certain conditions, functions of these processes are estimable. However, these functions are not themselves of great interest. When there is a set of parameters $\gamma = (\gamma_1,\ldots\gamma_K)$, where $K \ll n$, we then fit the complementary log–log binomial regression model incorporating covariates for these parameters.

2.9.3 Homogeneous mixing

We consider the case of homogeneous mixing, that is, $\lambda_{ij}(t) = \lambda$ for $i \neq j$, with $p(t;\mathbf{z}_i,\beta) = p_i = \exp(\beta_0 + \beta_1 z_i)$ for the case where z_i is a single dichotomous covariate. When the contact processes are not observable, the parameters λ and β_0 cannot both be estimated. The composite parameter $\lambda^* = \lambda \exp(\beta_0)$ is estimable and is interpretable as the average rate per unit of time at which one infective would tend to infect a susceptible with covariate equal to 0. The estimates for e^{β_1} for the different information levels and the corresponding estimated variances are given in Table 2.4. The estimator for Level I has the form of a log relative risk. Analyses IIA and IIB are the same since there are no contact covariates. The estimator for β_1 for Level II is similar to that for Level I except that a measure of exposure opportunity is substituted for a measure of actual exposure. The Cox regression estimator (Level III) does not have a closed form. The level IV estimator uses functions of the proportions infected in each group. If the probability of infection per contact is large, such as in measles or chickenpox, analysis I might be a better choice than analysis II (Figure 2.5). In this situation, knowledge of actual exposure, say a secondary attack rate study, provides a large improvement in the standard error over the use of expected exposure or exposure opportunity, say a study using Poisson regression. Knowledge of the actual amount of exposure, measured by contacts with infectives, leads to a large gain in efficiency when the absolute probability of transmission per contact of an infective with a susceptible is high. Infectious diseases such as measles and chickenpox have generally high transmission probabilities, but HIV has a low transmission probability, except perhaps during certain periods of infectiousness.

All of the models with the exception of level IV can be extended to accommodate individuals who are lost to follow-up or who enter the population after the study starts. A more complicated situation is introduced by the process letting $Y_j(t) = 1$ if person j is *present* in the population at time t, and 0 otherwise. This differs from standard usage in survival analysis where $Y_j(t) = 1$ indicates that the person is *under observation* at time t (Andersen and Gill 1982). A person who is not under observation but remains present in the population may influence the infection outcomes of other population members. This type of dependence is not seen in noninfectious disease studies.

Problems

2.1. In a vaccine efficacy study in which all participants are recruited at the same time, the time of onset of illness for all vaccinated and unvaccinated cases is observed. There is no loss to follow-up. No information on exposure to infection is observed.
(a) What level information is this about the transmission system?
(b) Which of the VE_S, in this case actually VE_{SP}, estimators can be computed from this study?

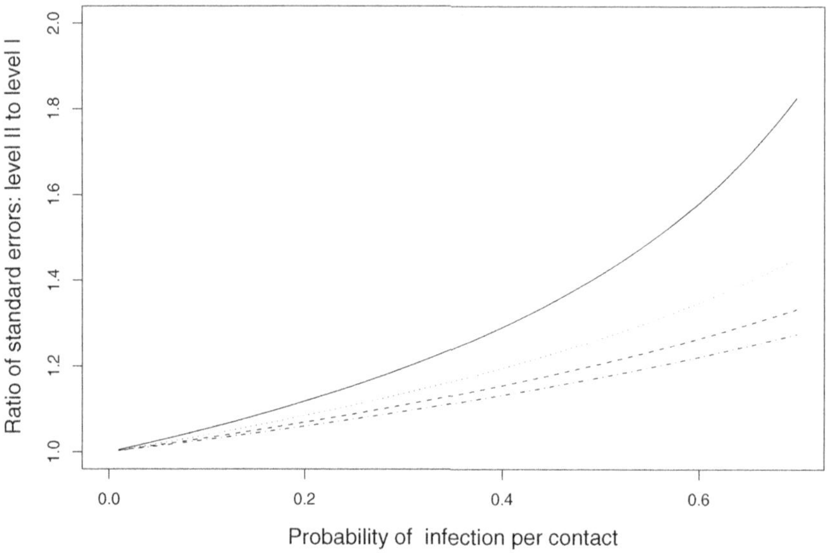

Fig. 2.5 Ratio of standard errors in the analysis at Level II compared to Level I by baseline transmission probability ($e^{\beta_0} = p_0$) and the covariate effect on the transmission probability, or transmission probability ratio ($TPR = e^{\beta_1}$) in group 1 compared to group 0. $TPR = e^{\beta_1} = 1$ (——), 0.5 (······), 0.25 (- - - -), and 0.1 (- · - ·). The ratios are based on the variances for β_1 at Levels I and II given in Table 2.4. The number of infections is assumed to be the same in each group, and therefore, cancel out (Rhodes et al, J R Stat Soc B 58:751-762, 1996, reprinted with permission of the Royal Statistical Society).

2.2. In a blinded, randomized controlled trial of an HIV vaccine, the estimated $VE_{S,\lambda}$ is 0.40. Using the dependent happening expression (2.7), compute by how much vaccinated individuals would need to increase their sexual contact rate to nullify the biological benefits of vaccination, assuming everything else remained the same.

2.3. From the data in Figure 1.3, compute $VE_{S,p}$ for the children with definite exposure in other households.

2.4. (a) Compute $VE_{S,CI}$ from the data in Table II of Figure 1.1.
(b) Compare the result with that in equation (2.6) and explain the difference.

2.5. Consider two populations of size $N = 1000$ as in Figure 2.4. In population A, 30 cases occur in the 600 vaccinated individuals, and 100 cases occur in the 400 unvaccinated individuals. In population B there are 700 cases.
(a) Compute VE_{direct}, VE_{IIa}, VE_{IIb}, and VE_{III}.
(b) What is the number of cases actually prevented in the vaccinated individuals

in population A? What number of cases prevented would one compute if the comparison population were taken to be the unvaccinated individuals in population A? Discuss the differences in the two results.

Chapter 3
Immunology and Early Phase Trials

The biological basis of successful vaccination is our own complex immune system and its response to pathogens. Vaccination can induce an immune response that mimics natural infection or tries to do even better than our response to a pathogen. Vaccination induces an immune response in the individual vaccinated. A population of hosts has a collective level of immunity that results from the level of immunity in the individuals that compose it. The collective immunological status of a population of hosts, as opposed to an individual host, with respect to a given pathogen is called herd immunity. Maintenance of individual immunity can depend on repeated boosting by natural infection. The level of transmission may be diminished by high levels of immunization or natural immunity in a population to the point that natural boosting of immunity does not occur. Thus for some infections, a complex interplay between individual and population level immunity is maintained through the dependent happenings.

The immune response is also the source of many safety considerations of vaccination. Before a vaccine can be shown efficacious against infection or disease in a large-scale field study, it must be shown to elicit an immune response and to be safe in smaller studies. The design and analysis of vaccine studies requires an understanding of immunology and vaccines that goes beyond the scope of this book. Our goal in this chapter is to present sufficient biological background and terminology that the other chapters of the book can be read and understood. The key ideas are the immunogenicity and safety of vaccines. Preclinical studies in animals and Phase I and II clinical studies in humans have the primary goals of assessing the immunogenicity and safety of vaccine candidates. Early phase studies as well as experimental challenge studies are discussed briefly in this chapter. Population-level considerations include herd immunity and natural boosting of immunity.

The book *Vaccines* by Plotkin, Orenstein, and Offit (2008), now in its fifth edition, is the standard reference book on vaccines. *Janeway's Immunobiology* by Murphy, Travers, and Walport (2008), seventh edition, is the standard reference book on immunology, with many sections on infectious diseases and vaccines. We recommend both of these books to anyone with further interest in the topic.

M.E. Halloran et al., *Design and Analysis of Vaccine Studies*, Statistics for Biology and Health, DOI 10.1007/978-0-387-68636-3_3,

3.1 Immunology and Infection

3.1.1 Innate and adaptive immune systems

The immune system is composed of a complex network of cells, molecules, and tissues with intricate interactions. The immune response can be divided into the innate immune response and the adaptive immune response. The elements of the innate immune system are encoded in a fixed way in our bodies. The innate immune system does not develop a specific response to an infectious agent. It relies on a limited and invariant repertoire of receptors to recognize microorganisms. The innate immune response can discriminate between self and nonself, and thus is able to decide when to launch an attack. Often the innate immune system can deal with invaders that breach the skin, the mucosa, or the airways. When it senses a foreign pathogen that it cannot contain, it mobilizes the adaptive immune system.

The adaptive immune system develops a specific response to a pathogen. B cells produce specific antibodies for antigens on the pathogens. An antibody is a protein that binds specifically to its antigen. An antigen is any substance that can be recognized and responded to by the adaptive immune system. T cells develop the ability to kill specific pathogens and to help B cells produce specific antibodies. Naive T cells move continuously around the body and through the various lymphoid tissues. Antibodies and T cells both bind antigens at receptors that are specific to the antigen. A nearly infinite range of specificities of antigen receptors of antibodies in B cells and in T cell receptors are encoded by a small set of genes by an irreversible rearrangement of segments of the genes. Each cell expresses a unique receptor specificity that stays with its offspring. Cells of at least 10^8 different specificities are available in an individual at any one time (Murphy et al 2008). The adaptive immune system has the ability to remember its first encounter with a pathogen. When the pathogen invades the body again, the secondary response is much more rapid and much more intense. The adaptive immune response and its memory provide the rationale for immunization. The general idea is to prime the body with immunization to be ready to meet the invader with a swift and aggressive response.

The five main types of pathogens are viruses (measles, mumps, yellow fever), bacteria (meningococcus, tuberculosis, pertussis, cholera, typhoid), uni- and multicellular organisms with nuclei (malaria, sleeping sickness), fungi (*Candida albicans*, *Pneumocystis carinii*), and worms (filariasis, river blindness, hookworm). All successful vaccines in humans up until now are directed against viruses and bacteria, which are also called microparasites. Different effector mechanisms are used to clear primary infections with different pathogens and to protect against subsequent infections. With some infectious agents, such as measles or smallpox, the immune response to natural infection is quite protective against further disease. For such infectious agents, it has been fairly easy to produce efficacious vaccines that simply induce an immune response similar to that of natural infection. For some infections, such as malaria, HIV, and many of the parasites, the immune response to natural infection is insufficient to protect against disease. For such infections, vaccines have to be designed that actually do better than our own natural immune responses.

3.1.2 Immune response to infection

What happens when a person is infected by a pathogen for the first time? The innate immune system begins acting immediately. Immature dendritic cells distributed throughout the body serve as sentinels of infection. Dendritic cells have long tentacles and migrate around the body and into tissues, continually ingesting large amounts of extracellular fluid. They can distinguish self from nonself in the material they ingest. When they encounter a foreign pathogen, several things happen (Murphy et al 2008). The dendritic cells develop into mature dendritic cells, capable of presenting the antigens of the pathogen to naive T cells. That is, the mature dendritic cell becomes an antigen-presenting cell, a link between the innate and adaptive immune system. Macrophages, literally "big eaters", and neutrophils are also cells that ingest and digest pathogens that are capable of presenting antigen to cells as part of the link between the innate and adaptive immune response. Sometimes the dendritic cells, macrophages, and neutrophils are able to contain small invasions in the immediate phase of the innate immune response.

Inflammation is another local response to infection of the innate immune system that occurs after a few hours (Murphy et al 2008). This part of the innate immune response is communicated by proteins secreted by the cells. Chemokines are proteins secreted by cells that attract other cells with chemokine receptors into the infected area. Cytokines are proteins secreted by cells that affect cells close by with the right receptors. In inflammation, the chemokines released by the macrophages recruit more cells of the innate immune system into the area. Once the antigen-specific cells of the adaptive immune system have been created, they too will follow the chemokines to the infected area to intensify the attack. Inflammation causes redness, soreness, swelling, and warmth around the area of infection. Local inflammation at the injection site is a common side effect of vaccination.

If some threshold of infection is passed and the innate immune system is not able to clear the infection, the adaptive immune response is triggered. Triggering of the adaptive immune response depends on the transport of the infectious agent to the lymphoid organs, such as a lymph node, then recognition and proliferation by the naive T and naive B cells situated there (Murphy et al 2008). The antigen-presenting cell, such as a mature dendritic cell, grabs the antigen at the site of infection and migrates with it to the local lymphoid organ that contains naive T and naive B cells. The dendritic cell then presents the antigen to the naive T cell. The naive T-cell turns into specific effector cells that multiply. They become either antigen-specific CD8 cytotoxic T cells or antigen-specific helper CD4 T cells. Some of the armed effector T cells, particularly the cytotoxic T cells, leave the lymphoid tissue following the chemokine trail back to the site of infection to kill the pathogens. Some of the effector T cells, particularly the antigen-specific helper T cells, stay in the lymphoid tissue to help activate B cells that are presenting the specific antigen on their cell membranes. Antigen-specific B cells generally do not get to work until they encounter antigen-specific helper T cells. The B cells grow exponentially for a couple of days and become the antibody-producing plasma cells. It takes about four days for the adaptive immune system to develop a specific response the first time an infectious agent invades a person.

Once an infection is cleared, most of the effector cells die, and a specific immunological memory is retained in memory T and memory B cells (Murphy et al 2008). Memory T cells last a very long time, virtually forever, and are responsible for the long-term protection after infection or immunization. The second time the pathogen infects a person, the specific memory T and B cells produce a much more rapid and stronger response. Antigen-specific memory B cells replicate and produce antibodies with higher affinity, that is, higher binding strength for its antigen, than the primary response.

In summary, the first encounter with an antigen produces a primary response. After a lag phase, antigen-specific antibody is produced. Primary immunization plays the role of the first infection with an infectious agent. If the primary immunization is followed by a secondary or booster immunization, the secondary antibody response occurs after a much shorter lag, much more antibody is produced, and the antibody has a higher affinity, or strength of binding, to the antigen. It is also possible that natural exposure to infection could serve as a booster.

3.1.3 Antibodies and epitopes

Antibodies deal with extracellular forms of pathogens and their toxic products. Antibodies circulate in the fluid component of the blood called plasma. The term humors was used for body fluids, so that antibody mediated immunity is called humoral immunity (Murphy et al 2008). Antibodies are Y-shaped and the ends of their two arms are highly variable, which provides the diversity needed to recognize specific antigens. The stem of the Y determines the class of the antibody. The antibodies are also called immunoglobulins, a particular family of proteins. There are five major classes. For understanding vaccine studies, the most important classes are IgG, IgM, and IgA. The IgG is the most abundant antibody in the plasma and the longest lasting of the antibodies. IgM is the first immunoglobulin to be secreted by the B cells and is a herald of early infection. IgA is the main antibody associated with mucosal immunity. Antibodies do three main things. They bind toxins, they bind pathogens in the blood, and they bind to pathogens in the extracellular space.

An antibody generally recognizes only a small part of a large antigenic molecule, such as a protein, polysaccharide (large, complex sugar), or glycoprotein (a protein with sugars attached to it), of a pathogen. An epitope or antigenic determinant is the small structure recognized by an antibody or an antigen receptor on a cell. A large molecule such as a protein, polysaccharide, or glycoprotein can have many different epitopes. A T-cell epitope is a small part of the pathogen that is recognized by a T-cell receptor. Effector T cells only recognize epitopes of a pathogen when they are presented to them bound to a particular type of protein on the surface of an antigen-presenting cell, such as a dendritic cell, macrophage, neutrophil, or B cell. These cell surface proteins that can hold the antigen while it is presented are encoded in a cluster of a couple hundred genes known as the major histocompatibility complex (MHC). In humans, the genes in this cluster are also called the human leukocyte antigen (HLA) genes. There are many genetic variants (polymorphisms) in each gene in the cluster across the human population. Thus, each person has his or her own set of cell-surface proteins that bind antigen to be recognized by the effector T cells. The MHC (HLA) provides a broad population-level genetic diversity as a defense against pathogens (Murphy et al 2008).

3.2 Vaccines

3.2.1 Smallpox

Edward Jenner is generally credited with having introduced, or at least made popular, at the end of the 18th century the use of cowpox inoculation as a protection against smallpox. The latin word for cow, *vacca*, and the vaccinia virus of coxpox, gave the name to vaccination. Smallpox was a widespread and serious, often lethal, disease. The pockmarks it left on the face could be severely disfiguring. Before vaccination for smallpox was introduced, smallpox virus itself was used intentionally via the skin to produce a protective immune response against smallpox, a process called variolization. Variolization generally, but not always, produced a milder case of smallpox than natural infection. The virus could be obtained either from fresh pustules or from the dried scabs from smallpox lesions. The practice was more widespread outside Europe. In the 18th century, it was introduced into Europe, but apparently with limited uptake (Buchan 1792).

Vaccination against smallpox with eradication of the disease nearly two centuries after introduction of the first vaccination is a great public health success story (Fenner et al 1988). Several characteristics of the disease and the vaccine, and the dedication of a generation of public health workers led to the success. The disease is only moderately transmissible, it has no animal reservoir, it causes typical skin lesions in nearly everyone who acquires the disease, and immunity to natural infection is complete and apparently life-long. It has a relatively long generation time, about two weeks, so that for a viral disease, it is pretty slow-moving. The vaccine was independent of the cold chain and easily administered subcutaneously with a bifurcated needle that held just the right amount of vaccine between its two prongs that were simply jabbed into the skin. To find the last cases towards the end of the international campaign, rewards were offered to people to turn in suspected cases. Then people in the surrounding area were vaccinated, a strategy that came to be called ring vaccination. Smallpox was declared eradicated by the WHO in 1980. Routine immunization against smallpox stopped by 1983.

3.2.2 Early development

After the introduction of the vaccine for smallpox, nearly a century passed before the next success (Table 3.1). In the early years of vaccine development, two main approaches were pursued (Plotkin and Plotkin 2008). One approach was based on attenuated live organisms that can stimulate protective immunity but not cause disease. The other approach was based on killed organisms or purified components of killed organisms. The latter have the advantage that they cannot cause disease or revert to wild-type, but because they cannot replicate, they do not stimulate the immune system in the same way as live attenuated organisms. Another consideration is that many live attenuated virus vaccines need to be kept either cold or frozen, making their widespread use dependent on a cold chain.

In the 19th century, scientists such as Louis Pasteur in Paris, among others, were experimenting with using an attenuated version of infectious agents to immunize individuals (Plotkin and Plotkin 2008). This approach was radically different from using a different less virulent pathogen, such as cowpox against smallpox. Louis Pasteur experimented with attenuated rabies virus vaccine. The idea of injecting a live virus into a human being, whether the virus was attenuated or not, shocked the public. Pasteur got into trouble for his experiments in humans with live rabies vaccine, but was later exonerated. Research in the latter half of the 19th century focused on developing vaccines using killed organisms. Several groups independently developed a typhoid vaccine, including A. E. Wright, who later had the argument with Karl Pearson (see Chapter 1.1) about efficacy of the typhoid vaccine. Killed cholera and killed plague vaccines were also developed near the end of the 19th century.

The serious diseases associated with tetanus bacteria and diphtheria bacteria are caused by specific protein toxins that they release. So it is sufficient for an immunization to induce antibodies against the toxins. The vaccines against tetanus and diphtheria, chemically weakened toxins, called toxoids, were available in the 1920s (Plotkin and Plotkin 2008).

The tuberculosis vaccine bacille Calmette-Guérin was developed by Albert Calmette and Camille Guérin by severe attenuation over 13 years of a bovine tubercle bacterium and introduced in 1927. BCG vaccine is a live attenuated bacterial vaccine. Today it is the most widely used vaccine in the world, though its efficacy is variable, partly due to variability of the BCG strains around the world (Plotkin and Plotkin 2008). The live virus yellow fever vaccine was available for human use in 1935.

Table 3.1 History of human vaccine development (Plotkin and Plotkin 2008)

Live, Attenuated	Killed Whole Organism	Protein or Polysaccharide	Genetically Engineered
		18th Century	
Smallpox (1798)			
		19th Century	
Rabies (1885)	Typhoid (1896) Cholera (1896) Plague (1897)		
		First Half 20th Century	
Tuberculosis (1927) (Bacille Calmette-Guérin) Yellow Fever (1935)	Pertussis (1926) Influenza (1936) Typhus (1938)	Diphtheria toxoid (1923) Tetanus toxoid (1926)	
		Second Half 20th Century	
Polio (oral) Measles Mumps Rubella Adenovirus Typhoid (*salmonella* Ty21a) Varicella Rotavirus reassortants Cholera	Polio (injected) Rabies (cell culture) Japanese encephalitis Tick-borne encephalitis Hepatitis A Hepatitis B (plasma derived)	Pneumococcus polysaccharide Meningococcus polysaccharide *Hemophilus influenzae* type b polysaccharide Meningococcal conjugate *H. influenza* conjugate Typhoid (Vi) polysaccharide Acellular pertussis Anthrax secreted proteins	Hepatitis B surface antigen recombinant Cholera (recombinant Toxin B)
		21st Century	
Cold-adapted influenza (CAIV) (2003) Rotavirus (attenuated and new reassortants) Zoster (2006)		Pneumococcal conjugates (2000) Meningococcal quadrivalent conjugates (2005)	Human papillomavirus recombinant (2006)

Whole cell killed pertussis vaccine became available in 1926. Safety concerns about the whole cell pertussis vaccine led to a search for an alternative. Natural immunity to pertussis induces antibodies to pertussis toxin, filamentous hemagglutinin, pertactin, and fimbrial antigens (Storsaeter et al 1992). Acellular pertussis vaccines containing pertussis toxoid and possibly one or more of the three other antigens became available in the 1990s.

The development of a safe and easy cell culture method to grow viruses, by John Enders, Thomas Weller, and Fred Robbins, started the golden age of vaccine development in 1949 (Plotkin and Plotkin 2008). The live oral polio vaccine (OPV) of Albert Sabin and the injected inactivated polio vaccine (IPV) of Jonas Salk were both developed in the early 1950s. The live virus measles, mumps, rubella and varicella vaccines followed in succession between the 1960s and the 1990s. Various killed influenza virus vaccines were available since the 1930s, and the live cold-adapted influenza virus (CAIV) vaccine was licensed finally in 2003 in the United States.

3.2.3 Recent developments and beyond

Many bacteria including meningococcus, pneumococcus, and *Hemophilus influenzae* have an outer capsule composed of polysaccharides (complex sugars) (Murphy et al 2008). The capsules are species- and type-specific. There are more than 90 serotypes of pneumococcal bacteria, a subset of which causes most of the disease. Important meningococcal bacteria types are A, B, C, W135, and Y. Vaccines are generally effective against only the types that they contain, although some cross-protection can occur. The best defense against bacteria with polysaccharide capsules is to coat them with antibody (opsonization). A bacterium, or other antigen, coated with antibodies is recognized as foreign by certain cells (phagocytes) that eat it and destroy it. Vaccination aims to elicit antibodies against the polysaccharide capsules. The first vaccines for these bacteria were made from the purified polysaccharide capsule. However, complex sugars are not as immunogenic as proteins, especially in very young children. The newer conjugate vaccines for such bacteria link the bacterial polysaccharide to a protein carrier to be able to elicit the innate immune response and the T-cell-dependent antibody response and be more strongly immunogenic.

Reassortant vaccines are produced by coinfection of cell culture with wild-type and attenuated virus strains so their genomes can mix. This approach can be used with viruses with segmented genomes, such as influenza and rotavirus (Murphy et al 2008). A modern approach to live attenuated vaccines is to use recombinant DNA technology to put mutations into the genes responsible for virulence in a way that makes reversion to wild-type nearly impossible.

Several new approaches to vaccines are being tried. DNA vaccination injects small bits of the DNA encoding an immunogenic part of the virus directly into the muscle. Surprisingly, the elicited immune response is able to protect against infection with the whole virus. Subunit vaccines contain only parts of the antigenic material of the pathogen. They induce a response against only some proteins in the pathogen. Vector-based vaccines integrate genes of the pathogen of interest into the DNA of another pathogen that serves as the vector. When the vector pathogen replicates in the host it expresses the genes of the pathogen of interest, inducing an immune response to that pathogen. Many more vaccines are in the pipeline, including vaccines against malaria, HIV, dengue fever, new vaccines against tuberculosis, and new generations of vaccines against numerous infectious agents for which vaccines already exist.

3.2.4 Adjuvants

Adjuvants are substances that enhance the ability of an antigen to induce an immune response (Murphy et al 2008). Many of the antigens used in vaccines by themselves do not produce a strong immune response, partly because they do not themselves induce the innate immune response needed to activate the naive T cells. Adjuvants are included in many vaccines to enhance the immunogenicity. Different adjuvants promote different types of immune response. Adjuvants are often made of bits of cell walls of bacteria, but may be too strong to be used in human vaccines. The pertussis toxin protein has adjuvant properties. In the combination vaccine diphtheria, pertussis, tetanus, the components of pertussis serve as an adjuvant.

3.3 Vaccine Safety

Prophylactic vaccines are generally given to healthy people, so that safety is a primary consideration at all phases of clinical testing and after licensure. Safety concerns of vaccination result partly from the immune response to foreign material in the body, either from the pathogen antigen of interest or the adjuvant. Unwanted reactions after vaccination are called side effects or adverse events or adverse experiences (AEs). Some adverse events could immediately follow vaccination, and others could appear over the next few days. Typical adverse events local at the injection site include inflammation with swelling, redness, soreness, and/or warmth. Systemic adverse events include fever, malaise, chills, or muscle aches. Serious adverse events (SAEs) include anaphylactic shock immediately following vaccination, serious ulceration or abscesses at the vaccination site, or death, among others.

Other safety issues arise with vaccines that contain whole attenuated or killed pathogens. Attenuated pathogens in vaccines can be shed. Shedding is not synonymous with transmission, but occasional transmission might occur. One transmission event of the cold-adapted influenza virus vaccine was documented, but without causing disease (Vesikari et al 2006). However, in some cases transmission of the vaccine virus to contacts can result in disease, such as with the live oral polio vaccine. Some attenuated pathogens can revert to wild-type and cause disease. In immunocompromised people, that is, people with weakened immune systems, such as people with HIV, on cancer chemotherapy, or for other reasons, live attenuated vaccine viruses can cause severe disease. For this reason, live attenuated vaccines are not supposed to be given to most immunocompromised people or close contacts of immunocompromised people.

If whole pathogens are not completely killed before being put into the vaccine, they could also cause disease. Shortly after the killed (Salk) polio vaccine trials in the United States, when manufacturing of the vaccine ramped up, vaccine from Cutter Laboratories contained virus that was not sufficiently inactivated. Over 200 paralytic polio cases were traced to vaccine from Cutter (Oshinsky 2005). The incident resulted in much stricter manufacturing requirements, but also damaged the public trust in being vaccinated against polio. Widespread immunization against swine influenza in the United States in 1976 caused several hundred cases of Guillain–Barré syndrome, resulting in several deaths from pulmonary complications (Neustadt and Fineberg 2005). A rotavirus vaccine was withdrawn shortly after introduction when a few cases of a rare type of intestinal obstruction occurred that might have been attributable to the vaccine (Murphy et al 2001). Perception of the safety of vaccination is also important for people to agree to be vaccinated or to have their children vaccinated. Safety of vaccines has become increasingly important as the threat of disease has been reduced.

3.4 Immune Assays

Measuring the immune response to vaccination is important to understand how immunogenic the vaccine is. For a vaccine to be licensed, evidence of its potency must be demonstrated. Potency is the specific ability or capacity of the vaccine as measured by a laboratory test. Increasingly, immune measures are being used as outcomes in definitive studies leading to licensure of vaccine candidates (Chapter 15).

3.4.1 Antibody assays

The most important assays measure the antibodies circulating in the plasma, the fluid part of the blood (Murphy et al 2008). Once blood is collected, it is allowed to clot. Serum is the fluid component of clotted blood, and when the antibodies in it are of interest, it is called antiserum. Assays make use of the high specificity of the antibody for its antigen. Assays for antibodies are also called serological assays and the use of antibodies called serology. Serial dilutions of the antiserum are performed, usually diluting at each step by half, a process called titration. The titer of an antiserum is the dilution at which binding of the antibody to its antigen falls to 50% of the maximum.

The enzyme-linked immunosorbent assay (ELISA) is one of the most common assays. It can be used to detect antibody or to detect antigens in viral infections. The assay relies on direct measurement of antibody binding to its antigen.

The hemagglutination assay is based on the ability of some viral surface or envelope proteins to agglutinate, or stick to human or animal red blood cells and cause them to clump. Hemagglutinin is the main surface protein of the influenza virus. Protective immunity against influenza is generally attributed to neutralizing antibodies directed against the hemagglutinin. The antibodies against hemagglutinin are measured by the ability to inhibit the hemagglutination assay. The titer, or dilution, in a person's antiserum at which this is measured is called the hemagglutination assay inihibition (HI or HAI) titer.

Immunoblots can be used to test sera for the presence of antibodies to specific proteins (Murphy et al 2008). Immunoblots, also known as Western blots, are used to separate proteins (antigens) of different sizes. Antibodies are then exposed to the size-separated proteins on the blots to allow them to bind to their specific antigens. The bound antibodies are then labeled so they can be seen. If a vaccine is composed of just parts, or subunits, of a pathogen, then the antibody response to the vaccine will look different from the antibody response to the whole pathogen. Thus, the response to natural infection can be differentiated from the response to a subunit vaccine because there will be fewer bands on the immunoblot in a person who did not have a natural infection.

Several statistical issues related to analyzing and interpreting assays are not discussed in this book. These include interval censoring of the titer measurements and interpretation of null results when the result may be positive but simply below the limits of detection of the assay. Gilks et al (1993) estimated the waning of antibody titers with a random-effects models for longitudinal data using Gibbs sampling. This approach can be used to determine schedules for booster shots if it is known what level of antibodies are protective.

3.4.2 T-cell assays

A number of assays can be used to characterize T cells (Murphy et al 2008). T cells are more difficult to characterize than B cells or their antibodies because there are different types of T cells with different functions. Also measurement of the T-cell receptors in the cell membrane is more difficult than measuring antibodies. Cytotoxic T cells can be measured by seeing if they kill specific target cells. CD4 help T cells can be measured by the amount of cytokines they release when exposed to the specific antigen. The ELISPOT assay is a modification of the ELISA assay that allows measurement of the frequency of T cells in a population of T cells that respond to a specific antigen. The ELISPOT can also be used to detect specific antibody secretion of B cells. T cell assays are available that allow identification of functional subsets of T cells, T-cell-receptor specificity, frequency of certain subsets of lymphocytes, and assessment of the diversity of the T-cell repertoire, among others. As vaccines are developed based on stimulation of cellular immunity, it would be important to include more discussion of the assays. In addition, evaluation of correlates of immunological protection are beginning to include assessment of cellular immunity.

3.5 Herd Immunity

Herd immunity describes the collective immunological status of a population of hosts, as opposed to an individual host, with respect to a given pathogen (Fox and Elveback, 1975; Anderson and May, 1982). Herd immunity can be thought of as a collective biological state of a population of hosts. Herd immunity of a population can be high if many people have been immunized or have recovered from infection with immunity or be low if most people are susceptible. The level of herd immunity can decrease if the proportion of susceptibles increases or vaccinated protection wanes in individuals. The term herd immunity is sometimes somewhat incorrectly used to refer to the threshold at which circulation of an infectious agent is essentially eliminated. We prefer the definition of herd immunity that considers it a continuum rather than a threshold. If herd immunity is high enough, then a threshold may be reached at which infectious hosts no longer contact enough susceptible hosts to maintain transmission.

Herd immunity can be measured in several different ways. Seroprevalence is the proportion of a population that has antibodies to a particular antigen. Seroprevalence of protective antibodies against an infectious agent is a measure of herd immunity. In Figure 3.1, the age-specific seroprevalences, that is, proportions of people with anti-hepatitis A virus (HAV) IgG and anti-hepatitis E virus (HEV) IgG in a collection of communities in Vietnam (Hau et al 1999) are plotted. Seroprevalence of anti-HAV IgG rises very quickly with age essentially reaching 1.00. Seroprevalence of anti-HEV IgG, on the other hand, is very low. The area under the bar graphs, adjusted for the varying sizes of the age groups, can be regarded as the level of herd immunity. The herd immunity for HAV is high and that for HEV is low. On average, 97% versus 16% of the people have antibodies against the two diseases. There is concern that the population is susceptible to an outbreak of HEV. Fine (1993) reviews herd immunity. Fine and Mulholland (2008) use the term community immunity, which is a useful alternative to herd immunity.

The indirect effects of vaccination are primarily due to herd immunity resulting from increased levels of protection in individuals. Recently impressive indirect and overall effects have been observed with the conjugate pneumococcal vaccines, meningococcal, and Hib vaccines, indicating important herd immunity (Chapter 13).

Mechanisms of immunity to the three stages of the malaria parasite can be roughly classified as infection-blocking, disease-modifying, and transmission-blocking. Naturally acquired immunity to malaria is transient and can be lost in the absence of

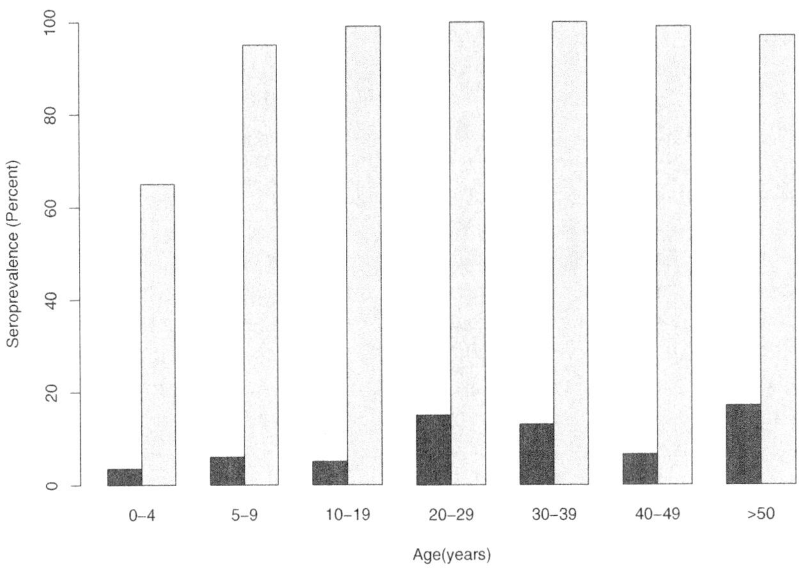

Fig. 3.1 Age-specific prevalences of anti-hepatitis E virus (black bars) and anti-hepatitis A virus (gray bars) immunoglobulin G in Vietnam. Data from Hau et al (1999).

frequent natural boosting by infective mosquito bites (Boyd 1949). The possible dynamic interplay of stage-specific immunity, duration of vaccine effectiveness, natural boosting, level of vaccine coverage, intensity of transmission, and the consequences for incidence and prevalence of malaria has excited speculation since the 1980s (Bruce-Chwatt 1987; Molineaux et al 1985). Because immunity to malaria decreases transmission, there is a negative feedback loop between the two. Vaccination programs suppressing transmission without eliminating it will alter existing host–parasite balances of both infection and disease, raising difficult public health questions. Halloran et al (1989) showed malaria vaccination could result in increased disease, either in the population as a whole, or in the unvaccinated portion of the population, depending on the antigenic stage of vaccination, the level of coverage, the duration of vaccine-induced immunity compared with naturally induced immunity, and the vaccination strategy.

With many other infectious diseases, such as measles, it is not well understood whether what appeared to be life-long immunity was dependent on continual re-exposure to infection before widespread immunization. Thus waning of vaccine-induced immunity could result in large portions of the adult population being susceptible to disease once again.

3.6 Early Phase Vaccine Studies

The early phase of vaccine development involves searching for candidate vaccine antigens. These include in vitro studies as well as testing in animals. Once a candidate antigen is found, then a vaccine is formulated. The decision to move from preclinical testing to Phase I, Phase II, and finally Phase III in humans is a complex process involving the immunogenicity and safety of the vaccine candidate, the cost and potential market for the vaccine, and many other factors (Sadoff and Wittes 2007).

If appropriate animals are available for that particular infectious agent, then the vaccine candidate will be tested in preclinical studies in animals. In preclinical vaccine studies in nonhuman primates, one wants to minimize the number of animals used, and at the same time, obtain sufficient information to reach valid conclusions. Sample sizes are small and exact inference is used. Albert (1996) considered three approaches to computing the sample size in preclinical studies of an AIDS vaccine. The vaccine candidate is evaluated for safety, immunogenicity, and possibly efficacy against experimental challenge with the infectious agent. In early preclinical studies, knowledge about the immune response may affect decisions about choice of antigen, broadness of coverage, and delivery systems. The immune response to antigens is often quite specific to the animal host, so that using animal immune responses to make conclusions about human responses is uncertain. However, immunogenicity in animals can give some help in making the decision to move a vaccine forward to clinical testing in humans (Sadoff and Wittes 2007).

If the vaccine candidate looks safe with possibly good immunogenicity, then a Phase I clinical trial in humans is conducted. In Phase I clinical trials, safety is the primary outcome of interest, but immunogenicity is also evaluated. Phase I trials are usually small and conducted in healthy adults generally not at risk to be naturally exposed to infection. Phase I trials may involve different vaccine candidates, doses, or schedules of administration (number and timing of doses).

Phase II studies are further safety and immunogenicity testing in humans. Decisions to move forward to the larger Phase II trials are based on the results of the safety and immunogenicity data in the Phase I studies. Phase II studies are often conducted in populations more similar to the target population for the final vaccine than Phase I studies. When an immune marker is or immune markers are considered to be a reliable measure of protection against disease, Phase II studies can be the definitive study for licensure with immune markers as outcomes. Examples include the meningoccal C vaccine in Great Britain (Balmer and Borrow 2004) and the current development of meningococcal A vaccine for Africa (Jódar et al 2003). The immune response is also used for licensing vaccines when the incidence of disease is very low, making vaccine field studies infeasible or for vaccines against biological threat agents. Concomitant use trials are designed to show that administration of two or more vaccines at the same time does not interfere with the immunogenicity of the antigens. For example, when varicella vaccine (V) was added to the measles, mumps, rubella vaccine (MMR) to make MMRV, it had to be shown that the varicella component would not interfere with the immunogenicity of the other three.

During and after licensure, immune responses allow generalization to populations that were themselves not tested for efficacy (Sadoff and Wittes 2007). We return to the topic of using immunological surrogates of protection as outcomes in vaccine studies in Chapter 15. Phase IIb studies are intermediate sizes trials, still Phase II studies, that are large enough that some information on vaccine efficacy may be available (Rida et al 1997). The preliminary efficacy results can also be used to expand enrollment to a full-scale Phase III field study.

During a clinical study, all adverse events and serious adverse events are recorded for study participants. A decision must be made whether the adverse event is due to the vaccine. For example, a person might have died in a car accident. Likely, the conclusion would be made that this SAE (death) was not due to the vaccine. Phase I and II trials can detect common adverse or serious adverse events. Some Phase III trials can detect relatively infrequent serious adverse events. Because usually several adverse events are recorded, the problem of multiplicity of tests is an issue. Sometimes serious adverse events do not become associated with a vaccine until millions of people have been vaccinated. These events are followed in post-licensure, or Phase IV, observational studies. Central registries have been set up in many countries to record adverse events and serious adverse events following vaccination. The problem with observational studies is to decide whether there is an increased rate of adverse events in people receiving the vaccine that is caused by the vaccine. Statistical methods have been developed to analyze such observational safety studies (Fine and Chen 1992; Farrington 1995). To handle the topic in depth lies outside the scope of this book.

3.7 Human Challenge Studies

Some pathogens have characteristics that make experimental infection in humans, called human challenge studies, to measure vaccine efficacy ethical and feasible. The pathogen should either not generally cause lethal infection or a very effective treatment must be available, or both. Human challenge studies have been conducted with malaria (Patarroyo et al 1987; Webster et al 2005), influenza (Clements et al 1984, 1986, 1990; Jones et al 2009), and other vaccines. Occasionally, such as in influenza, the challenge is with the attenuated vaccine virus (Belshe et al 2000).

Problems

3.1. What are the main differences of the innate immune response and the adaptive immune response?

3.2. How are safety issues of vaccination related to the immune response to vaccination?

3.3. What are the advantages and disadvantages of adjuvants for human vaccines?

3.4. Why were virus vaccines not developed until the second half of the 20th century?

3.5. Consider the role of natural boosting by exposure to infection to maintain immune protection against a disease such as malaria or measles. Explain how widespread immunization in childhood could result in increased disease in adults over the long-term.

3.6. How does a seroprevalence survey provide information about the level of herd immunity in a population?

3.7. (a) Assume a Phase II trial of a vaccine candidate provides evidence of good immunogenicity and safety. How would you decide to take a particular candidate forward to an expensive, large-scale Phase III vaccine field trial?
(b) How would you decide if you have similar evidence on three vaccine candidates?

Chapter 4
Binomial and Stochastic Transmission Models

4.1 Overview

How we think about the transmission dynamics of an infectious agent within a host population influences how we design, analyze, and interpret vaccine studies. It can influence our choice of interventions. In this chapter and the next we introduce transmission models necessary for estimating and understanding the effects of vaccination. In this chapter, we present the binomial model and the chain binomial model. These models are central to formulating statistical models for estimating transmission parameters and vaccine efficacy parameters. They form the basis of the models in Chapters 10 through 12. The binomial model is also the basic building block of the small- and large-scale stochastic simulation models of vaccination interventions in populations, that can also be used to produce data for design of vaccine studies. In a stochastic model, whether an event occurs is random, depending on a number produced by a random number generator described later.

In Chapter 5 we present simple differential equation transmission models that are generally deterministic. That is, every time the equations are solved, the same answer is obtained. This approach is essential to understanding large complex models of the population effects of vaccination programs, but less relevant to our purposes in this book. Much of theoretical discussion of the effect of vaccination on the basic reproductive number R_0 stems from the solution of differential equation models, so the chapter discusses R_0 and the effects of vaccination.

Without getting too formal, all of the models in this and the following chapters assume that people can be in discrete states, such as susceptible, infected but latent, infected and infectious, or recovered. The binomial models in this chapter are discrete event models, in that whole individuals become infected or recover. They are particularly interesting for analyzing data because the likelihood functions for the discrete events can be easily formulated. Binomial models can be formulated in discrete time or in continuous time as we show. In contrast, in the differential equation models, the number of people flowing from one state to another, such as from susceptible to infected, is continuous. That is, there can be 450.75 people in the in-

M.E. Halloran et al., *Design and Analysis of Vaccine Studies*, Statistics for Biology and Health, DOI 10.1007/978-0-387-68636-3_4,

fected compartment. We consider only differential equation models formulated in continuous time, although discrete time versions are sometimes used.

For all transmission models, whether for estimating parameters of interest or for simulating vaccine interventions, the underlying assumptions about how people mix and contact each other is central. We begin this chapter with a general introduction to mixing structures and population dynamics.

4.2 Contact Processes and Mixing Structures

Individuals make contact with other individuals before an infectious agent enters the population. What types of contacts and contact processes are of interest can depend on the infectious agent of interest. Contacts may be through the air or casual touching. Some models assume that people behave like gas molecules with the rate of contacts being determined by density. If people are pressed more closely together, as in an urban environment, they contact each other more often than if they were less densely distributed, as in a rural environment. Hence, for infections spread by air, droplet, or casual touching, such as measles, influenza, or mumps, population density plays a role in determining the value of R_0. Alternatively, for diseases spread by contacts made by choice, such as in sexual contacts or injection of intravenous drugs, the contacts may be determined more by social behavior. In many cases, both density and social choice will play a role in determining contact rates and mixing patterns.

4.2.1 Random mixing

Under the assumption of random mixing, every person in the transmission unit is assumed to make contact equally with every other person. Thus, an infective person will equally expose every other person in the transmission unit. In a model of the United States based on random mixing, every infective person in the population will expose every susceptible. In a model with small transmission units, such as households, schools, or day care centers, the assumption of random mixing implies that each person in the transmission unit makes contact with the others equally. We denote by c the constant contact rate that does not change over time in a randomly mixing population. Most populations do not mix randomly. We consider a few approaches to nonrandom mixing.

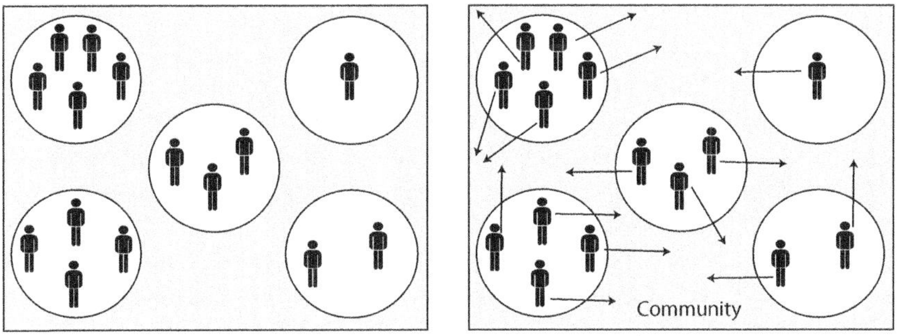

Fig. 4.1 Transmission units under different assumptions of their relation to one another. On the left, individuals are assumed to mix only within their transmission units. The transmission units are independent of one another. On the right, individuals can also mix in the community. The transmission units are assumed embedded within a community.

4.2.2 Transmission units within populations

Given an assumption of random mixing in small transmission units such as households, one can then make assumptions about the relation of the transmission units to one another. The transmission units can be assumed to be completely separate and independent of one another, as on the left in Figure 4.1. Under this assumption, an infected person in one transmission unit does not expose someone in another transmission unit. This is the assumption that underlies the simple chain binomial model discussed later. Alternatively, the individuals in the transmission units can be assumed to mix in the community at large as well and either expose each other to infection or be exposed to infection from some community source (right, Figure 4.1). When we define this community structure, it allows that a susceptible individual can become infected if exposed to an infected person within the household as well as the possibility of being infected in the community at large during the course of an epidemic or over the duration of a study. The transmission units could be households, sexual partnerships, schools, workplaces, or day care centers, for example. The assumption of transmission units in a community underlies the analyses in Chapter 11. The assumption of independent transmission units underlies the analyses in Chapter 12.

More complex mixing models can be formulated where an individual can belong to several overlapping transmission units and mix in the community at large as well. For example, a schoolchild can mix with family members at home, with other school children in the schools, and with people in the neighborhoods and community at large. People may be assumed to mix randomly within each mixing group. Network theory is used to study the contact patterns and social networks of actual populations and simulated populations formally (Morris and Kretzschmar 1997; Koopman et al 2000; Eubank et al 2004; Newman et al 2006; Meyers et al 2006; Kenah and Robins 2007a, b).

4.2.3 Mutually exclusive subpopulations

Rather than small transmission units, we may think of a population as divided into mutually exclusive subpopulations that mix with members of their own subpopulations differently than with members of other subpopulations. Quite commonly, the population is divided into mutually exclusive, nonoverlapping age groups when modeling infectious diseases such as measles (McLean et al 1991) and chickenpox (Halloran et al 1994a). The population could be divided into mutually exclusive groups with different activity levels, such as in models of sexually transmitted diseases (Hethcote and York 1984).

In a population composed of three mutually exclusive mixing groups, groups 1, 2, and 3, the contact pattern is described by a *mixing matrix* that has the same number of rows and columns as the number of mixing groups. The entries in the matrix represent the contact rates of individuals within and between the groups. The contact rate of individuals of group j with individuals of group i is denoted by c_{ij}. The mixing pattern of three groups is represented by the matrix

$$C = \begin{bmatrix} c_{11} & c_{12} & c_{13} \\ c_{21} & c_{22} & c_{23} \\ c_{31} & c_{32} & c_{33} \end{bmatrix} .$$

On the diagonal are the contact rates within groups, c_{11}, c_{22}, and c_{33}. The entries off the diagonal, for example, c_{12} and c_{32}, represent the contact rates between the groups corresponding to that row and column. Simple social contact data can be used to improve estimates of age-specific transmission parameters for infectious respiratory spread agents (Wallinga et al 2006; Halloran 2006).

The average number of new infectives that one infective will produce, R_0, will be highest in the group with the highest within-group contact rate, assuming that the transmission probability and infectious period are the same in all groups. If an epidemic occurs and there is contact between the three groups, the epidemic in the group with the highest contact rate will help drive the epidemic in the groups with the lower rates. The group with the highest R_0 would then serve as a *core population* for transmission (Hethcote and York 1984) . The existence of a core group has consequences for intervention programs. It may be easy to reduce the average R_0 for the whole population below 1, while R_0 in the core population remains above 1, so that transmission will persist. In infectious diseases, the chain is only as weak as its strongest link.

Hethcote and York (1984) examined different strategies for reducing gonorrhea taking into account sex workers who acted as a core group and their contacts within the general population. They found that an intervention program generally needs to be targeted at the subpopulation with the higher R_0, in this case, the core population of sex workers, to have most effect. In general, when planning interventions in situations with heterogeneous transmission or levels of infection, targeting therapy or prevention to the groups with the highest transmission or levels of infection is often most effective in reducing infection in the population at large.

4.2.4 Population dynamics

Transmission models can be formulated with open populations with vital dynamics or with closed populations. There are two ways to enter and two ways to leave a population. Individuals can enter a population by being born into it or immigrating. Individuals can leave a population by dying or emigrating. Open populations may include just birth and death with no immigration or emigration. Open populations may also include just emigration, analogous to loss to follow-up. Open populations are analogous to open or dynamic cohorts. In a closed population, there are no births, immigration, deaths, or emigration. The closed population is analogous to a closed cohort. Whether a transmission model is formulated with an open or closed population will depend on the circumstances and time frame of the study. Dynamic consequences of the assumptions are considered in Section 5.4.

4.3 Probability of Discrete Infection Events

We consider the simple binomial model of transmission for discrete contacts and discrete time and a simple model in continuous time.

4.3.1 Probability of infection in discrete time or contacts

The binomial model is often used to estimate the transmission probability as well as effects of covariates such as vaccination status. The basic idea of the binomial model is that exposure to infection occurs in discrete contacts, which can also be discrete time units of exposure. Generally it is assumed that each contact is independent of another. We have defined p as the transmission probability during a contact between a susceptible person and an infectious person or other source of infection, such as an infectious mosquito. The quantity $q = 1 - p$ is the probability that the susceptible person will not be infected during the contact, called the *escape probability*. For example, if the transmission probability for influenza is $p = 0.30$, then the escape probability for one contact is $q = 1 - p = 0.70$. If a susceptible person makes n contacts with infectious people, then, assuming all contacts are equally infectious, the probability of escaping infection from all of the n contacts is $q^n = (1-p)^n$. The probability of being infected after n contacts with infectives is $1 - q^n = 1 - (1-p)^n$.

Suppose a person has five successive contacts with someone who has influenza (Figure 4.2a). What is the probability that the person will have become infected by the five contacts? In this example, $n = 5$. The calculation proceeds by first calculating the probability that the susceptible person will escape infection from all five contacts. Then this number is subtracted from one to get the probability that the person is infected at least once. If the probability of escaping infection from the first exposure is $q = 0.7$, then the probability of escaping infection from the

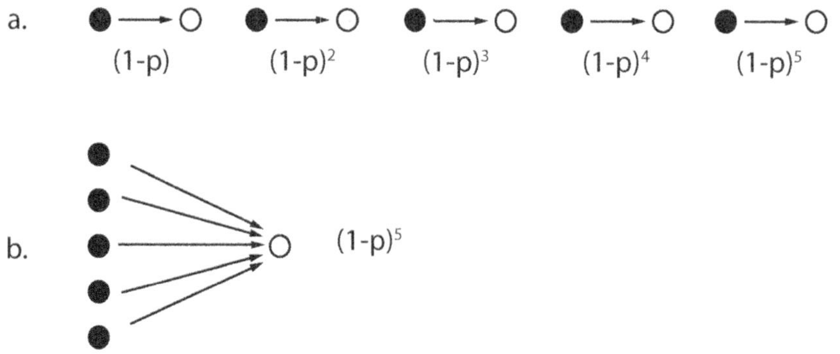

Fig. 4.2 (a) The escape probability with five consecutive contacts. (b) The escape probability with five simultaneous independent contacts, as in the Reed–Frost model. In both cases, the probability of infection is $1-(1-p)^5$.

second exposure is the probability of escaping the first one times the probability of escaping the second: $q \cdot q = 0.7 \cdot 0.7 = 0.49$. The probability of escaping infection from the third contact is similarly the probability of escaping infection from the first two contacts times the probability of escaping infection from the third, $q^2 \cdot q = 0.49 \cdot 0.7 = 0.34$. The probability of escaping infection from five successive contacts is $0.7^5 = 0.17$. The probability of becoming infected at least once is $1-(1-p)^n = 1-(0.7)^5 = 0.83$.

We have made an important assumption here. We assumed that each successive contact was not affected by any of the previous contacts. That is, the person did not develop immunity or become more susceptible as time went on. We also assumed that all of the contacts had the same risk of transmission. These assumptions may not be fulfilled. If so, the assumptions can easily be changed and a more complicated form of the binomial model developed. Becker (1989) discusses chain binomial models with random effects.

In a different problem, suppose a susceptible child attends school one day where five of the children simultaneously have influenza. What is the probability of becoming infected (Figure 4.2b)? Assume that the probability of becoming infected from one contact with one child with influenza is $p = 0.3$. Proceeding as before, the probability of escaping infection from one child is $q = 0.7$. Now we can calculate the probability of escaping infection from all five children, with $0.7^5 = 0.17$, so the probability of being infected on that day at school is $1 - q^5 = 0.83$.

Although the answers for the two examples are numerically the same, the biological assumptions in the two examples are different. In the example of influenza at school, it is assumed that each of the five *simultaneous* exposures to infection are the same, and that each additional child with influenza increases the probability of being infected independent of how many other infective children are present. The contacts and exposures to infection are assumed to operate the same as if they were successive and independent. The assumption of independence is commonly used in the binomial model, whether contacts are simultaneous or successive. This assumption is at the heart of the Reed–Frost model discussed below.

What if, however, biologically we think that once there is one infectious child in a classroom, then the room is saturated with infectious particles? Then adding more infectious children to the school will not increase the probability of becoming infected. We need to change our expression for the probability of becoming infected. If p is the probability of becoming infected from one infected person at school, then $q = 1 - p$ is again the escape probability from exposure to one infected. In contrast to the previous model, however, the probability of becoming infected from exposure to two or more infecteds at the same time is still p and the escape probability is still $q = 1 - p$. Under these biological assumptions, the probability of becoming infected from one child with influenza on one day is $p = 0.3$, and the probability of becoming infected from simultaneous exposure to five children with influenza on one day is also $p = 0.3$. The Greenwood model (1931) makes the assumption that the probability of infection on a given day does not change with increased number of infectives. The assumption is, however, seldom used in practice.

4.3.2 Other transmission models

Another way to model the probability of becoming infected is simply to multiply the number n of contacts with infectives times the transmission probability p, np. In the above influenza example, however, $np = 5 \cdot 0.3 = 1.5$. Because probabilities have to lie between 0 and 1, this approach obviously has limits. In particular, either n or p, or both, need to be small. Another commonly used expression for the probability of not becoming infected is e^{-np}, with the corresponding probability of becoming infected being $1 - e^{-np}$. In the influenza example above, then, the probability of not becoming infected is $e^{-5 \cdot 0.3} = e^{-1.5} = 0.22$ and for becoming infected is $1 - e^{-1.5} = 0.88$. Comparing this with the probability of being infected calculated from the binomial model, 0.83, we note that they are similar but not identical.

In the influenza example above, the transmission probability is high, and the product of np is large. If the transmission probability is much smaller or the contact rate is much smaller, or both, then the three methods for calculating the probability of becoming infected give similar answers. Suppose again that there are five infectious contacts in one day, but that the transmission probability of the infection in question is just $p = 0.001$. Then using the binomial model, the probability of becoming infected is $1 - (1 - p)^n = 1 - (.999)^5 = 0.00499$. Using the exponential expression, the probability of becoming infected is $1 - \exp(-5 \cdot 0.001) = 0.00499$, and based on the simple expression, $np = 5 \cdot 0.001 = 0.005$. There is little difference in the answers. In this example, the calculated np makes sense as the probability of becoming infected. The two simpler approaches are sometimes used as approximations for the binomial model. They are generally less time consuming to compute than the binomial model, which can be an issue in complex models. However, as we have just demonstrated, the approximation will not always be good. All three models require the same data for estimation of the parameters, namely the number of people who become infected, the number who do not, and the number of contacts made by each person up to when he or she becomes infected.

4.3.3 Probability of infection in continuous time

The above models assume discrete contacts or contacts within discrete units of time. Another approach to modeling the probability of becoming infected assumes that contacts occur in continuous time. The expression cp is the probability of being infected per unit time if all the contacts are with infectious persons, or c is the rate of infectious exposures and p is the transmission probability per exposure. Analogous to the discrete model, the expressions $\exp(-cp)$ and $1-\exp(-cp)$ are the probabilities of escaping infection or becoming infected per unit time, respectively. If the exposure occurs over some time period Δt, then the probabilities of escape or of infection in the time interval Δt are $\exp(-cp\Delta t)$ and $1-\exp(-cp\Delta t)$, respectively.

Another notation for the transmission rate per unit time of contact with an infective person is $\beta = cp$. Then the probabilities of escape or of infection in the time interval Δt are $\exp(-\beta\Delta t)$ and $1-\exp(-\beta\Delta t)$, respectively. Unless data are available on the contact rate separate from the transmission probability, in this model the transmission rate will be estimated from data on the time interval of exposure and infection status of each person in the study.

4.3.4 Contacts with persons of unknown infection status

Sometimes contacts are made with persons or sources of unknown infection status. We denote the probability that an individual with whom a contact is made is infectious by P. Then the probability of being infected from a contact of unknown infection status is $\rho = pP$. The quantity ρ is not a transmission probability in the strict sense, but a per-contact infection probability. The probability of escaping infection from contact with someone of unknown infection status is $1-\rho = 1-pP$. Under the binomial model, the probability of becoming infected after n such contacts is $1-(1-pP)^n = 1-(1-\rho)^n$.

Suppose as in the influenza example above that $p = 0.3$ but the contacts are with five individuals of unknown infection status. If the individuals are randomly chosen from a population where prevalence of influenza is $P = 0.4$, then the probability of being infected after five contacts is $1-(1-0.3\cdot 0.4)^5 = 0.47$.

An analogous expression can be developed for the continuous time model, because the hazard rate or incidence rate of infection as a function of the contact rate, the transmission probability, and the prevalence is $\lambda(t) = cpP$, the dependent happening expression (2.7). The probability of escaping infection within some period of time Δt is $\exp(-cpP\Delta t)$, and of being infected is $1-\exp(-cpP\Delta t)$, analogous

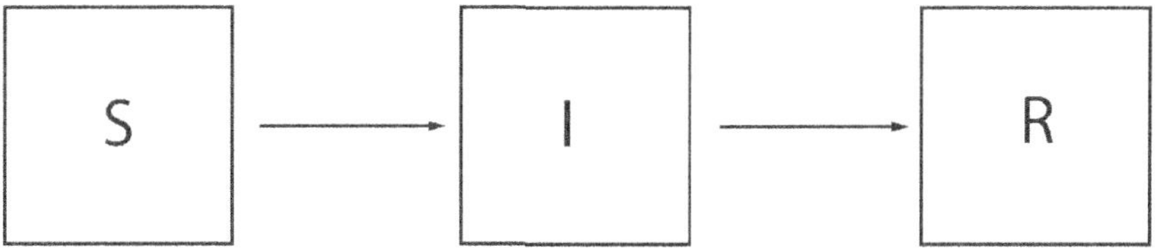

Fig. 4.3 Three states in the Reed–Frost chain binomial model: S, susceptible; I, infective; R, removed (immune).

to the cumulative incidence in a given time period Δt. These examples demonstrate some of the options and subtleties inherent in different approaches to modeling the transmission process.

4.4 Chain Binomial Models

Chain binomial models are dynamic models developed from the simple binomial model by assuming that infection spreads from individual to individual in populations in discrete units of time, producing chains of infection governed by the binomial probability distribution. To use the model, one needs to know the number of susceptibles and number of infectives in each generation. The expected distribution of infections in a collection of populations after several units of time can be calculated from the chained, that is, sequential, application of the binomial model. The Reed–Frost and Greenwood models are examples of chain binomial models. As mentioned above, the Reed–Frost model assumes that exposure to two or more infectious people at the same time are independent exposures. The Greenwood model assumes that exposure to two or more infectious people at the same time is equivalent to exposure to one.

The models are formulated in discrete time, with the time unit being approximately the generation time of the infectious agent. The generation time is about two weeks for measles and a few days for influenza.

In the Reed–Frost model, the assumption is made that people pass through three states (Figure 4.3). They start out susceptible, denoted by S, then become infected and infectious, denoted by I, after which they recover with immunity, denoted by R. Models of this type of infection process are called SIR models for susceptible, infected, recovered. Sometimes the notation XYZ is used for the three states. This simple model assumes that there is no latent period and that there are no asymptomatic infections. This model could be a simplified representation of influenza, measles, or chickenpox that ignores the latent period. In the simple Reed–Frost model, one assumes that the population size is constant N. If there are only three possible states, then each person in a population of N individuals is in one of these three states, where S_t is the number of susceptible people, I_t is the number of infectives, and R_t

Table 4.1 Chain binomial probabilities in the Reed–Frost model in households of size 3 with 1 initial infective and 2 susceptibles, $S_0 = 2, I_0 = 1$

Chain	Chain Probability	At p=0.4	At p=0.7	Final Number Infected
$1 \longrightarrow 0$	q^2	0.360	0.090	1
$1 \longrightarrow 1 \longrightarrow 0$	$2pq^2$	0.288	0.126	2
$1 \longrightarrow 1 \longrightarrow 1$	$2p^2q$	0.192	0.294	3
$1 \longrightarrow 2$	p^2	0.160	0.490	3
Total	1	1.00	1.00	

is the number of immune people at time t, where the subscript t denotes that the model is in discrete time. In contrast, in the continuous-time differential equation models in Chapter 5, the number of people in each state at the continuous time t is denoted by $S(t)$, $I(t)$, and $R(t)$.

As a simple example of the Reed–Frost chain binomial model, consider spread of infection in a transmission unit, such as a household, with three individuals, where one person is initially infected and the other two are initially susceptible (Table 4.1). The goal is to compute the probability of any of the possible chains. The model assumes that the initial infective is no longer infective after the first time unit. In the first time unit, one of three things can happen. One possibility is neither of the two susceptibles becomes infected. A second possibility is both of them become infected. A third possibility is just one of them becomes infected. The probability neither becomes infected is the probability both escape infection, or q^2. In this case, the chain ends, so the probability of this chain is q^2. If both susceptibles become infected in the first time unit, the chain also ends. The probability of both becoming infected from the first exposure is p^2.

The probability one person becomes infected from the first infected and the other does not is pq. This can happen two ways, so the probability of just one of the susceptibles being infected from the initial infective person in the first time unit is $2pq$. If one susceptible is infected in the first time unit, then this person is the new infective who exposes the last remaining susceptible. Exposure of the last remaining susceptible can result in two possible outcomes. Either she becomes infected or she does not, with probabilities p and q, respectively. The *chained probabilities* are then $2pq \cdot p = 2p^2q$ and $2pq \cdot q = 2pq^2$, respectively.

In Table 4.1 the chain probabilities are calculated for two different values of p, $p = 0.4$ and $p = 0.7$. In 1000 groups of size three with one initial infective, at $p = 0.4$, 360 of the groups would be expected to have just one infected, 288 to have two infected, and $192 + 160 = 352$ to have three infected at the end. Similarly, at $p = 0.7$, 90 would be expected to have one infected, 126 to have two infected, and 784 to have three infected. Because there are two different chains by which all three people become infected, if we were not able to observe the actual chains, we would not know which path the chain had taken. That is, we may only have data on the number of people who get infected in each transmission unit or household. So we would have only final value data and observe the final size distribution.

The R_0 in the Reed–Frost model, assuming that the duration of infectiousness is one time unit, or $d = 1$, is $R_0 = pN$, or sometimes $R = p(N-1)$, if there is one initial infective. More generally, $R = p(N - I_0)$, where I_0 is the number of initial infectives. In this example, if $p = 0.4$, then $R_0 = 0.4 \times 2 = 0.8$. If $p = 0.7$, then $R_0 = 0.7 \times 2 = 1.4$. In deterministic models, if $R_0 > 1$, the epidemic will always take off, and if $R_0 < 1$, the epidemic will never take off. An index that makes more sense in the probabilistic world of stochastic models is the probability that the epidemic will not take off.

Another index in stochastic models is the probability that an epidemic will not spread from the initially infected people, called the *probability of no spread*, denoted by P_{ns}. It can be calculated from the transmission probability p, or escape probability, $q = 1 - p$, the number of initially infected people in the population I_0, and the number of initially susceptible people S_0. The probability that a susceptible person escapes infection from all I_0 initial infectives is q^{I_0}. The probability that all S_0 of the initially susceptible people escape infection from all of the initial infectives is $P_{ns} = (q^{I_0})^{S_0}$. In the above example, with $p = 0.4$, the probability of no spread is $P_{ns} = (0.6^1)^2 = 0.36$. With $p = 0.7$, $P_{ns} = (0.3^1)^2 = 0.09$. The probability of no spread is the same as the probability that the infection chain ends with just the initial infectives.

4.4.1 The Reed–Frost model

Based on the definition of the Reed–Frost model above, we write the transition probability of getting $I_{t+1} = i_{t+1}$ new infectives at time $t+1$, given $S_t = s_t$ and $I_t = i_t$ susceptibles and infectives one time period before as

$$\Pr(I_{t+1} = i_{t+1} | S_t = s_t, I_t = i_t) = \binom{s_t}{i_{t+1}} \left(1 - q^{i_t}\right)^{i_{t+1}} q^{i_t(s_t - i_{t+1})}, \quad s_t \geq i_{t+1} . \tag{4.1}$$

Then, we can update the number of new susceptibles and recovered people by the equations

$$S_{t+1} = S_t - I_{t+1}, \tag{4.2}$$

$$R_{t+1} = R_t + I_t = \sum_{r=0}^{t} I_r. \tag{4.3}$$

Because the population is closed, $S_t + I_t + R_t = N$ for all t. The epidemic process starts with $I_0 > 0$, and terminates at stopping time T, where

$$T = \inf_{t \geq 0} \{t : S_t I_t = 0\} . \tag{4.4}$$

Table 4.2 Chain binomial probabilities in the Reed–Frost model in households of size 4 with 1 initial infective and three susceptibles, $S_0 = 3, I_0 = 1$

Chain	Chain Probability	Final Number Infected
$i_0 \to i_1 \to i_2 \to \ldots \to i_T$		R_T
$1 \longrightarrow 0$	q^3	1
$1 \longrightarrow 1 \longrightarrow 0$	$3pq^4$	2
$1 \longrightarrow 1 \longrightarrow 1 \longrightarrow 0$	$6p^2q^4$	3
$1 \longrightarrow 2 \longrightarrow 0$	$3p^2q^3$	3
$1 \longrightarrow 1 \longrightarrow 1 \longrightarrow 1$	$6p^3q^3$	4
$1 \longrightarrow 1 \longrightarrow 2$	$3p^3q^2$	4
$1 \longrightarrow 2 \longrightarrow 1$	$3p^3q(1+q)$	4
$1 \longrightarrow 3$	p^3	4

Equations (4.1–4.3) form the classical Reed–Frost model. Formal mathematical treatment of the model involves formulation of the discrete, two-dimensional Markov chain $\{S_t, I_t\}_{t=0,1,\ldots}$. I_t is the (binomial) random variable of interest, and S_t is updated using (4.2). The probability of a particular chain, $\{i_0, i_1, i_2, \ldots, i_T\}$, is given by the product of conditional binomial probabilities from (4.1) as

$$\begin{aligned} &\Pr(I_1 = i_1 \mid S_0 = s_0, I_0 = i_0)\Pr(I_2 = i_2|S_1 = s_1, I_1 = i_1)\cdots \\ &\Pr(I_T = i_T|S_{T-1} = s_{T-1}, I_{T-1} = I_{T-1}) \\ &= \prod_{t=0}^{T-1} \binom{s_t}{i_{t+1}} \left(1 - q^{i_t}\right)^{i_{t+1}} q^{i_t(s_t - i_{t+1})}. \end{aligned} \tag{4.5}$$

Table 4.2 shows the possible chains for a population of size 4 with one initial infective, ie, $S_0 = 3$, $I_0 = 1$.

In some cases, the distribution of the total number of cases, R_T, is the random variable of interest. We let J be the random variable for the total number of cases in addition to the initial cases, so that $R_T = J + I_0$. If we let $S_0 = k$ and $I_0 = i$, then the probability of interest is

$$\Pr(J = j|S_0 = k, I_0 = i) = m_{ijk}, \tag{4.6}$$

where $\sum_{j=0}^{k} m_{ijk} = 1$. Then, based on probability arguments (eg, see Bailey 1975; Becker 1989), we have the recursive expression

$$m_{ijk} = \binom{k}{j} m_{ijj} q^{(i+j)(k-j)}, \quad j < k, \quad m_{ikk} = 1 - \sum_{j=0}^{k-1} m_{ijk}. \tag{4.7}$$

Data are usually in the form of observed chains, $\{i_0, i_1, \ldots, i_r\}$, for one or more populations, or final sizes, R_T, for more than one population. If the data are in the form of observed chains, suppose we have N populations and let $\{i_{k0}, i_{k1}, \ldots, i_{kr}\}$ be the observed chain for the kth population. Then, from (4.5), the likelihood function for estimating $p = 1 - q$ is

$$\mathrm{L}(p) = \prod_{k=1}^{N}\prod_{t=0}^{r-1}\binom{s_{kt}}{i_{kt+1}}\left(1-q^{i_{kt}}\right)^{i_{kt+1}} q^{i_{kt}(s_{kt}-i_{kt+1})}. \tag{4.8}$$

Whether data are available on observed chains or just the final size distribution, the simple Reed–Frost model assumes that transmission units are independent of one another as in the left Figure 4.1. The initial infectives in the transmission unit somehow get infected, then the chain of infection unfolds within the transmission unit without any further introduction of infectives. Alternatively, one could assume that people, whether the initial infectives or the others in the transmission unit, are also exposed to infection outside the transmission unit in the community at large, as in the right Figure 4.1, or in other mixing places. Longini and Koopman (1982) modified the Reed–Frost model for the case where there is a constant source of infection from outside the population that does not depend on the number of infected persons in the population. Analysis of data assuming transmission units in a community is presented in Chapter 11. Becker (1989) gives details on different aspects of the Reed–Frost model and estimation of the parameters of interest from data. Bailey (1975) (Section 14.3) gives an example where (4.8) is used to estimate the transmission probability $\widehat{p} = 0.789 \pm 0.015$ (estimate ± 1 standard error) for the household spread of measles among children.

4.4.1.1 History

The probabilistic form of the Reed–Frost epidemic model was introduced by the biostatistician Lowell J. Reed and the epidemiologist Wade Hampton Frost around 1930 as a teaching tool at Johns Hopkins University. It was developed as a mechanical model consisting of colored balls and wooden shoots. Although Reed and Frost never published their results, the work is described in articles and books by others (see Chapters 14 and 18 in Bailey (1975) and Chapters 2 and 3 in Becker (1989). The model was first formulated and analyzed as a stochastic process by Abbey (1952) and Maia (1952). The first published computer simulation of the Reed–Frost model was by Elveback and Varma (1965). An excellent description of the early Reed–Frost model is given by Fine (1977). The deterministic version of the Reed–Frost model has been traced back to the Russian epidemiologist P. D. En'ko who used the model to analyze epidemic data in the 1880s (Dietz 1988). The Reed–Frost version of the chain binomial model and its extensions are used to study the dynamics of epidemics in small populations, such as families or day care centers, and to estimate transmission probabilities from epidemic data. See also Andersson and Britton (2000).

4.4.2 The Greenwood model

For the Greenwood model, the number of new infectives does not depend on the number of old infectives, but just on the presence of one or more infectives. Thus, the transition probability of getting $I_{t+1} = i_{t+1}$ new infectives at time $t+1$, given $S_t = s_t$ and $I_t = i_t$ susceptibles and infectives one time period before is

$$\Pr(I_{t+1} = i_{t+1} | S_t = s_t, I_t = i_t) = \left\{ \begin{matrix} \binom{s_t}{i_{t+1}} p^{i_{t+1}} q^{(s_t - i_{t+1})}, & s_t \geq i_{t+1}, \ i_t > 0 \\ 0 & \text{otherwise} \end{matrix} \right\}. \tag{4.9}$$

Analysis of the Greenwood model is similar to that of the Reed–Frost model.

4.4.3 Stochastic realizations of the Reed–Frost model

Realizations of epidemics according to the Reed–Frost model in equations (4.1)–(4.3) can be simulated using a random number generator. At each ti t, for each susceptible person exposed to I_t infectives, a random number between 0 and 1 is generated. If the random number is smaller than the infection probability $1 - q^{I_t}$, then the person becomes infected. If the random number lies between the infection probability and 1, then the person escapes infection in that time interval. The actually realized chain then depends on the series of random numbers that are generated, and varies from realization to realization. The probabilities in Tables 4.1 and 4.2 are the expected probabilities of particular chains if a large number of epidemics are simulated.

Tables 4.3 through 4.5 show realizations of stochastic epidemics in a population with 20 people at three different values of p. Table 4.3 shows epidemics in populations of size 20 and $p = 0.05$. Ten epidemics were run with one initial infective, $I_0 = 1$, $S_0 = 19$; the other ten epidemics were run with three initial infectives, $I_0 = 3$, $S_0 = 17$. The underlying Reed–Frost model is identical for both types of run, just the initial conditions are different. The $\mathrm{R}_0 = 1.0$, without taking into account the initial infectives. Taking into account the number of initial susceptibles, the initial reproductive numbers are 0.95 and 0.85, respectively. With one initial infective, the probability of no spread is $P_{ns} = (0.05^1)^{19} = 0.377$; with three initial infectives, $P_{ns} = (0.05^3)^{17} = 0.073$. The number of initial infectives is important to how long the chain is, whether any further infections occur, and the average number of final infectives. The chains in the table demonstrate the randomness of the epidemics and how in nature, given the same conditions, many different outcomes can occur merely by chance.

In Table 4.4, the transmission probability is increased to $p = 0.06$, so that $\mathrm{R}_0 = 1.2$. Taking into account the one initial infective, the reproductive number is 1.14, and the probability of no spread is $P_{ns} = (0.06^1)^{19} = 0.309$. The chains are noticeably longer than those with one initial infective and $p = 0.05$ in Table 4.3.

Table 4.3 Ten stochastic epidemics with the Reed–Frost model, 20 people, $p = 0.05$

	1 Initial Infective, $I_0 = 1$		3 Initial Infectives, $I_0 = 3$	
Epidemic	Final Infected	Chain	Final Infected	Chain
1	1	$1 \to 0$	8	$3 \to 2 \to 2 \to 1 \to 0$
2	1	$1 \to 0$	8	$3 \to 2 \to 1 \to 2 \to 0$
3	8	$1 \to 3 \to 3 \to 1 \to 0$	14	$3 \to 4 \to 3 \to 3 \to 1 \to 0$
4	1	$1 \to 0$	4	$3 \to 1 \to 0$
5	1	$1 \to 0$	11	$3 \to 2 \to 1 \to 4 \to 1 \to 0$
6	2	$1 \to 1 \to 0$	4	$3 \to 1 \to 0$
7	1	$1 \to 0$	4	$3 \to 1 \to 0$
8	1	$1 \to 0$	14	$3 \to 3 \to 3 \to 2 \to 2 \to 1 \to 0$
9	4	$1 \to 1 \to 1 \to 1 \to 0$	6	$3 \to 2 \to 1 \to 0$
10	1	$1 \to 0$	10	$3 \to 1 \to 3 \to 2 \to 1 \to 0$

Table 4.4 Ten stochastic epidemics with the Reed–Frost model, 20 people, $p = 0.06$

	1 Initial Infective, $I_0 = 1$	
Epidemic	Final Number Infected	Chain
1	1	$1 \to 0$
2	1	$1 \to 0$
3	2	$1 \to 1 \to 0$
4	8	$1 \to 2 \to 4 \to 1 \to 0$
5	10	$1 \to 2 \to 4 \to 2 \to 1 \to 0$
6	2	$1 \to 1 \to 0$
7	12	$1 \to 1 \to 3 \to 3 \to 1 \to 2 \to 1 \to 0$
8	8	$1 \to 2 \to 3 \to 2 \to 0$
9	9	$1 \to 3 \to 2 \to 1 \to 1 \to 1 \to 0$
10	14	$1 \to 3 \to 3 \to 2 \to 2 \to 2 \to 1 \to 0$

In Table 4.5, the transmission probability is increased to $p = 0.1$, so that $R_0 = 2.0$. Taking into account the one initial infective, the reproductive number is 1.9, and the probability of no spread is $P_{ns} = (0.1^1)^{19} = 0.135$. A clear bimodal distribution has emerged at this higher transmission probability. Two of the epidemics produce only one more infective, but in the other eight, most of the population becomes infected. In general, there are three different shapes for the final size distribution of the Reed–Frost epidemics depending on the R_0 and the number of initial infectives (Figure 4.4). In the illustration, there are 500 realizations at each R_0 with just one initial infective in each population of 200 people. With R_0 near or less than 1, most of the epidemics do not take off, but in a few, more than 50 people are infected. With a moderate R_0, the distribution is U-shaped or bimodal, with many of the epidemics not taking off, but in many most of the population becomes infected. With a higher R_0, nearly all of the people are infected in most of the epidemics. The terms *minor* and *major* epidemics distinguish situations in which there is a little spread from

Table 4.5 Ten stochastic epidemics with the Reed–Frost model, 20 people, $p = 0.1$

	1 Initial Infective, $I_0 = 1$	
Epidemic	Final Number Infected	Chain
1	2	$1 \to 1 \to 0$
2	16	$1 \to 3 \to 2 \to 2 \to 3 \to 3 \to 2 \to 0$
3	17	$1 \to 1 \to 3 \to 5 \to 6 \to 1 \to 0$
4	17	$1 \to 1 \to 1 \to 2 \to 3 \to 3 \to 4 \to 1 \to 1 \to 0$
5	17	$1 \to 2 \to 4 \to 6 \to 4 \to 0$
6	16	$1 \to 1 \to 2 \to 2 \to 4 \to 5 \to 1 \to 0$
7	14	$1 \to 1 \to 2 \to 4 \to 6 \to 0$
8	19	$1 \to 3 \to 3 \to 6 \to 3 \to 3 \to 0$
9	17	$1 \to 1 \to 3 \to 4 \to 4 \to 3 \to 1 \to 0$
10	2	$1 \to 1 \to 0$

the initial infectives from situations in which an epidemic gains momentum and is self-sustaining. See also Rida (1991).

Because quite often an epidemic might not take off even in the absence of an intervention, Halloran et al (2002a) defined the *epidemic prevention potential*, EPP, to be a function of the relative probability that an epidemic takes off in the absence of intervention and that an epidemic takes off in presence of an intervention program. The EPP of an intervention program compared to no intervention program is

$$\text{EPP} = 1 - \frac{\text{probability to take-off with no intervention}}{\text{probability to take-off with intervention}}. \tag{4.10}$$

4.5 Stochastic Simulation Models

The simple Reed–Frost model is the basic building block of small- and large-scale stochastic simulation models of infectious disease spread and studies of interventions. Such models need to include (1) the natural history of the infection of interest, (2) the demographics of the relevant population, (3) the contact structure and assumptions about where and how transmission occurs, and (4) models of the interventions and assumptions about how they will affect transmission, natural history, or the contact structure. Halloran et al (2002b) and Longini et al (2007a) examined vaccination strategies for smallpox. Several studies of interventions for pandemic influenza have made use of such simulation models (Longini et al 2004, 2005; Germann et al 2006; Ferguson et al 2006; Halloran et al 2008). Here we present one example of a stochastic simulation model used to examine potential indirect, total, and overall effects of cholera vaccination.

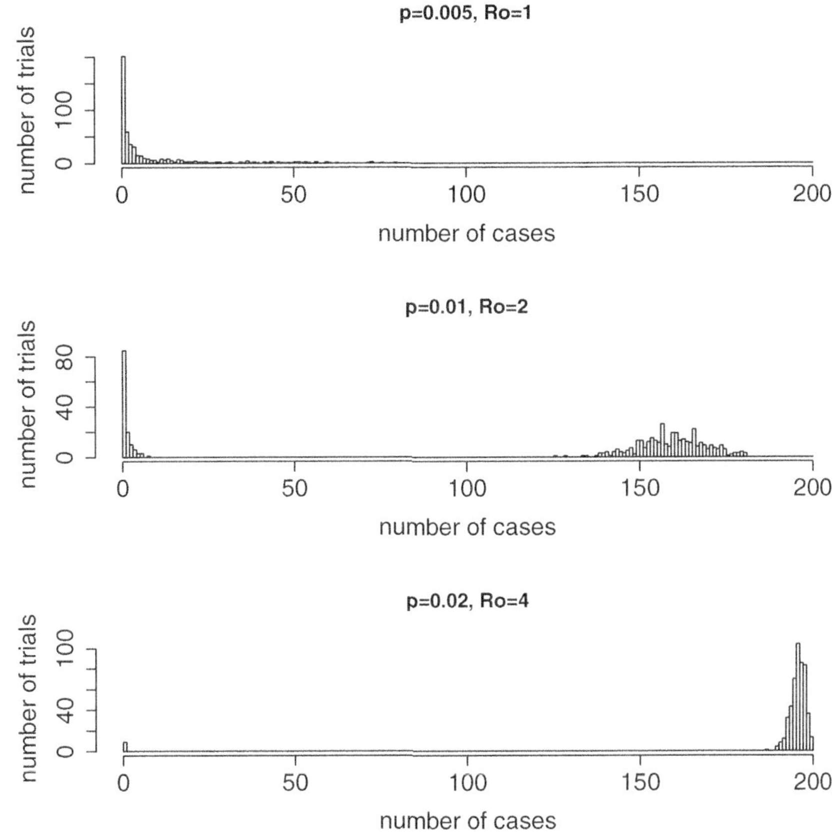

Fig. 4.4 Reed–Frost chain binomial model at three values of R_0. Populations of size 200 had one initial infective. Each histogram has 500 realizations of the epidemic.

4.5.1 Endemic cholera and vaccination

In the mid 1980s, a randomized vaccine trial with oral cholera vaccine in Matlab, Bangladesh, yielded an estimated 70% direct vaccine efficacy for up to two years (Clemens et al 1990; Durham et al 1998). Information about Matlab, Bangladesh was used to construct a model of the population as it was in 1985, consisting of 183,826 subjects (Longini et al 2007b). These subjects were mapped into families and families were distributed in baris, patrilineally related household clusters. In the model, baris are further clustered into subregions of about 6 square km in size considered to be the geographic cholera transmission areas with local sources of water. The model represents the number of contacts that a typical person makes with sources of potential cholera transmission in the course of a day. The age and bari size distributions of the population are based on data from Ali et al (2005).

Women and children are assumed to come into contact with sources of infection in the subregion where they live. Working males are assumed to make contact with infective sources in the subregion where they live as well as where they work.

The model included natural history assumptions about cholera. The model was calibrated to cholera illness incidence data from a large cholera vaccine trial in the Matlab field area of the International Centre for Diarrhoeal Disease Research, Bangladesh (ICDDR,B), that took place from 1985–1989 (Section 13.2.5). Oral cholera vaccine or placebo (killed *E. coli*) was offered to children 2–15 years old and women greater than 15 years old.

An infection function was defined that gives each susceptible person's daily probability of infection from all possible sources of infection created by infected people excreting cholera vibrios into the environment or through more direct contact similar to that in the Reed–Frost model with environmental exposure outside the transmission units. The probability of infection is proportional to the number of vaccinated and unvaccinated people in the subregion where contact is specified to occur. The model of vaccine effect assumed that immunity resulted in a proportional reduction in the probability of infection per contact with an infectious source, that is, a leaky vaccine. Results were averaged over all the subregions within vaccination coverage strata.

As described in Chapter 2, the indirect, total, and overall vaccine effectiveness measures were based on the reduction in infection rates when comparing the appropriate groups within a subregion with no vaccination to a comparable subregion with a fraction $f > 0$ of the population vaccinated (Figure 4.5). Let r_{ij} denote the cholera infection rate for people in subregion j with vaccination status i, where $i = 0$ for unvaccinated and $i = 1$ for vaccinated. The indirect effect of vaccination is measured by comparing the infection rates between the unvaccinated in the two subregions. Thus, the indirect vaccine effectiveness IVEF (VE_{IIa}) when comparing subregion 1 to 2 is $IVEF_{12} = 1 - (r_{01}/r_{02})$. The overall effect of vaccination is measured by comparing the average (over the vaccinated and unvaccinated groups) infection rates between the two subregions. Thus, the overall vaccine effectiveness, OVEF (VE_{III}), is $OVEF_{12} = 1 - (r_{.1}/r_{.2})$, where the $\cdot$ indicates averaging over the vaccinated and unvaccinated. The total effect of vaccination is measured by comparing the infection rate in the vaccinated in subregion 1 to the unvaccinated in subregion 2. Thus, the total vaccine effectiveness, TVEF (VE_{IIb}), is $TVEF_{12} = 1 - (r_{11}/r_{02})$. The direct effectiveness compares the vaccinated to the unvaccinated within a subregion. The direct vaccine effectiveness, DVEF(VE_{direct}), is $DVEF_1 = 1 - (r_{11}/r_{01})$.

The vaccine coverage levels in the target population and the effective coverage in the entire population from the trial are summarized in Table 4.6 (see also Table 13.5). The estimated reproductive number was 5.0 with a standard deviation of 3.3. Vaccine efficacy for susceptibility was set to $VE_S = 0.7$ (Clemens et al 1990; Durham et al 1998) and for infectiousness to $VE_I = 0.5$. Figure 4.6 shows the number of cases over time comparing the unvaccinated to the vaccinated populations for different levels of coverage.

For effectiveness measures, a comparison is made between the intervention subregions to hypothetical subregions that receive no vaccine, where $f = 0$. Table 4.7

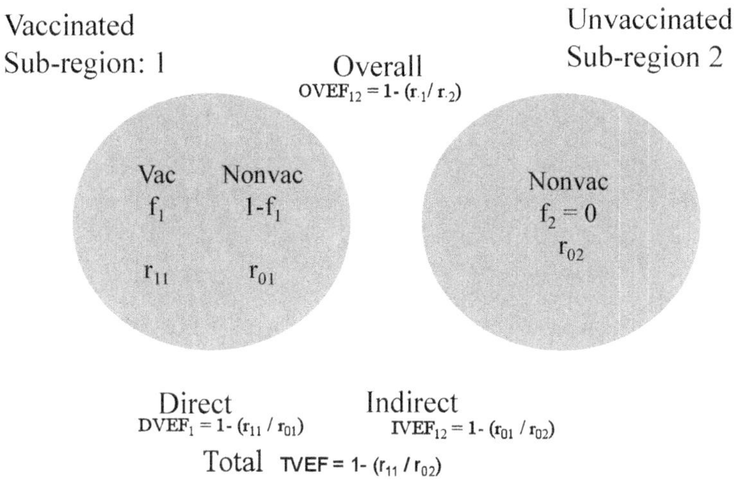

Fig. 4.5 Schematic of effectiveness comparisons for two subregions. Subregion 1 has a fraction $f_1 > 0$ people vaccinated, and the comparison subregion 2 has nobody vaccinated, so that $f_2 = 0$ (from Longini et al 2007b)

Table 4.6 Vaccination coverage, average incidence rates, and direct effectiveness (calibration runs) (Longini et al 2007b)

Vaccination Coverage (%)		Mean Cases/1,000 (95% CI)				Mean Direct Effectiveness (%)(95% CI)	
Population Target	Overall	Vaccinated Observed	Vaccinated Simulated	Placebo Observed	Placebo Simulated	Observed	Simulated
14	9	2.7 (1.9 to 3.5)	2.8 (0.5 to 6.1)	7.0 (6.5 to 7.5)	7.8 (1.9 to 14.8)	62	65 (52 to 77)
31	20	2.5 (2.0 to 3.0)	1.7 (0.3 to 3.8)	5.9 (5.4 to 6.4)	4.7 (0.9 to 10.2)	58	65 (55 to 76)
38	25	4.7 (1.2 to 2.0)	1.3 (0.2 to 3.4)	4.7 (4.2 to 5.2)	3.8 (0.8 to 8.6)	67	65 (54 to 77)
46	30	2.3 (1.9 to 2.7)	1.0 (0.1 to 2.5)	4.7 (4.2 to 5.2)	2.8 (0.5 to 6.8)	52	66 (54 to 79)
58	38	1.3 (1.0 to 1.6)	0.6 (0.1 to 1.8	1.5 (1.2 to 1.8)	1.8 (0.3 to 4.8)	14	66 (51 to 50)

shows the indirect, total, and overall effectiveness results for possible coverage levels when comparing coverages in the entire population, two years of age and older, ranging from 10% to 90% compared to no vaccination. For example, the average indirect effectiveness, comparing a population with a coverage of 30% to one with no vaccination is 70%. This indicates that on average, the cholera incidence among unvaccinated people in a population with 30% coverage would be reduced by 70% compared with a completely unvaccinated population.

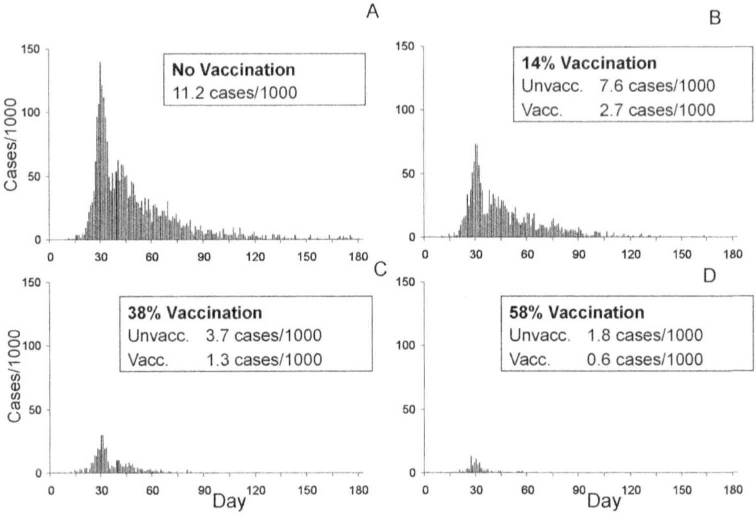

Fig. 4.6 Simulated number of cholera cases/1000 over a 180-day period in the Matlab study population for a single stochastic realization: (A) No vaccination; (B) 14% vaccination coverage of women and children; (C) 38% vaccination coverage; (D) 58% vaccination coverage (from Longini et al 2007b).

Table 4.7 Average indirect, total,and overall effectiveness of vaccination, and cases prevented per 1000 two-dose regimens (Longini et al 2007b)

Vaccination	Mean Effectiveness (%) (95% CI)			Mean Cases Prevented per
Coverage (%)	Indirect	Total	Overall	1000 Dose Regimens (95%)
10	30 (−39 to 83)	76 (47 to 95)	34 (−30 to 84)	40 (−34 to 97)
30	70 (31 to 93)	90 (76 to 98)	76 (44 to 95)	30 (17 to 36)
50	89 (72 to 98)	97 (91 to 99)	93 (82 to 99)	21 (19 to 23)
70	97 (91 to 99)	99 (97 to 100)	98 (95 to 100)	16 (15 to 17)
90	99 (98 to 100)	100 (99 to 100)	100 (99 to 100)	13 (12 to 14)

From Table 4.6, the simulated direct effectiveness at all coverage levels resulting from the simulations is about 66%, and the vaccine efficacy for susceptibility, VE_S ,is preset at 70%. This small underestimation is due to the model assumption that the vaccine effect is a leaky effect, a 70% reduction in the risk of infection per contact with an infective source, but the risk ratio estimator of vaccine effectiveness over the entire cholera epidemic is used (Chapter 7).

4.5.2 Use in study design

In general, stochastic simulation models are useful for generating simulated data with variability so that methods of analysis can be used and compared. Stochastic computer simulations are especially useful in helping to design studies and to develop new methods of analysis (see for example, Halloran et al 2002a; Golm et al 1999; Longini et al 1999). Deterministic models do not generally generate variability, but can be used to understand properties of the transmission system.

Problems

4.1. Compute the average number of people infected in the four examples of 10 epidemics in Tables 4.3 through 4.5. Make histograms of the number of people infected in each set of 10 epidemics and compare the shapes of the histograms.

4.2. (a) Compute the final size distribution from equation (4.7) for households of size 4 with one initial infective when $p = 0.4$.
(b) Compare it to the final size distribution obtained using the chain probabilities in Table 4.2.

4.3. (a) Let the transmission probability be $p = 0.4$, and the number of contacts $n = 6$. Compute the probability of being infected and the probability of escaping infection using the three approaches compared in Section 4.3.2.
(b) Do the same assuming that $p = 0.002$. Compare and explain the results of the different calculations.

4.4. (a) Compute the probability of no spread, P_{ns}, in a population with 3 initial infectives and 17 initial susceptibles if $p = 0.06$.
(b) Compute the same assuming $p = 0.01$.

4.5. In a population with prevalence of infectives of 0.2, and transmission probability $p = 0.005$, what is the probability that a person becomes infected after contact with 10 randomly selected partners in the population?

4.6. Consider a child who makes contact in a day at home with four other household members and at school with 20 other classmates. Assume that the transmission probability within the home is $p_h = 0.1$ and at school is $p_c = 0.05$. Assuming the Reed–Frost model, what is the probability the child becomes infected in a day if at home one person is infectious and at school 3 classmates are infectious?

4.7. (a) Write a stochastic computer simulation program for the Reed–Frost model that allows for different size of the population N, number of initial infectives I_0, and transmission probability p. The output can contain the realizations of individual chains, the realized final size distribution, the basic reproductive number R_0, and the probability of no spread P_{ns}. Explore the behavior of the system.

(b) Write a similar stochastic computer simulation for the Greenwood model.
(c) Compare the behavior of the two models for fixed values of N, I_0, and p.

Chapter 5
R_0 and Deterministic Models

5.1 Basic Reproductive Number

The basic reproductive number, R_0, is defined as the expected number of new infectious hosts that one typical infectious host will produce during his or her infectious period in a large, completely susceptible population. For example, if $R_0 = 5$ for mumps in a human population, then one infectious person in that population would be expected to produce five new secondary infectious cases if the population were completely susceptible. If he produced three additional cases who were not infectious, R_0 would still be 5.

For microparasitic infections such as viruses and bacteria, R_0 can be thought of as the product of the contact rate c, the duration of infectiousness d, and the transmission probability per contact with the infectious person, p:

$$R_0 = \begin{array}{c}\text{number of}\\ \text{contacts per}\\ \text{unit time}\end{array} \times \begin{array}{c}\text{transmission}\\ \text{probability}\\ \text{per contact}\end{array} \times \begin{array}{c}\text{duration}\\ \text{of}\\ \text{infectiousness}\end{array} = cpd\ .$$

R_0 summarizes many important aspects of an infectious agent in a host population in one parameter. It allows comparison of seemingly disparate diseases from the viewpoint of population biology. A value of R_0 is not specific to an infectious agent, but to an infectious agent population within a particular host population at a particular time. Contact rates relevant for respiratory transmission will be lower in rural areas than in urban areas. So, for example, we expect the R_0 of mumps to be lower in rural than in urban areas. The R_0 of malaria may be low during the season of low mosquito density, but high during the season in which mosquitoes are plentiful. The R_0 of HIV in a sexually active population of single people might be much higher than it is in a population of fairly monogamous married couples.

R_0 is dimensionless. It represents the number of new infectious cases per infectious case. Without further information about the magnitude of the quantities composing R_0, we cannot conclude much about the time frame of an epidemic, the transmissibility of the infectious agent, or the contact rate. R_0 is about 2 to 3 for influenza in some populations and also about 2 to 3 for HIV in some populations.

M.E. Halloran et al., *Design and Analysis of Vaccine Studies*, Statistics for Biology and Health, DOI 10.1007/978-0-387-68636-3_5,

Influenza has a relatively high transmission probability and short duration of infectiousness. The influenza virus spreads on a different time scale than HIV, which has a low transmission probability and longer duration of infectiousness. If we knew only that $R_0 = 3$ for both, then we would know that they both could easily produce epidemics, but we would not be able to draw conclusions about the relative time frames of the two.

The serial interval, T_g, or generation time, provides information about the time frame of the epidemic. The serial interval is the average time from the infection of a primary case to the new infections that result from exposure to the primary case (Svensson 2006; Fine 2003; Cauchemez et al 2006a) The rate of growth of an epidemic is determined approximately by the ratio R_0/T_g (Fraser et al 2004). For an infection with a given R_0, the rate of growth will be much faster if the generation time is two to three days, such as influenza, rather than two weeks, such as smallpox.

If the recovery rate v is constant, then the duration of infectiousness equals the reciprocal of the rate of recovery from infectiousness, so that $d = 1/v$. If $d = 4$ days, $v = 1/(4 \text{ day}) = 0.25 \text{ day}^{-1}$. The product of the contact rate times the transmission probability, cp, can also be expressed as a transmission coefficient β that includes both terms and can be defined as the average number of adequate contacts of a person per unit time. Then, alternate expressions for R_0 are $R_0 = cp/v$ or $R_0 = \beta/v$. As presented above, the expression assumes that everyone who gets infected becomes infectious. A term could be included for the probability of becoming infectious after infection or for reduced infectiousness in asymptomatic people.

Compare the expression $R_0 = cpd$ with the dependent happening expression (2.7) $\lambda(t) = cpP(t)$. The product cp of the contact rate times the transmission probability occurs in both, representing the dynamic underlying transmission system. We might consider that R_0, the number of new infectious individuals one infective produces, views the dynamics from the point of view of the infectious individual. On the other hand, the hazard rate of infection views the dynamics from the point of the view of the susceptible individuals, and it depends on what proportion of the people with whom they make contact are infectious.

The R_0 for indirectly transmitted diseases depends on the product of the two components of transmission. Indirectly transmitted diseases are those in which a parasite is transmitted between two different host populations. An example is the vector-borne disease malaria, which is transmitted from humans to mosquitoes and back to humans. Another example is heterosexual transmission of sexually transmitted diseases where infection is transmitted from a man to a woman and back to a man.

The definition of R_0 assumes all contacts are with susceptibles. In real populations, however, some people might be immune to an infectious agent. Under these circumstances, the expected number of new cases produced by an infectious person is less than R_0 and is called the *effective reproductive number*, denoted by R. If x is the proportion of a randomly mixing, homogeneous population that is susceptible, R is the product of R_0 times the proportion x of the contacts made with susceptibles:

$$R = R_0 x . \tag{5.1}$$

Suppose that $R_0 = 3$ for influenza in a population and that one-half of the population is immune. Then, the effective reproductive number for influenza is $R = 3 \times 0.5 = 1.5$. A case of influenza would produce on average only 1.5 new secondary cases rather than three in this population.

5.1.1 R_0 and public health

Under what conditions will an epidemic occur? In general, for an epidemic to occur in a susceptible population, R_0 must be greater than one. If R_0 is less than one, an average case will not reproduce itself, so an infectious agent will not spread. Because R_0 is an average, a particular infectious person could produce more than one infective case, even when $R_0 < 1$, so there may be a small cluster of cases. We would not, however, expect a self-sustaining outbreak.

Under some circumstances an infectious agent will invade and establish itself in a susceptible host population, with an ensuing epidemic, then die out again. Some infectious agents will invade, however, and after an initial epidemic, persist. It becomes endemic, with either fairly stable, possibly seasonal transmission, or other epidemic patterns. When an infectious agent has established itself and is endemic so that, over time, the average incidence does not change, then each infectious case must be producing on average one infectious case, that is, replacing itself. Otherwise the average incidence would either be increasing or decreasing. Thus, at equilibrium, on average, $R = 1$.

Figure 5.1 shows the epidemic curves at four different values of R_0 for a given infectious agent. For a given generation time and host population, the higher the R_0, the faster the epidemic, the higher the peak incidence, and the higher the final attack rates.

From the public health perspective, the role of vaccination is to reduce R, which will slow spread, reduce peak incidence, decrease the overall attack, and increase effectiveness of other intervention programs through synergy. Slowing spread and reducing peak incidence is important if planning capacity to respond to a potential epidemic. For example, in Figure 5.1, vaccination before the epidemic might change R so that an epidemic that would have behaved as represented by the curve at $R_0 = 2.4$ might be changed to produce the curve at $R_0 = 1.6$, which would be a great public health benefit. If vaccine efficacy and coverage are both high enough, it might be possible to prevent spread of the epidemic or eliminate transmission. In the next section, we study the effects of vaccination on R_0 and R.

5.2 Vaccination and R_0

How might we reduce or eliminate an infectious agent from a host population? Viewing the components of R_0, an intervention might reduce the contact rate,

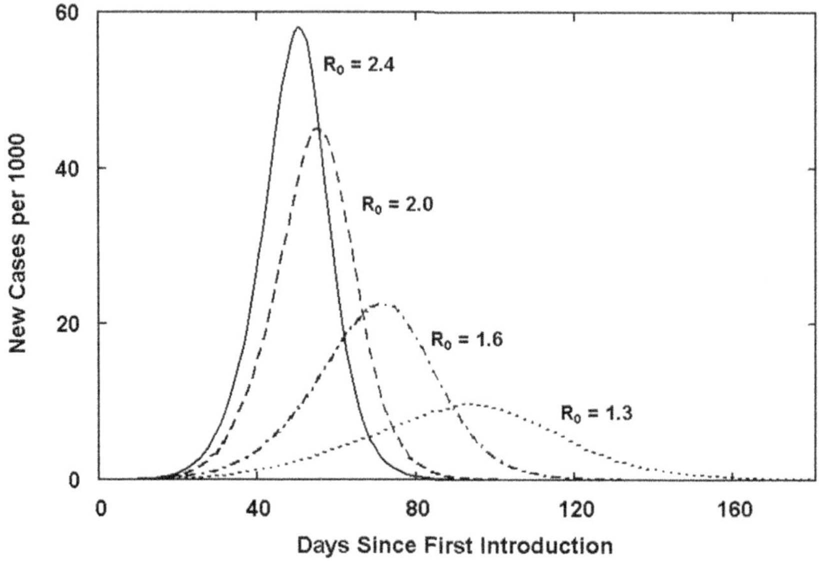

Fig. 5.1 Four epidemic curves at four different values of R_0. For a given generation time and population, the higher the R_0 is, the faster the epidemic, the higher the peak incidence, and the higher the final attack rates.

shorten the duration of effective infectiousness, or reduce the transmission probability. Our focus is on vaccination in this book. Vaccination can reduce the transmission probability either by reducing susceptibility or infectiousness of the two individuals in a contact, or reduce the potential for transmission by shortening the duration of infectiousness. Vaccination might even have the unwanted effect of increasing the contact rate because people feel protected by vaccination. If we want to reduce transmission so that the infectious agent will die out, then we must keep the average number of secondary cases produced by one infectious case below 1, $R < 1$.

5.2.1 The critical vaccination fraction and R_0

If the fraction of susceptibles is low enough, the probability that an infective host has contact with a susceptible host before recovering will be very low. The infectious agent will not be able to persist. The fraction f^* required to be vaccinated to eliminate transmission is called the critical fraction. What fraction f^* of the population do we need to vaccinate to produce enough immune people that the infective people will not be able to infect on average one other person?

Let $R_f(t)$ be the reproductive number at time t when the fraction f of the population is vaccinated with a particular vaccine. Thus $R_1(t)$ is the reproductive number at time t if everyone is vaccinated. $R_{0.75}(t)$ is the reproductive number if 75% of the population is vaccinated. The effect of a vaccination strategy in a population can be measured by the relative reduction in the (basic) reproductive number after the campaign compared with that before the vaccination campaign

$$VE_{R,f}(t) = 1 - \frac{R_f(t)}{R_0} . \tag{5.2}$$

$\mathrm{VE}_{R,f}(t)$ is an example of an overall effect of a vaccination strategy in a population, VE_{III}. In all of the following, we assume a simple homogeneously mixing population.

First we consider simple computation of R_f and the critical vaccination fraction when the vaccine only affects becoming infected, VE_S. Suppose that a vaccine confers complete protection against infection in everyone vaccinated, so that $\mathrm{VE}_S = 1.0$, and that vaccination confers long-lasting immunity. Substituting $1 - f^*$ for x in expression (5.1) for R, in principle, we need to vaccinate a fraction f^* such that

$$R_f = R_0(1 - f^*) < 1 , \tag{5.3}$$

to eliminate transmission. The fraction that needs to be immunized to eliminate transmission is

$$f^* > 1 - 1/R_0 . \tag{5.4}$$

Assume that $R_0 = 3$ for influenza in a population. Under the assumption of random mixing, the fraction that needs to be immunized before the age of first infection is $f^* = 1 - 1/R_0 = 1 - 1/3 = 0.67$. A higher R_0 requires immunization of a higher fraction to eliminate transmission. If $R_0 = 4$, then $f^* = 1 - 1/4 = 0.75$.

With a leaky vaccine, the vaccine might reduce the probability of being infected if exposed, so that the probability of being infected upon exposure is just the fraction θ of what it would be without vaccination. In this case, $\mathrm{VE}_S = 1 - \theta$. Everyone is still susceptible to being infected, but vaccinated people are less susceptible than unvaccinated people. With leaky vaccines, the assumptions about VE_I and VE_P are important, because vaccinated people can become infected. At high values of VE_S, the assumptions about VE_I and VE_P will have less effect on transmission effects than at low values of VE_S. In this example, we assume that the vaccine affects only the susceptibility to infection, VE_S. Because θ multiplies the transmission probability p, then $R_1 = c\theta pd = \theta R_0$. The fraction θ is the *näive susceptible equivalent* contribution to overall transmission of a vaccinated person compared to an unvaccinated person (Halloran et al 1994c). If a fraction f is vaccinated, then $R_f = (1 - f)R_0 + f\theta R_0$, and

$$f^* > \frac{1}{1-\theta}\left(1 - \frac{1}{R_0}\right). \tag{5.5}$$

If in the influenza example the transmission probability per contact in the vaccinated people is reduced so that $\text{VE}_S = 1 - \theta = 0.90$, then the relative probability of infection in the vaccinated is just the factor $\theta = 0.10$ of that in the unvaccinated. If $R_0 = 3.0$ and everyone is vaccinated, then $R_1 = 0.10 \cdot R_0 = 0.30$. The vaccine would likely be successful in preventing the spread of influenza. If the protective efficacy is $\text{VE}_S = 1 - \theta = 0.50$, then $\theta = 0.50$. Even if everyone is vaccinated, $R_1 = 0.50 \cdot 3.0 = 1.50$. Because $R_1 > 1$, we would not expect to eliminate transmission with this vaccine.

Suppose as in an all-or-none vaccine, that vaccination completely protects the proportion α, and it fails in the fraction $1 - \alpha$, so that $\text{VE}_S = \alpha$. In this situation, it does not matter what VE_I and VE_P are, because people who are protected by the VE_S do not get infected, and the others have no protection. (See Chapter 7 for more details.) If the fraction f of the population is vaccinated, the fraction protected by immunization is αf, and $R_f = R_0(1 - \alpha f)$. The critical vaccination fraction to eliminate transmission is

$$f^* > \frac{1}{\alpha}\left(1 - \frac{1}{R_0}\right). \tag{5.6}$$

Assume as in the above influenza example that $R_0 = 3$. If vaccination fails completely in the fraction $1 - \alpha = 0.15$ while conferring complete and long-lasting protection in the other fraction $\alpha = 0.85$, the critical vaccination fraction f^* to eliminate transmission increases from 0.67 to

$$f = \frac{1 - 1/R_0}{\alpha} = \frac{0.67}{0.85} = 0.79\,. \tag{5.7}$$

If the vaccine fails in the fraction 0.40 of the vaccinated people, then the fraction that must be vaccinated is $0.67/0.60 > 1.0$. With such a vaccine at the high failure rate, elimination of transmission would not be possible even if everyone were vaccinated.

Both the leaky and the all-or-none models in equations (5.5) and (5.6) can be expressed as

$$f^* > \frac{1}{\text{VE}_S}\left(1 - \frac{1}{R_0}\right). \tag{5.8}$$

Further technical discussion of the reproductive number can be found in Diekmann et al (1990), Hill and Longini (2002), Becker and Hall (1996), and Farrington (2003) among many others.

5.2.2 R with VE_S and VE_I

We now consider the effect of a vaccine that has both a VE_S and VE_I effect. In the simplest case, assume that $\text{VE}_S = 1 - \theta$ and $\text{VE}_I = 1 - \phi$ have multiplicative and symmetric effects on the transmission probability. If everyone is vaccinated, then

$R_1 = \theta\phi R_0$. To eliminate transmission if everyone is vaccinated requires $\theta\phi < 1/R_0$. In this case, the combined vaccine efficacy is

$$\mathrm{VE}_C = 1 - \frac{R_1}{R_0} = 1 - \theta\phi. \tag{5.9}$$

A number of papers discuss the effects of VE_S and VE_I on R_0. Halloran et al (1994c) called the resulting ability of the vaccinated person to contribute to R_0 the *naive susceptible equivalent*. Longini et al (1998) provided a formula for vaccine effectiveness based on the reproductive number for homogeneously mixing populations. Becker and Starczak (1998) extended the model for the relation between the reproductive number when the individual response to the vaccine is described by a bivariate random variable, one for relative susceptibility and one for relative infectiousness. Farrington (2003) generalized the models to accommodate arbitrary mixing patterns with just one level of mixing, eg, an age-dependent mixing pattern.

5.2.3 R_0 and influenza vaccination

Basta et al (2008) consider the more complex example of influenza. In influenza, a proportion k of infected persons are assumed to develop symptoms. That is, pathogenicity is assumed to be k. The proportion $(1-k)$ remains asymptomatic. Asymptomatic influenza infections may be less infectious than symptomatic cases, with relative infectiousness of the factor m. The basic reproductive number has a more complex form even when no one is vaccinated because people who are asymptomatic are less infectious. The basic reproductive number is a weighted average of the number of new infections that a typical symptomatic infective and a typical asymptomatic infective would produce. Let r_0 be the basic reproductive number for an unvaccinated infectious symptomatic person. Then the overall basic reproductive number for influenza is

$$R_0 = (1-k)mr_0 + kr_0 = ((1-k)m + k)r_0. \tag{5.10}$$

In addition to having efficacies $\mathrm{VE}_S = 1-\theta$ and $\mathrm{VE}_I = 1-\phi$, influenza vaccination may reduce the probability of developing symptoms. Denote the vaccine efficacy for pathogenicity by $\mathrm{VE}_P = 1-\psi$.

When a fraction of the population is vaccinated, all three vaccine efficacies enter into the new formula for the reproductive number. The reproductive number with the fraction f vaccinated is

$$R_f = r_0\{(1-f)((1-k)m+k) + \theta\phi f((1-\psi k)m + \psi k)\} \tag{5.11}$$

based on the largest eigenvalue of the next generation matrix (Basta et al 2008). Rida and Sandberg (2009) accounted for loss of protection as well in the expression for R_f. Vaccine efficacy based on the relative reduction of R_0 when the fraction f is

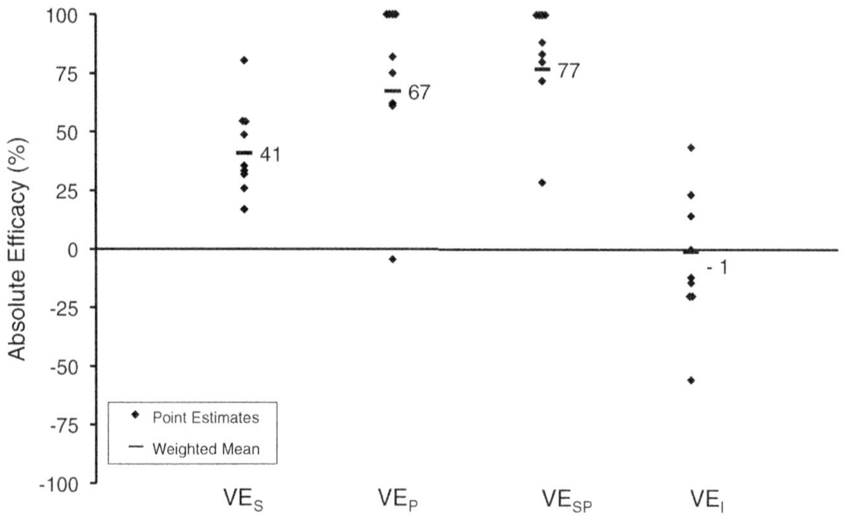

Fig. 5.2 Estimates of VE_S, VE_P, VE_{SP}, and VE_I from human challenge studies of live attenuated influenza virus vaccine (from Basta et al 2008, Am J Epidemiol, 168:1343–1352. Reprinted with permission).

vaccinated is

$$VE_{R,f} = 1 - \frac{R_f}{R_0} = 1 - \frac{(1-f)((1-k)m+k) + \theta\phi f((1-\psi k)m+\psi k)}{(1-k)m+k}.$$

This measure is analogous to the predicted effectiveness (Farrington 2003). If everyone in the population is vaccinated, then $f = 1$, and the combined efficacy, VE_C, measured by the reproductive number is

$$VE_C = 1 - \frac{R_1}{R_0} = 1 - \frac{\theta\phi((1-\psi k)m+\psi k)}{(1-k)m+k}. \tag{5.12}$$

VE_C is a useful index because it assesses the combined effect of all three vaccine efficacy components, $VE_S = 1-\theta$, $VE_I = 1-\phi$, and $VE_P = 1-\psi$.

Using human challenge studies, Basta et al (2008) estimated VE_S, VE_P, VE_{SP}, and VE_I for live attenuated influenza virus vaccine. VE_S was computed from infection, using serology or viral shedding to determine infection in the vaccinated and unvaccinated groups. VE_{SP} was based on the probability of developing symptoms. VE_P was based on the probability of developing influenza illness given infection. VE_I was based on the viral shedding conditional on being infected as a surrogate for transmission. Figure 5.2 shows the estimates of VE_S, VE_P, VE_{SP}, and VE_I from human challenge studies.

Figure 5.3 demonstrates the complete vaccine efficacy, VE_C, for influenza vaccination in equation (5.12) as a function of VE_S and VE_P with $VE_I = 20\%$ held

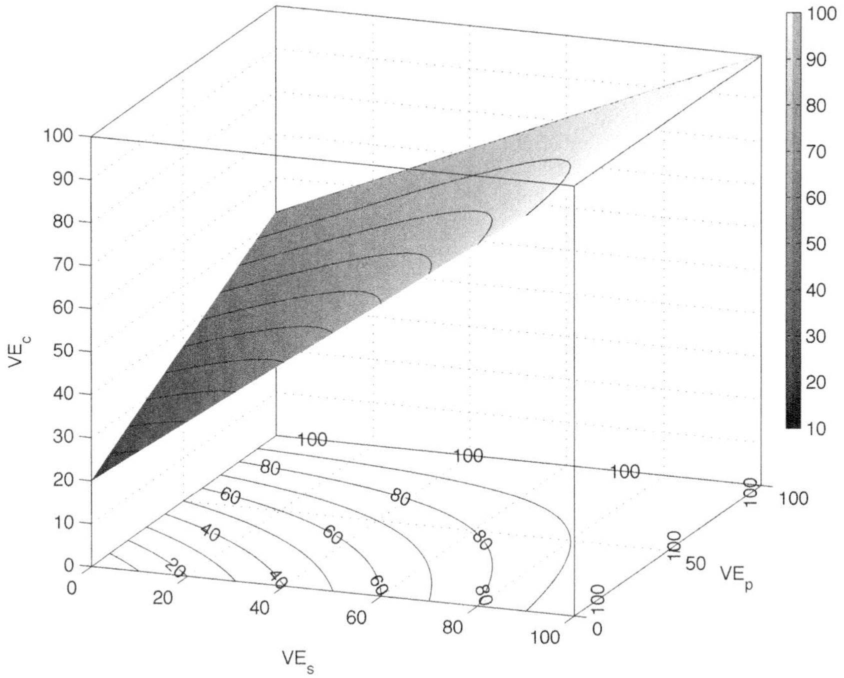

Fig. 5.3 Combined vaccine efficacy as a function of VE_S and VE_P with $VE_I = 20\%$. The contour lines represent values of VE_S and VE_P where VE_{SP} is constant.

constant. The natural history parameter pathogenicity was set to $k = 0.67$ and relative infectiousness in asymptomatic infected people was assumed to be $m = 0.50$. As discussed in Chapter 2, in this situation, $VE_{SP} = 1-(1-VE_P)(1-VE_S) = 1-\psi\theta$. The contour lines represent values of VE_S and VE_P where VE_{SP} is constant. Under this model of influenza natural history and the three assumed efficacies, the combined VE_C is not uniquely determined by a value of VE_{SP}, but is a function of the VE_S and VE_P. If $VE_S = 100\%$, then $VE_C = 100\%$. However, at $VE_P = 100\%$, VE_C is between 50 and 60%, because asymptomatic people still are infectious. In both cases, VE_{SP} is the same. That is, in both combinations of VE_S and VE_P that yield $VE_{SP} = 100\%$, no clinical cases would appear. From a clinical point of view the efficacy of the vaccine would seem to be 100%. However, transmission would be much different under the two different combinations. One could imagine an extreme case in which the vaccine has no effect on infection or infectiousness, but prevented all clinical disease in infected individuals. In this situation, circulation of the infectious agent would continue just as before vaccination in the community, but no clinical illness would be observed.

Table 5.1 Quantities for the R_0 for malaria in the Ross–Macdonald model

N is the size of the human population.
M is the size of the female mosquito population.
$m = M/N$ is the number of female mosquitoes per human host.
a is the rate of biting on humans by a single mosquito (bites per unit time).
b is the transmission probability from infective mosquito to human;
c is the transmission probability from infective human to mosquito.
r is the recovery rate for humans.
μ is the mortality rate for mosquitoes.
τ is the latent period of the malaria parasite in the mosquito.

The influenza model makes particular assumptions about the natural history and the VE_P. The VE_P reduces the probability of developing symptoms, and because of the assumption that asymptomatic people are less infectious, also reduces the infectiousness separately from an explicit VE_I effect. The choice of VE_P depends highly on the natural history of the infectious agent and how the vaccine is expected to work. In an HIV model, VE_P is sometimes assumed to lengthen the period between infection and development of AIDS symptoms. In this situation, if VE_I and VE_S are assumed to equal 0, then a positive VE_P will increase transmission, and VE_C will be negative. VE_C may be further negative if people increase their risk behavior because they think that they are protected (Halloran et al 1994b). In a TB model, once people are infected, the model might assume that people experience one of two possible natural histories. In the first, the people progress rapidly and have a high probability of developing TB disease within a short period of time. In the second, the people are slow progressors and have a low life-time probability of developing TB. A possible model for VE_P in this situation is that if a person becomes infected, he has a higher probability of becoming a slow progressor, and thus has a much lower probability of developing TB disease. VE_C would be a complex function of these different assumptions and pathways.

5.3 Other Aspects of R_0

The basic reproductive number has many other uses. It can be used to compare the relative strength of potential intervention programs. Historically, the concept of R_0 played an important role in the choice of malaria intervention campaigns against the anopheline mosquito vectors. Malaria is an indirectly transmitted disease in that it is transmitted from human to human via female anopheline mosquitoes. We can also say it is transmitted from mosquito to mosquito via the human. Thus, the R_0 expression is composed of two parts, the part from mosquito to human and the part from human back to mosquito. The variables in R_0 based on the Ross–Macdonald model of malaria (Ross 1911; Macdonald 1957; Aron and May 1982) are shown in Table 5.1. The expression for R_0 in the Ross–Macdonald model is

$$R_0 = \frac{ac}{r} \times \frac{mabe^{-\mu\tau}}{\mu} = \frac{ma^2bce^{-\mu\tau}}{r\mu}. \tag{5.13}$$

The abundance of mosquitoes enters linearly, the rate of biting in humans rather than other hosts quadratically, and the probability of surviving through the extrinsic incubation period of the malaria parasite in the mosquito decreases exponentially with an increase in mosquito mortality rate in the Ross–Macdonald expression for the R_0. The malaria parasite has to mature in the mosquito before the mosquito can infect the next person it bites. Often malaria mosquito vectors tend to bite people indoors, then rest on the walls while they excrete some of the blood fluid. This behavior makes spraying walls with insecticides, called residual indoor spraying, a potentially powerful intervention.

5.3.1 Evolution and R_0

R_0 can be used to quantify evolutionary concepts. *Virulence* is a measure of the speed with which a parasite kills an infected host. We denote the disease-dependent death rate, or virulence, by α. If ν is the recovery rate from infectiousness, and α the virulence, then the duration of infectiousness is $d = 1/(\nu+\alpha)$ and $R_0 = cp/(\nu+\alpha)$. Since R_0 is a function of the time spent in the infective state, R_0 could decrease as virulence increases. If the infectious agent is highly virulent so that it kills its host quickly, then R_0 could be less than 1, and the infectious agent will die out. For example, suppose that the infectious agent does not kill the host and that the host usually recovers from infectiousness in about $d = 10$ days. Then $\nu = 0.1$ per day. If $R_0 = 3.0$ for this disease, then $cp = \nu R_0 = 0.1 \times 3.0 = 0.3$. If instead the infectious agent kills the host on average in a little over three days if the host does not recover first, then $\alpha = 0.3$ per day, and $R_0 = 0.3/(0.1+0.3) = 0.75$. In this case $R_0 < 1$, so the infectious agent will not be successful. If, on the other hand, the infectious agent kills the host only after about 10 days on average if the host does not recover first, then $R_0 = 0.3/(0.1+0.1) = 1.5$. In this case, $R_0 > 1$. Viewed in this way, there is evolutionary pressure on infectious agents to become less virulent and to develop a more benign relation to the host.

In some diseases, hosts become more infectious when they become sicker, so the transmission probability increases at the same time virulence increases. Thus, R_0 could increase as virulence increases, putting evolutionary pressure on the parasite to increase virulence. The balance depends on the particular infectious agent. In the above example, suppose that even though the infectious agent kills the host on average after about three days, the transmission probability p also increases by a factor of two. Then $R_0 = (c2 \cdot cp)/(\nu+\alpha) = (2 \cdot 0.3)/(0.1+0.3) = 1.5$. In this case, $R_0 > 1$, so we would expect the infectious agent to be successful. The increased virulence was offset by the increased transmission probability to keep $R_0 > 1$.

The *case fatality ratio* is the probability of dying from a disease before recovering or dying of something else. In the notation used here, the case fatality ratio is $\alpha/(\nu+$

α). If virulence is $\alpha = 0.3$ per day, and the recovery rate is $v = 0.1$ per day, then the expected case fatality ratio is $0.3/(0.1+0.3) = 0.75$. This means that 75% of the people die before recovering. As virulence increases, the case fatality ratio increases.

5.3.2 Estimating R_0 in real-time

Estimating R_0 of an emerging infectious disease in real-time is important to determine the probability of epidemic or pandemic spread (Yang et al 2007a, 2007c) and to assess the efficacy of intervention measures (Wallinga and Teunis 2004; Cauchemez et al 2006b; White and Pagano 2008). Estimating R_0 during an outbreak is an important growing area, especially since the begin of the novel H1N1 influenza pandemic early in 2009.

5.3.3 Caveats

R_0 is a conceptually useful measure that provides a summary of several aspects of an infectious disease. However, the simple relations described above usually do not hold. Heterogeneities in the contact rates, transmission probabilities, and infectious periods produce different values of R_0 in different subgroups. If members of a group who live near each other are not immunized, transmission could occur in that group, even when transmission has been eliminated in other segments of the population. Contact rates can increase locally if people move into crowded conditions, such as into college dormitories, military barracks, or refugee camps. Especially when transmission is tenuous or near elimination, heterogeneities and stochastic variation (Chapter 4) play important roles in determining whether an infectious agent can or will persist in a population. R_0 is a relatively static concept. Further understanding of infectious diseases in populations requires study of transmission dynamics.

5.4 Deterministic Transmission Models

Here we present a simple deterministic SIR model of the spread of infection in a closed population similar to the Reed–Frost model in equations (4.1–4.3). Similar to the Reed–Frost model, people pass through three states (Figure 4.3). They start out susceptible, denoted by S; then become infected and infectious, denoted by I; after which they recover with immunity, denoted by R. There are two main differences. First, the model is formulated in continuous rather than discrete time. Second, fractions of people can move from one state to the next, rather than discrete individuals. The model is based on the mass action principle, in which people all mix with others. We briefly discuss other simple and and more complex models. One advantage of deterministic models is that they are more amenable to theoretical analysis than stochastic models. They require less computational power than large stochastic models. A purely deterministic model always gives the same answer. Characteristics of epidemics using deterministic models were studied by Hamer (1906), Ross (1911, 1915), Kermack and McKendrick (1927), and Soper (1929) in the early 20th century.

5.4.1 Simple deterministic SIR model

Let $S(t)$, $I(t)$, and $R(t)$ be the number of susceptible, infected, and immune people at time t. We consider a closed population of N initially susceptible people who are assumed to be mixing randomly with contact rate c. In this closed population, the size of the population N is constant, and $N = S(t) + I(t) + R(t)$. The population is analogous to a closed cohort. The dynamics of the epidemic are described by three differential equations that express the rate of change of the number of people in each of the three states:

$$\begin{aligned} \text{change in susceptibles}: \quad & \frac{dS(t)}{dt} = -cp\frac{S(t)I(t)}{N} \\ \text{change in infectives}: \quad & \frac{dI(t)}{dt} = cp\frac{S(t)I(t)}{N} - \nu I(t) \\ \text{change in immunes}: \quad & \frac{dR(t)}{dt} = \nu I(t). \end{aligned} \tag{5.14}$$

The expression for the basic reproductive number in model (5.14) is $R_0 = cp/\nu$. As described in Section 5.1, one can use different parameters for essentially the same model, such as $R_0 = \beta/\nu$, if β were used rather than cp, or $R_0 = cpd$. R_0 is formally derived as the largest eigenvalue of the next generation matrix from the set of differential equations describing a deterministic transmission model (Diekmann et al 1990).

The rate at which people leave the susceptible compartment S and become infected at time t is simply the incidence rate, the hazard rate or force of infection. Prevalence of infectives at time t, $P(t)$, is the number of infectious people $I(t)$ divided by the size of the population N, or $I(t)/N$. Thus the dependent happening expression for the hazard rate $\lambda(t)$ as a function of prevalence in equation (2.7) in the epidemic model is

$$\lambda(t) = cpP(t) = cp\frac{I(t)}{N} . \tag{5.15}$$

The change in the number of susceptibles, the population-at-risk to become infected, per small interval of time dt at time t equals the hazard rate $\lambda(t)$ times the size of the population-at-risk, $dS(t)/dt = -\lambda(t)S(t)$. The change in the number of infectives, $dI(t)/dt$, is the difference between the number of new infections and the number of

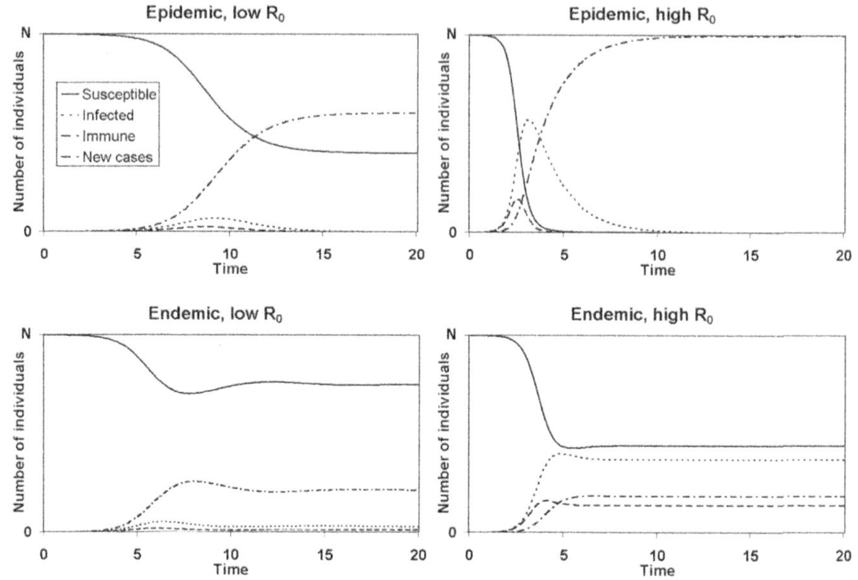

Fig. 5.4 Comparison of epidemic and endemic curves at low and high R_0. The infectious agent is introduced into a population of N susceptible people. Susceptible people become infected and infectious, then develop immunity. In the top two figures, the population is closed, so the epidemic dies out. In the top left figure with a low R_0, fewer people become infected than in the top right figure with a higher R_0. In the bottom figures, the population is open with birth of new susceptible people and death of people from the susceptible, infectious, and immune compartments at a constant rate independent of being infected. Prevalence of susceptible, infected, and immune people achieves a dynamic equilibrium.

infectives developing immunity. The change in the number of immunes, $dR(t)/dt$, is the number of infectives recovering (developing immunity) at rate v in the small time interval.

5.4.2 Dynamics of an epidemic

Assume to begin that all N people are susceptible, and that an infectious agent is introduced so that someone (possibly a fraction of a person in this model) becomes infectious, entering state I. The top two plots in Figure 5.4 show two SIR epidemics in a closed population at a low and higher R_0, both greater than 1. If $R_0 > 1$, the epidemic will always take off in a deterministic model. The infection spreads from the first infective to the average number R_0 of susceptibles. In Figure 5.4, the number of infectives $I(t)$ initially increases. As the epidemic spreads, the number of susceptibles $S(t)$ decreases, and the number of people with immunity in $R(t)$ begins to increase. Incidence of new cases and prevalence of infection will increase until the number of susceptibles available becomes a limiting factor. Then the number of new cases and prevalence begin to decrease until the infectious agent dies out and no people are left in the infective compartment $I(t)$. An infectious agent in a closed population where people recover with long-lasting immunity will inevitably die out, because the key to persistence in a host population is a continuous supply of susceptibles. The susceptibles can be produced either by births or immigration into the population, by recovery without immunity, or by waning of immunity after it is acquired. In this example of a closed population, however, no new susceptibles are produced.

We can associate aspects of the epidemic process with the usual epidemiological measures. An estimate of the incidence rate, hazard rate, or force of infection, $\lambda(t)$, provides an estimate of $cpI(t)/N$. A cross-sectional study to estimate prevalence $P(t)$ of current infection would yield an estimate of $I(t)/N$. The number of new infections in an interval of time dt estimates $[cpI(t)/N]S(t)dt = \lambda(t)S(t)dt$. The epidemic process of a disease producing long-lasting immunity in a closed population is always either increasing or decreasing, except at the turning point. An important consequence for conducting studies in epidemics in closed populations is that there is no stationary state of the disease process. Thus epidemiological methods, study designs, or analytical methods that assume stationarity of the disease process are not applicable under epidemic conditions.

The epidemic process depends on R_0. The expected number of new cases per infective host decreases from R_0 to $R(t) = R_0 x(t)$, where $x(t) = S(t)/N$, the proportion still susceptible at time t. $R(t) > 1$ while the epidemic is increasing. The epidemic peaks when $R(t) = 1$, then decreases when $R(t) < 1$. The latter occurs when $S(t)/N < 1/R_0$, that is, the proportion of the population still susceptible becomes less than the reciprocal of the basic reproductive number. Not all the susceptibles need to become infected before the infectious agent dies out. The greater R_0 is, the fewer susceptibles will be left when the epidemic peaks and the fewer susceptibles will be left at the end of the epidemic. (Compare the two top figures in Figure 5.4.) Thus, the cumulative incidence, or attack rate, after an epidemic provides information on R_0. If an intervention reduced some aspect of R_0, then the intervention would result in the epidemic peaking when a greater proportion of the population had not yet been infected, and fewer people would become infected before the epidemic died out.

5.4.3 Other simple models

Other combinations of states are available for dynamic transmission models, whether discrete event as in Chapter 4 or continuous, as discussed here. An SEIR model allows people to pass through a latent period in a state denoted by E. In an SI model, people become infectious, but never recover. Other examples include SIS models, in which people recover without immunity to become susceptible again, and SIRS models, in which people acquire immunity, but lose it again to become susceptible. Hethcote (1976) gives a thorough analysis of the deterministic versions of these models.

In a closed population, there are no births, immigration, deaths, or emigration. An infection that confers long-lasting immunity will always die out in such a population. An open population can have people entering or leaving or both. In an open population, the susceptibles form a dynamic cohort with the population-at-risk changing over time. In an open population, if the replenishment of susceptibles is fast enough compared with the dynamics of the infectious agent, then the infectious agent will not necessarily die out. The infectious agent can invade the population, establish itself, persist and become endemic. The bottom two graphs in Figure 5.4 show an SIR model with the infectious agent introduced into an open susceptible population. The subsequent epidemic is followed by endemic persistence of the infectious agent. At the higher R_0, the initial epidemic and the prevalence of infected people is higher than at the lower R_0. Although the lines in the graphs look flat, this is a dynamic equilibrium, in which people are being born and dying, and new infections and recoveries are occurring. At equilibrium, $R = 1$, so that on average, each infectious individual produces one further infectious case. It is possible, however, that the infectious agent will die out if the replenishment of susceptibles is not fast enough in comparison to the spread of immunity to the infectious agent.

In the SIS and SIRS models, the susceptibles are replenished even in close populations, so that persistence would be possible under some circumstances. Infectious agents can also persist by hopping from one population to another, then returning to one where the susceptibles have had time to replenish themselves.

When an infectious agent is first introduced into a population, there will be a period when the dynamics are not stationary, as seen in Figure 5.4. Epidemiological methods that assume stationarity of the disease process cannot be used during the epidemic phase. If the parasite has achieved a dynamic equilibrium, however, then some relations might be applicable. This open population with the dynamic cohort at risk for infection is amenable to many of the study designs standardly used in dynamic cohorts. In choosing study designs and methods of analysis, we need to consider whether the dynamics of transmission are at equilibrium or changing over time.

5.4.4 Within host dynamics

The dynamics of the infectious agent within a host also can be described by dynamic models (Antia et al 1996; Pilyugin et al 1997; Antia et al 1998). These models describe the interaction of the infectious agent with the immune cells or antibodies that might attack it, and its target cells within the host. Similar concepts from population theory are used to model the within host dynamics of the infectious agent and to model the infectious agent circulating in the human populaton. For example, R_0 for a virus within a host describes the number of new viral particles successfully produced by one viral particle. The various compartments of immune cells such as T cells, B cells, and memory cells can be included in the dynamic models.

5.5 Modeling Vaccination Programs

The different concepts of vaccine efficacy translate naturally into deterministic transmission models. The values of VE_S, VE_I, and VE_P are inputs into the models. Then the indirect, total, and overall effects expected at different vaccination coverage levels or using different vaccination strategies can be computed. Many questions of interest require more complex models than we can present here. What are the age-related changes in infection and disease? Will natural immunity wane if transmission is too low, so that boosting of immunity does not occur? If many people are vaccinated, the incidence of infection will decrease, so that the average age of infection in the susceptibles will increase. Some diseases, such as mumps, chickenpox, and rubella, are more serious if acquired at older ages. Thus, the total number of cases could decrease due to a vaccination program at the same time that the number of serious cases would increase. For example, rubella is a mild disease in children, but it can result in congenital defects if a pregnant woman becomes infected. If many young people are vaccinated, but not all, then transmission will be reduced. The people who were not vaccinated will acquire rubella at a later age than if no one were vaccinated (Knox 1980; Ukkonen and von Bonsdorff 1988). Thus, it is possible that the number of babies born with congenital defects could increase, even though fewer people contract rubella.

In the United States, the question was raised whether varicella vaccination, especially if the fraction vaccinated was not high, could increase the number of primary chickenpox cases in older age groups who have more severe morbidity. Halloran et al (1994a) found that vaccination would likely not result in a greater number of severe cases. Complex models including age (Schenzle 1984) and mixing structures are required to study complex questions such as this one. The general rule is that a model has to contain the characteristics related to the question you are asking or you cannot get an answer.

Several caveats should be kept in mind in considering the results of complex models and computer simulations. Regardless of how complex the models are, they are always a simplification of reality. Someone made choices in choosing what would be included in the model. These choices affect the results produced by the model. Models are excellent at forcing us to make both our assumptions and our ignorance explicit. Often too few data are available to estimate the parameters and the results usually underestimate the uncertainty of the knowledge. Regardless of these caveats, models are useful in sharpening our thinking and especially in gaining qualitative understanding of complex processes. Comprehensive treatments of deterministic transmission models are found in Anderson and May (1991), Diekmann and Heesterbeek (2000), and Keeling and Rohani (2008).

Problems

5.1. Plot the critical vaccination fraction as a function of R_0 from equation (5.4).

5.2. Consider a vaccine that has a multiplicative leaky effect with $\mathrm{VE}_S = 0.80$, and a vaccine that has an all-or-none effect with $\mathrm{VE}_S = 0.80$. Vaccination is administered to infants. Both confer long-lasting immunity. (a) What would the age-distribution of vaccinated cases compared with unvaccinated cases over the long-term be with the leaky vaccine?
(b) What would the age-distribution of vaccinated cases compared with unvaccinated cases over the long-term be with the all-or-none vaccine?

5.3. (a) Write out the equations for an SIR model (5.14) allowing for birth into the $S(t)$ at a rate b proportional to N, and death that is not disease-dependent from each of the compartments at the rate δ.
(b) What is R_0 for this model?
(c) Expand the equations from (a) to allow that the fraction f is born vaccinated with a leaky vaccine with $\mathrm{VE}_S = 1 - \theta$.
(d) Expand the equations from (a) to allow that the fraction f is born vaccinated with an all-or-none vaccine with $\mathrm{VE}_S = \alpha$.
(e) Compare the two sets of equations in (c) and (d).

5.4. (a) Starting from the SIR model (5.14), derive an expression for the final attack rate as a function of R_0 and the final attack rate. That is, the final attack rate appears on both the left and right side of the equation.
(b) Plot the final attack rate as a function of R_0.

5.5. In a county in the United States, an active campaign to vaccinate school children with live attenuated influenza vaccine resulted in high level of coverage before the start of the influenza season. The investigators observed that the influenza season in that county started more slowly and peaked later than in other counties in the state and than in the United States as a whole. What is one plausible explanation for this observation? (Hint: see Figure 5.1).

5.6. Two hypothetical investigators who conducted separate studies of gonorrhea in a heterosexual population of men and women come to different conclusions. The subscripts m and f denote men and women. The first investigator conducted a study in clinics using a sound sampling scheme with good ascertainment. The results showed that the incidence rate and number of new clinical cases of gonorrhea is higher in men than women, $I_m > I_f$. The investigator concluded that gonorrhea is a greater problem in men than women. The second investigator conducted a population-based study that was also well designed, and found that the prevalence of gonorrhea infection is higher in women than in men, $P_f > P_m$. She concluded that the problem is greater in women. How can transmission concepts help us think about this paradox? (Hint: Assume that duration of infectiousness is longer in women than in men.)

Chapter 6
Evaluating Protective Effects of Vaccination

6.1 Overview

Evaluating the direct protective effects of vaccines in the individuals who were vaccinated has been the focus of vaccine studies over the past century. Generally, interest has been in the ability of vaccination to prevent or to ameliorate disease rather than to prevent infection (Clements-Mann 1998). Ascertainment of cases is often done by finding suspected cases in the population under study in people who exhibit a set of symptoms. The suspected cases are then tested for biological confirmation of the infectious agent of interest. Alternatively, surveillance can ascertain cases reported in central registries. However they are ascertained, with most vaccines, clinical disease is the primary outcome of interest. When ascertainment is on clinical cases, most asymptomatic infections may go undetected. A different situation arises when infection is the primary outcome. To ascertain infections in asymptomatic people, an active follow-up method of testing asymptomatic people is needed.

In this chapter we consider estimation and inference for direct protective effects of vaccination, VE_S and VE_{SP}, in studies that do not condition on exposure to infection. We consider aspects of the design of such studies. Several examples of randomized, double-blind (double-masked) controlled vaccine trials illustrate the standard approach to design and analysis of such studies. Our choice of studies to present was motivated largely because of their use as illustrations in other sections of the book. Most randomized and pivotal studies of vaccines have been based on VE_{SP} or VE_S. Much has been written on studies to meet the approval of the regulatory agencies, and the design of clinical trials generally. Our goal here is to consider how VE_S and VE_{SP} relate to other measures of vaccine effects within the dependent happening context, and consider a few design considerations. Because VE_S and VE_{SP} do not condition on exposure to infection, assumptions about the relative exposure opportunity in the vaccine and control groups are important.

We have generally distinguished VE_S, the vaccine efficacy for susceptibility to infection, from VE_{SP}, the vaccine efficacy for susceptibility to disease. However, in this and the following chapters, ascertainment is most often on disease rather

M.E. Halloran et al., *Design and Analysis of Vaccine Studies*, Statistics for Biology and Health, DOI 10.1007/978-0-387-68636-3_6,

than infection. In both instances, the population at risk is individuals susceptible to infection. In a sense, one can imagine a continuum after randomization that includes infection, development of symptoms, and possibly development of severe disease. Most of the methods apply equally well if ascertainment is on infection or clinical disease. In this and the next two chapters, we use VE_S often to denote situations where the primary outcome can be either infection or disease. Which one is meant is clear from the context. Any outcome that is the first cut after randomization will provide a statistically valid assessment of the effect of the vaccine on that outcome.

This is in contrast to VE_P, the vaccine efficacy for progression or post-infection outcomes. In this situation, the vaccine effect of interest is in an outcome that occurs only in those people who become infected. The methods of analysis and potential for biases are different for VE_P. In Chapter 7, we discuss different conceptual models of protective effects of vaccine and the consequences for choosing and interpreting protective efficacy estimates. The chapter also discusses methods to estimate waning vaccine effects. In Chapter 8 we present further topics in evaluating protective effects. The evaluation of the effect of vaccination on post-infection outcomes is considered in Chapter 9.

6.2 Estimating VE_S

The vaccine efficacy measures of interest in this chapter are the Levels II, III, and IV parameters in Table 2.2 that do not condition on exposure to infection. The Level IV measure $VE_{S,CI}(T)$ is defined using the cumulative incidence or attack rates at the end of the study:

$$\begin{aligned} VE_{S,CI}(T) &= 1 - \frac{\text{vaccinated infection events/persons–at–risk}}{\text{unvaccinated infection events/persons–at–risk}} \\ &= 1 - \frac{CI_1(T)}{CI_0(T)}. \end{aligned} \tag{6.1}$$

The Level II parameters $VE_{S,IR}$ based on the incidence rates and $VE_{S,\lambda}$ based on the hazard rates require knowledge of the infection times:

$$\begin{aligned} VE_{S,IR}(T) &= 1 - \frac{\text{vaccinated events/person-time}}{\text{unvaccinated events/person-time}} \\ &= 1 - \frac{IR_1(T)}{IR_0(T)}. \end{aligned} \tag{6.2}$$

The $VE_{S,\lambda}$ based on the hazard rate ratio is

$$\mathrm{VE}_{S,\lambda}(t) = 1 - \frac{\lambda_1(t)}{\lambda_0(t)}. \tag{6.3}$$

The Level III parameter VE_{PH} based on the proportional hazards model requires only the ordering of the infection times:

$$VE_{S,PH} = 1 - \exp(\beta). \tag{6.4}$$

where β is the log hazard ratio. In Chapter 2 we showed the intrinsic relationship of the parameters to one another based on the dependent happening relation (2.7). We also showed they form a hierarchy based on the amount of information required for their estimation.

In this chapter, we treat $VE_{S,IR}(T)$, $VE_{S,\lambda}$, and $VE_{S,PH}$ somewhat interchangeably. The interpretation of $VE_{S,CI}(T)$ and $VE_{S,IR}(T)$ ($VE_{S,\lambda}$, $VE_{S,PH}$) differ substantially. $VE_{CI}(T)$ is related to the number of cases saved over the period of the study, and $VE_{IR}(T)$ and the other two parameters measure a relative improvement in incidence rate or hazard, whereby both are underestimates if dependent happenings are not taken into account (Section 2.8.1). The choice between $VE_{CI}(T)$ and a vaccine efficacy based on incidence or hazard ratios could be influenced by the distribution of vaccine protection (Chapter 7).

6.2.1 Absolute versus relative efficacy

The control arm in a planned study is often another active vaccine assumed not to have an effect on the disease of interest. In the pneumococcal conjugate vaccine study below, a meningococcal conjugate vaccine is the control. In these studies, the goal is to show that the active vaccine of interest is superior to the control in preventing the primary outcome of interest. If a licensed (and recommended) vaccine is available for the disease of interest, it is generally unethical to use a placebo or vaccine against a different disease in the control arm. Then the study must compare two (or more) active vaccines against the same disease. The relative rather than the absolute efficacy can be computed. The relative efficacy is the relative reduction in disease risk or incidence by the one vaccine compared with the other. An example is the pertussis vaccine study in Senegal presented below. The whole cell pertussis vaccine was recommended for infants in Senegal, so the acellular pertussis vaccine could not be compared to a placebo. In contrast, in Sweden, the whole cell pertussis vaccine had been discontinued, so there was no licensed pertussis vaccine in Sweden when they conducted the study of the acellular pertussis vaccine. In the Swedish study, the control was the diphtheria–tetanus toxoid without the pertussis component.

As new generations of vaccines are introduced, it is more common to be comparing a new vaccine candidate with an existing vaccine. If both vaccines are fairly efficacious and or the outcome of interest is fairly rare, then the size of the field study becomes prohibitively large and expensive. For example, the pneumococcal vaccines are highly efficacious against invasive disease, so that field studies of new pneumococcal vaccines with invasive disease as the primary outcome are not feasible. In this setting, the hunt for immunological surrogates of protection becomes imperative. In the case of pneumococcal vaccines, there is also interest in developing pneumococcal nasopharyngeal carriage as a primary outcome for vaccine field study (Chapter 15).

Even when individuals cannot be randomized to a placebo, there may be individuals under surveillance who do not enroll in the trial, and thus do not receive either vaccine. The absolute efficacy of both vaccines can be computed by comparison with the individuals who happened not to be in either study arm. The study is then an observational cohort study, not a randomized study. The Senegal pertussis vaccine study included surveillance of cases in people not in the study, so was able to compute the absolute efficacy of both vaccines, although with the potential biases inherent in observational studies. With two active vaccines, the trial may be planned in a way to show that the efficacy of the new vaccine is not worse than the already licensed vaccine (a noninferiority study) or that the new vaccine has a higher efficacy than the other vaccine (a superiority trial), the usual approach in vaccine trials that compare a vaccine to a control.

6.2.2 Types of studies

Cohort studies for evaluating vaccines follow groups of people over time, some of whom are vaccinated, some of whom are not. Randomized vaccine studies are examples of cohort studies in which the vaccine has been randomly allocated. Cohort studies can be used to estimate any of the unconditional VE_S parameters if certain conditions are met. If all of the vaccine was administered before the beginning of the observation period, then the cohort is a fixed cohort. If, in addition, there is no loss to follow-up during the observation period, the cohort is a closed cohort. Then $VE_{S,CI}(T)$ can be estimated by the cumulative incidence or attack rates. More generally, open or dynamic cohorts allow people to join and leave the population under study and to change their vaccination status. From these studies in dynamic cohorts, estimates can be based on either cases per person-time at risk, the incidence rate, or using survival analysis methods in which the risk set can change over time. $VE_{S,IR}$ and $VE_{S,\lambda}$ can be estimated from either closed or open cohorts. Primary vaccine efficacy studies often report $VE_{S,IR}$ based on relative events per person-time, or Level II information.

In a case-control study, cases are ascertained and controls selected from a source population. The goal of the case-control study is to estimate the same unconditional estimands of vaccine efficacy as in the cohort studies. The method of sampling the controls and the method of analysis determine whether the case-control study will provide good estimates for $VE_{S,IR}$, $VE_{S,\lambda}$, or $VE_{S,CI}(T)$. A case-control study can be thought of as a sample of data from a hypothetical cohort study. The cohort can also be thought of as a source population that gives rise to the cases (Chapter 8).

6.2.2.1 Randomized versus observational cohort studies

Greenwood and Yule (1915) stated three conditions for valid inference in vaccine studies:

1. The persons must be, *in all material respects,* alike.
2. The effective exposure to the disease must be identical in the case of inoculated and uninoculated persons.
3. The criteria of the fact of inoculation and of the fact of the disease having occurred must be independent.

The conditions for a valid comparison are essentially met under randomization. Randomization is supposed to ensure that potential confounders are balanced between the two groups. Observational studies that do not assign vaccine randomly need to examine the three criteria carefully. The criteria can be thought of in terms of exposure to infection versus susceptibility to infection. First, randomization is supposed to ensure that the groups being compared are in all relevant aspects alike. Relevant covariates can include pre-existing immune levels such as antibody titer, prior vaccination, prior disease history, age, and gender, among others.

Second, randomization is supposed to ensure that effective exposure to infection of the two groups is the same. The two groups having the same exposure to infection is not the same as every person in the groups having the same exposure to infection. Even if, on average, exposure in the two groups is comparable, there may be heterogeneity of exposure to infection within the groups. Some participants might not be exposed at all to the infectious agent of interest. Because in field trials, exposure to infection is not under control of the investigator, in studies that do not condition on exposure to infection, the assumption of equal exposure in the two groups is a strong one, especially if a study is not randomized. For example, children of a higher socioeconomic status may be less exposed to a certain infection. If these children also tend to get vaccinated, then a study of the effect of vaccination will overestimate vaccine efficacy. Potential relevant covariates related to exposure to infection could include distance from potential environmental sources of infection, number of people living in the household, use of bednets, behavioral covariates such as number of sexual contacts or handwashing habits, among others. Going to work rather than working at home or attending school rather than either being too young to attend school or remaining at home for other reasons can affect exposure to infection.

Third, the chance of being vaccinated cannot be associated with the probability of developing disease. Some of these elements are similar to those in the first group related to susceptibility to infection and disease. As an example, children of a higher socioeconomic status may have better nutrition, and therefore better immune systems and better resistance to infection or disease if exposed. If children of higher socioeconomic status also tend to be vaccinated, then a study of the effect of vaccination will overestimate the vaccine efficacy. In both of these situations, socioeconomic status could be used as a proxy covariate for either exposure or for susceptibility to infection.

Table 6.1 Number of individuals, number of cases, and number of person-time at risk in vaccinated and control groups

	Number of Persons in Group	Number of Cases of Disease	Person-Time at Risk
Vaccinated	N_1	c_1	Y_1
Control	N_0	c_0	Y_0

If these three criteria are met, any differences in the rate of developing disease in the two groups is likely due to the biological effects of the vaccine. It is important to collect information on relevant covariates and potential confounders in both randomized and observational studies. Potential confounders will depend on the particular infectious agent of interest and the setting of the study. Reports of randomized cohort and case-control studies usually include a comparison of the vaccine and control groups on any covariates considered relevant.

Nonrandomized cohort and case-control studies need to address these potential sources of bias. Although propensity scores (Rosenbaum 1995) and marginal structural models (Robins et al 2000a) could be used to adjust for confounding in vaccine studies, these approaches have not found much use thus far. Further details of epidemiologic study design can be found in Rothman et al (2008). Interactions of preexisting immunity and level of exposure to infection can confound interpretation of vaccine efficacy estimates even when the study is randomized (Chapter 14).

6.2.3 Estimation and inference

The statistical methods for analyzing the studies described in this chapter are fairly standard. Consistent with the philosophy of this book, estimation with a measure of uncertainty such as confidence intervals, likelihood intervals, or a Bayesian posterior distribution is the focus rather than hypothesis testing. Our interest is in the estimate of vaccine efficacy and the interpretation of the estimate. Consider a vaccine study with N_1 individuals in the vaccine group and N_0 in the control group, and $N = N_0 + N_1$. The cohort can be observed either at time 0 and time T or over the interval $[0, T]$. The number of cases observed in the unvaccinated group is c_0 and in the vaccinated group is c_1. The total person-time at risk in each group is denoted by Y_0 in the unvaccinated group and Y_1 in the vaccinated group (Table 6.1).

Estimating $\text{VE}_{S,CI}(T)$ based on the cumulative incidence or attack rates requires only information about whether persons are infected by the end of the study at time T, that is, final value data:

$$\text{VE}_{S,CI}(T) = 1 - \frac{c_1/N_1}{c_0/N_0} \,. \tag{6.5}$$

Estimation of $VE_{S,CI}(T)$ based on the simple relative proportions of cases in each group assumes that there is no loss to follow-up, that is, no censoring.

Chick et al (2001) consider correcting for bias in risk ratio and vaccine effect estimators, especially when the number of cases is small. The standard maximum likelihood vaccine effect estimators are consistent, but they are biased because they are nonlinear functions of other estimators. The bias is small when the number of cases is relatively large, say >70 in the placebo arm. However, with small numbers of cases, the bias can be substantial. Chick et al (2001) propose various bias correction options, including one suggested by Jewell (1986). Bias of both the $VE_{S,CI}$ under an all-or-none model and the $VE_{S,CI}$ under the leaky model are explored. Of the options considered, the best was to add one to the positive count in the control population, both to the case count and the population count. For example, they recommend using

$$\widehat{VE}_{S,CI}(T) = 1 - \frac{c_1/N_1}{(c_0+1)/(N_0+1)}. \tag{6.6}$$

This addition in the control population increases the $VE_{S,CI}(T)$ estimates. As they point out, it may seem to "corrupt the data." However, for small studies, the simulations are convincing. Clearly when c_0 is large, the addition of one count will have a small effect. They also provide bias corrections for Bayesian vaccine effect estimators, for VE_I and VE_S based on the secondary attack rates, and for the vaccine effect of the susceptibility and infectiousness effects on the reproductive number.

$VE_{S,IR}(T)$ based on relative incidence rates is estimated by

$$VE_{S,IR}(T) = 1 - \frac{c_1/Y_1}{c_0/Y_0}. \tag{6.7}$$

The usual assumption is that the numbers of events follow a Poisson distribution. Similarly, from time-to-event data, to estimate $VE_{S,\lambda}$ investigators may estimate the instantaneous hazard rates in the vaccinated and unvaccinated $\lambda_1(t)$ and $\lambda_0(t)$, respectively, using survival analysis methods. When covariates such as age and gender are added, the analyses are stratified by the covariates or Poisson regression can be used.

Under the assumption that the effect of the vaccine is multiplicative, constant, and homogeneous, the Cox proportional hazards model can be used to estimate $VE_{S,PH}$. In this case, it is not necessary to estimate the hazard rate in the unvaccinated group, but only the relative hazard rate. Covariates including time-dependent covariates can easily be incorporated using standard software. The proportional hazards model with covariates can be used to investigate possible confounding factors. Because the proportional hazards model assumes that the baseline hazard is the same in both the vaccinated and the unvaccinated groups, for studies including different communities, it may be possible to include a covariate for each community. The model could then assume that the incidence varies by community, but the vaccine effect is the same in each community (Section 6.4.1).

Several approaches are available for the confidence interval for $\text{VE}_{S,CI}(T)$. O'Neill (1988) favored the method based on the log of the ratio of two binomial random variables (Katz et al 1978) because of its simplicity of interpretation and the symmetry of the confidence interval on the log scale. Let $\theta(T) = CI_1(T)/CI_0(T)$, so that $\text{VE}_{S,CI}(T) = 1 - \theta(T)$, and let $\beta(T) = \ln\theta(T)$. Assume for now that the follow-up is over the interval T, so that we can drop the T from the notation. The estimate of θ is $\hat{\theta} = (c_1/N_1)/(c_0/N_0)$ and $\hat{\beta} = \ln\hat{\theta}$. An estimate of the variance of β is

$$\sigma^2 = \frac{N_1 - c_1}{N_1 c_1} + \frac{N_0 - c_0}{N_0 c_0} = \frac{1}{c_1} + \frac{1}{N_1} + \frac{1}{c_0} + \frac{1}{N_0}. \tag{6.8}$$

In vaccine studies, N_0 and N_1 are usually large, so that the variance of β is approximated by a function of the number of cases in the vaccinated and unvaccinated groups, $1/c_1 + 1/c_0$. The $100(1-\alpha)$ percent confidence interval for $\text{VE}_{S,CI}(T) = 1 - \theta$ is

$$[1 - \exp(\hat{\beta} + z\hat{\sigma}), 1 - \exp(\hat{\beta} - z\hat{\sigma}], \tag{6.9}$$

where z is the $(1-\alpha)$ percentage point of the standard normal distribution. One can also use Taylor series approximations (Hightower 1988). Ewell (1996) compared Bayesian posterior regions with frequentist exact and large sample confidence intervals for intermediate (Phase IIb) trials. Koopman's (1984) method for the ratio of two binomials is also used. Generally two-sided intervals are recommended, and even required by some journals. The lower confidence bound on the vaccine efficacy estimate is sometimes of primary interest, especially in proof-of-concept studies, or Phase IIb studies.

An approximate confidence interval for $\text{VE}_{S,IR}$ can be obtained similarly as in (6.9). An estimate of the approximate variance of the log of the ratio of the incidence rate in the vaccinated group and the incidence in the unvaccinated group is again

$$\hat{\sigma}^2 = \frac{1}{c_1} + \frac{1}{c_0}. \tag{6.10}$$

If now $\theta = (c_1/Y_1)/(c_0/Y_0)$ and $\beta = \ln\theta$, then the $100(1-\alpha)$ percent confidence interval for $\text{VE}_{IR} = 1 - \theta$ is

$$[1 - \exp(\hat{\beta} + z\hat{\sigma}), 1 - \exp(\hat{\beta} - z\hat{\sigma}], \tag{6.11}$$

where z is the $(1-\alpha)$ percentage point of the standard normal distribution.

If there is loss to follow-up, then $\text{VE}_{S,CI}(T)$ also requires knowledge of the time of onset of cases. In a hepatitis B vaccine study, Szmuness et al (1980) calculated cumulative attack rates using a life-table method. The statistical significance of the differences between observed numbers of trial endpoints in different groups was calculated from the life tables by the log-rank summary chi-square test. In another hepatitis B vaccine study, Francis et al (1982) also used a life-table approach based on person-months of follow-up to get cumulative attack rates. Hudgens et al (2004) suggest using nonparametric maximum likelihood estimators of CI_1 and CI_0 in the presence of censoring (Kaplan and Meier 1958; Peto 1973). Standard survival analysis methods can be used for inference for $VE_{S,\lambda}$ and $VE_{S,PH}$:

$$\widehat{VE}_{S,PH} = 1 - \exp(\hat{\beta}). \tag{6.12}$$

where $\hat{\beta}$ is the partial likelihood estimate of the log hazard ratio (Cox 1972). The methods for the above analyses in this chapter are available on most statistical analysis packages.

When the number of cases in the study is small, exact confidence intervals may be used. Again, many approaches are available for exact confidence intervals. Randomized trials in this chapter used the Clopper–Pearson (1934) or Koopman's (1984) method. Agresti and Coull (1998) compare exact and approximate confidence intervals and find that sometimes approximate intervals are better than exact. Specialized software is available for most exact computations.

6.3 Design Considerations

In this section, we consider some of the design considerations of a vaccine study, with the studies in the next section serving as illustrations.

6.3.1 Vaccines and vaccination schedule

The vaccine of interest and the comparison, whether active control, placebo, or nothing, need to be specified. If active administration of vaccines is part of the study design, the number of doses, and the schedule for administering the doses need to be specified. Many vaccines require two or more doses for complete vaccination. For example, usually complete pertussis vaccination requires three doses. It is important when possible to record the number of doses of a vaccine that a person has received to determine if the person has complete or incomplete vaccination. In addition, the immune response requires some time to develop. Thus, many studies include only cases in the analysis that occur a certain time interval after the completion of vaccination. In a randomized study, participants who receive the number of doses according to protocol are included in the per-protocol analysis. In the intent-to-treat analysis, any person randomized to a particular arm regardless of how many doses received is included in the analysis. Analyses can also be broken down by the actual number of doses received.

In observational studies, the study can specify what the recommended dose schedule is for that vaccine, then ascertain the extent to which participants are vaccinated according to the recommended schedule.

6.3.2 Study population

The study needs to specify the usual person, time, and place of any field study, whether randomized or observational. Eligibility and exclusion criteria need to be specified.

6.3.2.1 Recruitment and vaccination

Recruitment into a vaccine study can be through a population-based study, a local census, by attendance at clinics or physician's offices, schools, workplaces, health maintenance organizations or public advertisements. The method of recruitment will depend on the societal context and the target age of vaccination. Vaccination can take place in clinics or by teams going to the field for vaccination.

6.3.3 Case definition

The case definition is an essential element for the study. In randomized studies, there will usually be a primary endpoint for the primary analysis. The case definition can be defined by clinical criteria alone or require biological confirmation of evidence of the infectious agent of interest. Several secondary endpoints may be based on different case definitions, other clinical endpoints related to the infectious agent of interest, or laboratory endpoints related to either the immune response or the course of the infection. Hudgens et al (2004) reviewed endpoints in vaccine trials.

6.3.4 Ascertainment of cases

Methods for ascertaining potential clinical cases include active surveillance such as through phone calls at specified intervals or visits to the homes. Suspect cases may be ascertained in clinical settings, whereby only cases that seek medical attention will be ascertained. If the case definition includes biological confirmation, then the relevant tests will be performed. Ascertainment of infected people rather than clinical cases requires testing of all of the study participants at regular intervals.

6.3.4.1 Safety and Immunogenicity

If a study actively administers vaccine, usually study participants will be directly observed for a period of time for short-term adverse events such as anaphylactic reaction. Parents or adults can be given diaries to keep track of adverse events. Investigators may make visits or phone calls to the homes of participants to register any adverse events. Immunogenicity of the vaccine could be measured on all or a subset of participants. It may not be measured on anyone. In observational studies, immunogenicity measures may not be available.

6.3.5 Sample size calculations

It happens often that vaccine studies go to the field, then suddenly there is no or little transmission, so there are few events. Someone once said that for vaccine studies, one should calculate the sample size then multiply by 5 or possibly 10. Here are a few formulae for simple sample size calculations as guidelines, but most sample size calculations for vaccine studies will need computer simulations. Careful, sometimes lengthy, baseline studies to understand the local epidemiology and transmission of the infection, seasonal and yearly variation in incidence, and other characteristics may be required before sample size calculations can be considered reliable.

Hayes and Bennett (1999) provide simple formulae for individually randomized studies which we summarize here as well as parallel design cluster randomized studies (Chapter 13). Let $z_{\alpha/2}$ and z_β be the standard normal distribution values corresponding to upper tail probabilities of $\alpha/2$ and β. The corresponding sample size will give a power of $100(1-\beta)\%$ of obtaining a significant difference ($P < \alpha$ on a two-sided test), assuming that the true (population) rates in the vaccine and control groups are λ_1 and λ_0. If the outcome is based on person-time, let y denote the person-time of follow-up in each group. Then the amount of person-time required in each group is (Smith and Morrow 1996; Hayes and Bennett 1999)

$$y = (z_{\alpha/2} + z_\beta)^2 \frac{\lambda_0 + \lambda_1}{(\lambda_0 - \lambda_1)^2}. \tag{6.13}$$

If the outcome is based on proportions, let π_0 and π_1 be the true population proportions in the presence and absence of the intervention. Let n be the number of individuals in each group. Then the number of individuals required in each arm is

$$n = (z_{\alpha/2} + z_\beta)^2 \frac{\pi_0(1-\pi_0) + \pi_1(1-\pi_1)}{(\pi_0 - \pi_1)^2}. \tag{6.14}$$

If the outcome is based on a continuous response, such as malaria parasite density, then the objective is to compare the mean of that variable in the intervention and control groups. Let μ_1 and μ_0 be the true population means and σ_1 and σ_0 be the standard deviations of the outcome variable in the vaccine and control groups. Let n be the number of individuals in each group. Then the number of individuals required in each arm is

$$n = (z_{\alpha/2} + z_\beta)^2 \frac{\sigma_0^2 + \sigma_1^2}{(\mu_0 - \mu_1)^2}. \tag{6.15}$$

Fay et al (2007) consider sample size calculations for testing differences in means between two samples and allowing for different variances in the two groups. The approach accounts for two sources of variability. One source of variability is in parameter estimates that are estimated from prior data. The second source of variability is if the vaccine fails in some of the people who are vaccinated. The sample size calculation needs to take the possible failure of the vaccine into account. The research was motivated by the design of a Phase II trial of a *Plasmodium falciparum* blood-stage malaria vaccine candidate in Africa. Baseline data on malaria in children had been gathered in a village in Mali in 1999 and 2000. Children were visited weekly and blood smears were done monthly. Data on malaria symptoms and blood smears were available. Several different primary endpoints for the trial were explored. The goal of vaccination was to elicit an immune response comparable to the immune response in older children, all of whom had had repeated exposure to malaria infection. For each candidate primary endpoint, the effect measure was defined as the difference in the malaria outcome in the older compared to the younger children. Instead of choosing an effect size arbitrarily, the observational data were used to estimate the standardized effect size and variances. The variability in the variance estimate can be accounted for simply by using a slightly larger nominal power in the usual sample size calculation, called calibrated power. Fay et al (2007) provide a table of calibrated power by sample size.

The second problem in designing the trial was that some of the children might not respond to the vaccine, for genetic or other reasons, An example would be an all-or-none distribution of protection. For the second problem, the proportion expected not to respond to the vaccine could be obtained from expert opinion, as in traditional sample size computations. Fay et al (2007) provide simple closed form sample size calculations. In general, the sample size will be greater if a proportion of the population does not respond to the vaccine than if all respond to the vaccine.

6.4 Examples of Randomized Trials

6.4.1 Relative efficacy of pertussis vaccines in Senegal

A randomized, double-blind trial comparing a diphtheria–tetanus–acellular pertussis vaccine (DTaP) (pertussis toxoid and filamentous hemagglutinin) with a whole cell vaccine (DTwP) was conducted in the Niakhar area of Senegal (Simondon et al 1997). (See Section 10.2.3 for more details about the area.) The comprehensive ongoing surveillance in the Niakhar area allowed a prospective, nested case-contact study and a cohort study to be conducted during the trial to estimate absolute efficacy of each vaccine.

Eligible infants were those born between February 1, 1990, and April 30, 1994 to mothers residing in the Niakhar area who attended the vaccination sessions. From 1990 through 1994, 4181 children were randomized to receive one of the vaccines at 2, 4, and 6 months. Surveillance by weekly home visits looked for cough illness persisting more than 7 days in all children under 15 years of age, including children not in the study. Adverse events were screened in the first two weekly visits following each vaccine dose using a standardized questionnaire. Any positive answer was followed up by a physician. The physicians doing the examinations took samples for culture and serological testing blinded to vaccination status. The primary protocol definition of a case of pertussis was defined as 21 or more days of cough confirmed by (a) positive bacterial culture from nasopharyngeal aspirates, (b) serology (IgG against pertussis toxoid and filamentous hemagglutinin), or (c) contact with a culture-confirmed person in the same compound and coughing had started within 28 days before or after onset of illness in the culture-confirmed child (epilink). Polymerase chain reaction (PCR) amplification was used to detect *B. pertussis* DNA in nasopharyngeal aspirates.

The study sample size had been determined assuming that the efficacy of the whole cell vaccine was 75% and allowed detection of the relative ratio of 1.5 in the two arms of the study at the 0.05 significance level. The overall ratio of pertussis incidence in the DTaP group relative to the DTwP group ($RR_{ac/wc}$) and confidence interval were estimated in a proportional hazards model with calendar time as the time scale and stratified by village. Pertussis is epidemic and the proportional hazards model assumes that the baseline hazard is equal in the comparison groups. The model allows the incidence to vary by village, but assumes that the rate ratio is the same across villages. A multivariate proportional hazards model was used to investigate confounding factors. A secondary intent-to-treat analysis included all children receiving at least one dose of the study vaccines. After the study began, the WHO recommended that the case definition be 21 or more days of paroxysmal cough, not just cough. For each child, surveillance ended either at the onset of pertussis, additional pertussis immunization, emigration, death, or refusal to continue in the investigation. All surveillance for the study ended December 31, 1994.

Comparability between children receiving three doses was checked for age at inclusion, gender, weight at first dose, rank of birth number, age of mother, number of persons in the compound, and the number of persons <15 years of age in the compound. No significant differences were found. During the period of surveillance, physicians confirmed at least one episode of >7 days cough in 837 of 2567 compounds reporting such episodes to field workers. The total duration of follow-up was 3165 person-year at risk in the DTwP group and 3193 person-year at risk in the DTaP group. Table 6.2 contains the number of cases and incidence rate ratios for different case definitions. The primary analysis considered cases that occurred ≥28 days after the third dose. The overall ratio of pertussis incidence in the DTaP group relative to the DTwP group ($RR_{ac/wc}$) using the protocol case definition was 1.54 (95% CI, 1.23–1.93). A multivariate proportional hazards analysis including the comparability factors revealed that children in compounds with more than 30 members had a higher rate of pertussis, but the value of $RR_{ac/wc}$ did not change.

In a cohort analysis of 229 unvaccinated children, using the same proportional hazards model and the protocol case definition, absolute efficacy was 66% (95% CI, 46–78) for DTwP and 48% (95% CI, 18–66) for DTaP. Using the WHO case

Table 6.2 Incidence rate ratio of DTaP (acellular pertussis) vaccine compared with DTwP (whole cell pertussis) vaccine for different case definitions in the Niakhar, Senegal study (Simondon et al 1997)

	No. of Cases		
	Whole Cell Vaccine	Acellular Vaccine	Incidence Rate Ratio [95% CI]
≥21 days of cough (protocol definition)			
Protocol confirmation criteria	123	197	1.54 [1.23–1.94]
Intention-to-treat	162	233	1.43 [1.16–1.74]
With PCR	65	128	1.87 [1.38–2.52]
≥21 days of paroxysmal cough (WHO definition)			
Protocol confirmation criteria	16	41	2.42 [1.35–4.34]
Intention-to-treat	23	49	2.06 [1.25–3.39]
With PCR	10	31	2.80 [1.36–5.74]

definition, the absolute efficacies were 91% (95% CI, 81–96) for DTwP and 79% (95% CI, 58–89) for DTaP.

This study illustrates several points. First, vaccine studies sometimes report the relative risk or rate ratios rather than the vaccine efficacies. Vaccine efficacy has the awkward property that it ranges from 1 to $-\infty$. The relative risk or rate ratios range from 0 to ∞ with the value of 1 being associated with no relative effect. Second, different case definitions can substantially alter the estimates. In the comparison of the DTaP to DTwP, the point estimates of the rate ratios were higher with the WHO definition, although the confidence intervals overlap. The absolute efficacy of both vaccines in the cohort analysis was higher with the WHO definition. The choice of case definition in pertussis is the subject of ongoing international discussion. The pertussis study in the next section uses a slightly different definition.

6.4.2 Absolute efficacy of pertussis vaccine in Sweden

Because of its limited efficacy, the Swedish-made whole cell pertussis vaccine was withdrawn in 1979. After that, Sweden had no licensed pertussis vaccine, so it was possible to conduct a randomized, placebo-controlled trial (Trollfors et al 1995). Infants were randomly assigned to receive DT toxoids or the same DT toxoids with pertussis toxoid (DTaP toxoids). The vaccine contained only the single component of the pertussis toxoid. About 99% of children in Sweden visit publicly financed child health clinics, where information about the study was given to the parents of infants. Full-term healthy infants in the Göteberg area were eligible if the family had a telephone and at least one parent spoke Swedish. The vaccinations and follow-up were performed at five study sites. The parents of 3450 of 5964 eligible children

Table 6.3 Pertussis vaccine efficacy, $VE_{S,IR}$, of DTaP compared with DT for different case definitions during the main period of follow-up (30 days after the third vaccination until the end of the study in the Swedish study)(Trollfors et al 1995)

	No. of Cases		
	DTaP Vaccine ($n = 1670$)	DT Vaccine ($n = 1665$)	Vaccine Efficacy [95% CI]
≥21 days of cough			
WHO definition	96	245	63 [52–71]
Göteberg confirmed	77	241	69 [60–77]
Göteberg confirmed + probable	99	252	62 [52–71]
≥21 days of paroxysmal cough			
WHO definition	72	240	71 [63–78]
Göteberg confirmed	58	236	77 [69–83]
Göteberg confirmed + probable	75	246	71 [62–78]
≥7 days of cough			
WHO definition	121	251	54[43–63]
Göteberg confirmed	98	244	62 [51–70]
Göteberg confirmed + probable	125	258	54 [42–63]

agreed to participate. Of these 1724 and 1726 were randomly assigned to DTaP and DT toxoids. There were 817 recipients of DTP toxoids and 850 recipients of DT toxoids with one or more older siblings.

The three vaccine doses were administered intramuscularly at 3, 5, and 12 months. First vaccinations occurred between September 1991 and September 1992, third vaccinations between May 1992 and July 1993. There were 52 children withdrawn from the study for various reasons. Coughing episodes between the first vaccination and July 24, 1994 were included in the study analysis. The surveillance period for each child was divided in two parts. The first part was between the first vaccination until 29 days after the third during which time the children were considered to be incompletely vaccinated. The second part began at the end of the first part for each child and lasted until July 24, 1994. Parents were asked to monitor adverse events for seven days, after which they were interviewed. They were contacted once a month by telephone for further surveillance of adverse events.

Parents were asked to contact the study nurse if anyone in the family coughed for seven or more days. Biological confirmation was done by culture or PCR of a nasopharyngeal sample and serology. Follow-up of each case continued for at least 60 days or until the cough ended. PCR was able to distinguish pertussis from parapertussis. The case definitions were similar to those of the Niakhar study, but the Göteberg group had their own classifications in addition to the WHO criteria. Essentially the Göteberg group allowed that household contacts for the epilink could be confirmed either by culture or serology, whereas the WHO definition allows only culture. The Göteberg group also distinguished two levels of biological evidence. Confirmed cases required two confirmation criteria, and probable cases required only one (Trollfors et al 1995). To measure immunogenicity, serum was obtained from 3361 children at least four weeks after the third vaccination. IgG antibodies against pertussis toxin and toxin-neutralizing antibodies were measured.

Vaccine efficacy, $VE_{S,IR}$, was based on the ratio of the incidence rates in the DTaP compared to the DT group. Confidence intervals were estimated by an exact calculation based on the conditional binomial distribution that follows from the assumption of a Poisson distribution for cases in each group (Clopper and Pearson 1934). Proportions were compared using a two-sided Fisher's exact test.

Of the 2037 coughing episodes lasting at least seven days, 465 (160 in the DTaP-toxoids group and 305 in the DT-toxoids group) met the criteria for confirmed or probable pertussis, including 368 that met the WHO definition. Another 14 children had clinical pertussis without laboratory confirmation. Thirty days after the third vaccination, 1670 and 1665 recipients of the DTaP and DT toxoids were still at risk for pertussis. The incidence of pertussis according to the WHO definition was 2.96 cases per 100 person-years among the DTaP toxoids recipients and 10.32 cases per 100 person-years in the DT toxoids recipients. The efficacy of the pertussis vaccine was 71% (Table 6.3).

As in the Niakhar pertussis study, the number of cases and the vaccine efficacy estimates vary with the case definitions. The estimates using $\geq$21 days of paroxysmal cough had the highest estimates, $\geq$21 days of any cough the middle estimates, and $\geq$7 days of cough the lowest estimates, reflecting the differing specificity of the case definition. Depending on the case definition used, over 15% of the children in the DT toxoids group developed pertussis during the trial. Although not discussed in detail in this book, the pertussis-toxin testing for defining a case had much lower sensitivity in recipients of DTP toxoids than in recipients of DT toxoids because the DTP-toxoid recipients already had high values for IgG antibodies against pertussis toxin in the acute-phase serum samples. Cultures and PCR were also less sensitive in vaccinated children. A study to estimate the indirect effects of vaccination was nested in this trial (Sections 10.2.5 and 12.5.1)

The acellular pertussis component of the vaccine in the Trollfors et al (1995) study had just the pertussis toxoid. Further acellular vaccine candidates were developed that contained additional antigens. Pertussis toxoid (PT) was included. Other antigens included were filamentous hemagglutinin (FHA), pertactin (PRN), and fimbriae types 2 and 3 (FIM). Two coordinated trials were conducted in Sweden as part of an international effort. Trial I was conducted during the years 1992–1995 (Gustafsson et al 1996). Two acellular pertussis vaccines, one whole cell pertussis vaccine, and one placebo were used. The placebo group ($n = 2574$) received diphtheria and tetanus toxoid (DT). The second group ($n = 2566$) received DTaP2 with two antigens, PT and FHA. The third group ($n = 2587$) received DTaP5 with PT, FHA, PRN, and the two FIM antigens. The fourth group received DTwP. A study to evaluate immunological surrogates of protection after household exposure to pertussis was nested in the primary efficacy study Trial I (Storsaeter et al 1998) (Section 15.3.2).

Trial II was conducted during the years 1993–1996 (Olin et al 1997) with no placebo group. The DTaP5 contained higher amounts of PT and FHA than the

DTaP5 of Trial I. The DTaP2 had the same composition as in Trial I. The source for DTwP in Trial II was different from that in Trial I.

6.4.3 *Absolute efficacy of live attenuated influenza vaccine in children*

Belshe et al (1998) conducted a randomized, double-blind placebo-controlled multicenter study of the efficacy of live attenuated cold-adapted trivalent influenza virus vaccine in children. Healthy children who were 15 to 71 months of age at time of recruitment and who had no contraindication were enrolled. The vaccine contained that year's recommended strains of influenza A (H1N1), influenza A (H3N2), and influenza B. Children were randomized 2:1 to receive vaccine or placebo. Vaccine was given either as a one- or two-dose regimen, with some of the sites using one or the other. Vaccine and placebo were administered with an intranasal spray applicator.

To evaluate side effects of vaccination, parents were asked to monitor and to record certain symptoms for 10 days after vaccination. They were given a thermometer to measure the temperature. Serious adverse events were followed throughout the trial. Strain-specific immunogenicity of the vaccine was measured in a substudy of 203 participants, approximately the first 21 children recruited at each site. The serum samples were assayed for presence of hemagglutination-inhibiting antibodies to the three viral strains contained in the vaccine.

The primary efficacy endpoint was the first episode of culture-confirmed influenza for subjects who became ill 28 days or more after the receipt of the first dose of vaccine or placebo or at any time after the second dose during the influenza season. Parents were contacted by telephone every two to three weeks until the beginning of an influenza outbreak in their community. Then weekly contact was made to remind the parents to report any relevant symptoms as soon as possible. Study staff attempted to collect specimens for culture for influenza virus confirmation within four days of the onset of symptoms. A case of influenza was defined as any illness detected by active surveillance that was associated with a positive culture for wild-type influenza virus.

The analysis was based on the $\mathrm{VE}_{S,CI}(T)$, using the observed proportions of cases in vaccine recipients and placebo recipients. Koopman's (1984) method for the ratio of two binomials was used to estimate 95% confidence intervals. A logistic generalized estimating equation (Liang and Zeger 1986) with an exchangeable covariance matrix was used to rule out the possibility of an effect within families on the results, because more than half the children in the study were in households with at least two children in the household.

Enrollment began in August 1996 with 1314 children enrolled in the two-dose cohort and 288 in the one-dose cohort. Surveillance ended April 1997 at the end of the influenza outbreaks at the study sites. Among children in the immunogenicity substudy, younger children were more likely to be seronegative before entering the

Table 6.4 Efficacy, $VE_{S,CI}(T)$, of one or two doses of live attenuated, cold-adapted influenza virus vaccine for the prevention of culture-confirmed influenza (Belshe et al 1998)

Influenza Type	Assigned to One Dose			Assigned to Two Doses Who Received Two Doses			All Participants		
	No. of Cases		Efficacy	No. of Cases		Efficacy	No. of Cases		Efficacy
	Vaccine ($n = 189$)	Placebo ($n = 99$)	[95% CI]	Vaccine ($n = 849$)	Placebo ($n = 410$)	[95% CI]	Vaccine ($n = 1070$)	Placebo ($n = 532$)	[95% CI]
A(H3N2)	2	8	87 [47–97]	4	49	96 [90–99]	7	64	95 [88–97]
B	1	6	91 [46–99]	6	31	91 [78–96]	7	37	91 [79–96]
Any	3	14	89 [65–96]	10	74	94 [88–97]	14	95	93 [88–96]

study than older children. Only 29% of children one or two years of age had antibodies to influenza A (H3N2) compared with 70% of children three years of age or older. Pre-existing antibody to influenza in an influenza vaccine study is considered an important potential confounder. Of the 3009 illnesses in the study subjects, 71 cases of influenza A (H3N2) and 44 cases of influenza B were confirmed. No cases of wild-type influenza A (H1N1) were identified in the study participants or the communities at large during the 1996–1997 influenza season. Table 6.4 shows the results. Vaccination was quite effective against culture-confirmed influenza. Although the data are not presented here, the spectrum of illness in the vaccinated children who developed influenza was milder than that in unvaccinated children.

In influenza vaccine studies for vaccines directed against annual influenza, there is generally an attempt to get all of the participants vaccinated before the beginning of the influenza season. Then given the short duration of the season, influenza vaccine studies can often use an analysis based on the simple cumulative incidence or attack rates. The trial continued beyond the first year. Longini et al (2000) analyzed the first and second year of the trial, allowing for site-specific attack rates. There was some evidence that study sites with high attack rates the first year had lower attack rates the second year and vice versa, suggesting a possible herd immunity effect.

6.4.4 Live attenuated influenza vaccine in adults without biological confirmation

A randomized, double-blind, placebo-controlled trial of live attenuated trivalent influenza virus vaccine in healthy adults was conducted from September 1997 through March 1998 in 13 centers across the United States (Nichol et al 1999). Three of the main outcome measures were episodes of febrile illness, severe febrile illness, and febrile upper respiratory tract illness. Cultures were not performed for confirmation of influenza illness and culture-confirmed influenza was not an outcome in contrast to the Belshe et al (1998) study in young children. Nichol et al (1999) called this an effectiveness study, not an efficacy study. Participants were enrolled mid-September

Table 6.5 Efficacy (effectiveness) of live attenuated, cold-adapted influenza virus vaccine for the prevention of some clinical outcomes (not culture-confirmed influenza) in adults (Nichol et al 1999)

Outcome	Vaccine Group		Placebo Group			
	Total Episodes No. (n=2833)	Rate per 1000 Persons per 7-Week Outbreak	Total Episodes No. (n=1420)	Rate per 1000 Persons per 7-Week Outbreak	Reduction in Rates, % [95% CI]	*p*-value
Febrile illness	406	151.3	225	168.1	10.0 [−2.1–20.7]	.10
Severe febrile illness	298	111.0	183	136.7	18.8 [7.4–28.8]	.002
Febrile upper resp tract illness	248	92.4	162	121.0	23.6 [12.7–33.2]	<.001

to mid-November 1997. Recruitment strategies varied across sites. Persons were eligible if they were 18 to 64 years old, worked at least 30 hours per week outside the home, had health insurance, and were reachable by telephone. There were the usual exclusion criteria. The vaccine contained the three viruses corresponding to those recommended for the 1997–1998 influenza season in the United States. Vaccines were administered intranasally between September 18 and November 15, 1997.

Participants were randomized 2:1 to receive the vaccine or placebo in the fall of 1997. A total of 3041 adults received vaccine and 1520 received placebo. Reactogenicity and safety were assessed by asking each participant to keep a record of daily symptoms on the evening of vaccination and seven days afterwards. Participants were called at day 28 to identify serious adverse events. Assessment of any serious adverse events continued to the end of the study. Influenza virus surveillance is conducted in many places across the United States. The surveillance identifies the influenza season and the strains of circulating wild-type virus. Nichol et al (1999) identified two influenza outbreak periods. The first was the site-specific peak outbreak, using the modal week at each site to begin an algorithm that identified the weeks in which at least 80% of the positive influenza isolates for the season were included. The total outbreak period was identified by a panel of experts from the surveillance information from all of the sites. The motivation for choosing the site-specific outbreak period was that the identified cases would have a higher probability of being influenza.

Bivariate comparisons for the proportions of subjects experiencing study outcomes were conducted using the Cochran–Mantel–Haenszel test controlling for site. Generalized linear models were used to calculate the variance of the event rates.

At the different sites, peak outbreak periods lasted from 4 to 12 weeks. The surveillance cultures revealed that nearly all of the isolates that year were influenza A (H3N2), 80% of which were a drifted variant of the vaccine strain, so that the vaccine was not well matched to a large portion of the circulating viruses.

Table 6.5 contains the results for three of the main outcome measures. For the most specific case definition of febrile upper respiratory tract illness, the efficacy of the vaccine is 23.6% (95% CI, 12.7–33.2), much lower than in the Belshe et al (1998) study the previous year in young children (Table 6.4). There are three possible explanations for the lower efficacy. First, the circulating strain was a drifted variant of the vaccine strain. Second, some investigators believe that adults do not respond to the intranasal live attenuated vaccine as well as children. Third, the case definition is not confirmed influenza, so that many of the illnesses captured in the analysis are likely not influenza, causing the efficacy estimates to be much lower than efficacy estimates of culture-confirmed influenza. This latter reason certainly played an important role. In Chapter 8 we show how to estimate vaccine efficacy for a biologically confirmed outcome when only a small subsample of the nonspecific cases are biologically confirmed.

6.4.5 Relative efficacy of live and killed influenza vaccine in young children

Soon after universal vaccination of children 6 to 59 months of age was recommended by the U.S. advisory bodies, a double-blind randomized trial in infants and young children to compare live attenuated influenza vaccine with inactivated influenza vaccine was conducted (Belshe et al 2007).

The study was conducted at 249 sites in 16 countries in the United States, Europe, the middle East, and Asia. The sites were physicians' offices and primary care clinics. Children were randomly assigned on a 1:1 basis to receive one of the two vaccines. Subjects were stratified in the randomization to age on receipt of the first dose, presence or absence of previous influenza vaccination, presence or absence of wheezing, and country of residence. The usual exclusion criteria applied. Children with mild or moderate asthma or wheezing more than 42 days before the trial were included. Children not previously vaccinated for influenza received two doses of the assigned study vaccine. To preserve blinding, children assigned the intranasal live attenuated vaccine received an intramuscular injection of salt solution, and analogously for children assigned the intramuscular killed vaccine.

Parents recorded local and systemic reactions until 42 days after vaccination. Medically significant events were collected throughout until the end of the surveillance period, May 31, 2005. Study staff contacted the parents every 7 to 10 days during the surveillance period. Nasal swabs for viral cultures were obtained either at the child's home or at the study site. The study was powered assuming a 3.0% attack rate in children receiving killed vaccine and a 1.8% attack rate in the children receiving live attenuated vaccine, for a relative efficacy of 40%. Assuming that 90% of the children would be able to be included in the per-protocol analysis, 8500 children would be needed for 90% power to demonstrate superiority of the live attenuated to the inactivated vaccine. The primary endpoint was the relative efficacy in preventing culture-confirmed influenza-like illness caused by well-matched influenza strains.

Table 6.6 Relative reduction in attack rate with live attenuated, cold-adapted influenza virus vaccine compared to inactivated vaccine regardless of match for the prevention of culture-confirmed influenza in infants and young children (Belshe et al 2007)

Virus	Live Attenuated Vaccine (n=3916)		Inactivated Vaccine (n=3936)		Reduction in Attack Rate
	Cases No.	Attack rate %	Cases No.	Attack Rate %	With Live Vaccine % [95% CI]
All	153	3.9	338	8.6	54.9 [45.4–62.9]
A/H1N1	3	0.1	27	0.7	89.2 [67.7–97.4]
A/H3N2	37	0.9	178	4.5	79.2 [70.6–85.7]
B	115	2.9	136	3.5	16.1 [−7.7–34.7]

The definition of influenza-like illness was an oral temperature of 37.8°C or higher or the equivalent in the presence of cough, sore throat, or runny nose or nasal congestion occurring on the same or consecutive days. Secondary endpoints included relative efficacy against mismatched influenza viruses and all influenza viruses, as well as several other clinical outcomes, such as otitis media.

From October 20 to October 29, 2004, a total of 8475 children were enrolled. Of these, 7852 were included in the per-protocol analysis. Table 6.6 shows the overall number of cases regardless of match of the vaccine with the circulating strains. The paper presents analysis by well matched vaccine, well-matched by age group, well matched by previous vaccination status, and not well matched. In this trial, of the 3936 children who received inactivated vaccine, 338 developed culture-confirmed cases of influenza. Of the 3916 children who received live attenuated vaccine, 153 cases developed. Relative reduction in attack rate by the live vaccine compared to the killed vaccine was 54.9% (95% CI 45.4–62.9).

6.4.6 Oral cholera vaccines in Bangladesh

Interest in oral cholera vaccines developed because parenteral vaccination had not been very successful. Cholera is a disease in the intestine, so it seemed that local mucosal immunity stimulated by an oral vaccine might be better. A randomized, double-blind trial of two oral killed cholera vaccines and one placebo arm was conducted in the Matlab field studies area of the International Centre for Diarrheal Research, Bangladesh (ICDDR,B) (Clemens et al 1986). The oral vaccines consisted of killed cholera whole cells (WC) either with or without the B subunit (BS) component of cholera toxin. The placebo arm received a heat-inactivated *E.coli* K12 strain.

Potentially eligible subjects for the trial were the 124,035 persons aged 2 to 15 years and females aged over 15 years residing in the vaccine trial area at the onset of vaccination. These are the groups at highest risk for cholera in Matlab. After exclusion criteria, 89,596 persons took at least one dose of vaccine or placebo. A census

Table 6.7 Occurrence of cholera and $VE_{S,CI}(T)$ during the first year of follow-up after the third dose among participants who ingested three complete doses of the vaccine or placebo assigned (Clemens et al 1988)

	Group				
Outcome	BS-WC No.	VE %	WC No.	VE %	K12 No.
Cholera	41	62	52	53	110
No cholera	20,664		20,691		20,727
Total	20,705		20,743		20,837

of the vaccine trial population was conducted three months prior to vaccination. Persons were randomized in the census to one of the three groups before teams went to the field. Vaccination occurred in three six-week rounds starting in January, 1985, with a short one-week round in May, 1985. Vaccines and placebo were delivered by 69 vaccination teams who were assigned to particular villages and visited people in their homes. The estimated fraction of the oral dose swallowed was recorded. Physicians in the trial area were stationed during vaccination to manage side effects.

Surveillance for diarrhea was maintained at the three diarrheal treatment centers serving the Matlab population. Stool samples or rectal swabs were processed to identify *V cholerae* 01, and to determine the biotype (El Tor or classical) and serotype of each isolate. To be considered fully vaccinated, a person needed to have three doses, and have swallowed all of the first dose and at least 3/4 of the second and third doses. Later follow-up analyses focused on those participants who had completely ingested all three doses (Clemens et al 1988; Clemens 1990). The case definition was that the participant presented for treatment of diarrhea whose onset was $\geq$14 days after receipt of the third dose, had various diarrheal symptoms not detailed here, *V. cholerae* was isolated, and a field check at the person's home confirmed that the person had indeed sought treatment on the specified date.

The vaccine efficacy measure after one year of follow-up was based on the proportion of vaccinees compared to the proportion of controls becoming ill with cholera, $VE_{S,CI}(T)$ (Clemens et al 1988). Table 6.7 presents the analysis of one year of follow-up. Cases were those presenting with onset between 14 and 365 days after the third dose. In this analysis, only those who ingested three complete doses were included. Of those initially enrolled in the study, 62,285 participants took three complete doses of either placebo, whole cell, or B-subunit whole cell vaccine, with 20,837, 20,743, and 20,750 in each group. The group reported one-sided confidence intervals, which are not included in Table 6.7 (see Problem 6.1 and Table 7.3). In subsequent years of follow-up, the efficacy of the vaccines appeared to wane. In Section 7.3 we present a method to analyze vaccine efficacy that wanes over time using the example of the cholera vaccine trial.

6.4.7 Pneumococcal conjugate vaccine in California

A randomized, double-blind trial of a heptavalent pneumococcal vaccine was conducted at 23 medical centers within Northern California Kaiser Permanente (NCKP), a health maintenance organization (Black et al 2000). Healthy infants were randomized 1:1 to receive either heptavalent pneumococcal conjugate or the meningococcus type C conjugate vaccine at 2, 4, 6, and 12 to 15 months of age. Infants with specific risk factors were excluded. The heptavalent vaccine contained saccharides of the serotypes 4, 9V, 14, 18C, 19F, 23F, and 6B conjugated to a protein carrier made of nontoxic mutant diphtheria toxin. At that time, the seven serotypes were responsible for 83% of invasive disease in children younger than 4 years of age. The control meningococcal conjugate vaccine had the same carrier.

The primary endpoint was invasive pneumococcal disease caused by the vaccine serotypes. Secondary endpoints included otitis media. The outcome pneumonia was reported separately from the primary analysis. Active surveillance for cases in the study population was conducted using automated clinical and laboratory databases of the NCKP system. Invasive pneumococcal disease was defined as a positive culture of *Streptococcus pneumoniae* from a normally sterile body fluid (blood, spinal fluid) obtained from a child presenting with an acute illness compatible with pneumococcal illness.

Between October 1995 and August 1998, 37,868 children were enrolled into the trial. Of the 18,927 children who received at least one dose of pneumococcal conjugate, 17,174 received at least two doses, 15,565 received at least three doses, and 10,940 received at least four doses. Of the 18,941 children who received at least one dose of meningococcal conjugate, 17,196 received at least two doses, 15,536 received at least three doses, and 10,995 received at least four doses.

In this trial, protective efficacy was estimated by 1 minus the ratio of the number of cases of invasive disease in the pneumoccal vaccine arm compared to the meningococcal arm. In other words, the computation does not use the denominators. Efficacy was evaluated with the binomial test of the null hypothesis that the vaccine has no efficacy for the seven serotypes. The analysis incorporated a sequential design. An interim analysis had been planned when 17 cases had occurred. The null hypothesis was to be rejected if the case split was 15:2 or more favorable, $p = 0.0023$, with a final evaluation planned when 26 cases had occurred and an overall two-tailed p value of <0.05. Exact binomial confidence intervals were calculated by the Clopper–Pearson (1934) method. An intent-to-treat analysis included all invasive disease caused by a pneumococcal serotype regardless of number of doses completed. Safety of the vaccine was assessed by telephone follow-up on subsets of the study population, one receiving DTwP, one receiving DTaP. The computerized utilization data of the NCKP was also used to compare rates of events in the two groups. Immunogenicity of the conjugate vaccine was evaluated in a subset of children receiving DTwP concurrently and in a subset given DTaP in the first year of life. Serum IgG to the seven serotypes was measured using ELISA from samples collected before the first vaccination and one month after the third dose.

Table 6.8 Efficacy of heptavalent pneumococcal vaccine against invasive pneumococcal disease results as of April 20,1999 (Black et al 2000)

Analysis for Serotypes Contained in the Vaccine	Cases Split Control: Pneumococcal Vaccine Groups	Efficacy % [95% CI]	*p*-value
Per protocol fully vaccinated	39:1	97.4 [82.7–99.9]	<0.001
Intent to treat	49:3	93.9 [79.6–98.5]	<0.001
Partially vaccinated only	7:1	85.7 [0–100]	0.05
All cases regardless of serotype	55:6	89.1 [73.7–95.8]	<0.001

At the interim analysis, all 17 of the cases of invasive disease in fully vaccinated children were in the control group. At the interim intent-to-treat analysis of children receiving at least one dose, all 22 cases were in the control group. The Study Advisory Group recommended termination of the trial at the interim analysis because of the high efficacy. Enrollment was discontinued at the end of August 1998. Blinded follow-up and per-protocol vaccination of the two groups continued until April 20,1999. After that, all children in the control group were offered pneumococcal conjugate vaccine. The vaccine was highly efficacious against invasive pneumococcal disease (Table 6.8). During the trial, concern grew that there would not be enough events for the definitive analysis. This motivated the design and implementation of the grouprandomized study to estimate the total effects of using the pneumococcal vaccine (Section 13.4.2).

6.5 Report of a Study

In the preceding examples we have not included every aspect of the report of the studies. A report should tell the type of study, whether randomized, cohort, or case-control. The entities that reviewed the study protocol should be listed. These could include local institutional review boards, regulatory bodies, such as the U.S. Food and Drug Administration, medical products committees, and ethics boards. Details of the vaccines and placebos, their manufacturers, the lots, and any other relevant aspect such as storage should be included. Details of the route and schedule for administering the vaccines are needed. The study description should include the usual person, time, and place. The study population, the eligibility for inclusion, the dates for eligibility, exclusion criteria, how cases were ascertained, the case definition(s), the follow-up period, and where the study took place all should be included. The surveillance for side effects or adverse events, the laboratory methods if any for biological confirmation of cases, reasons for loss to follow-up, and immunogenicity tests, should be described. The statistical analysis and possibly how the sample size was chosen should be described. The results usually include a descriptive comparison of the groups on important potential confounders. Reports of randomized controlled trials can follow the Consolidated Standards of Reporting Trials (CONSORT) Statement (Moher et al 2001; Altman et al 2001).

6.6 Reduction in Burden of Illness

Most of the studies of VE_S presented in this chapter have a case definition that is a 0,1 dichotomous outcome. Although several different case definitions, some more and some less severe, may be considered in separate analyses, they are all scored 0,1 in any given analysis. Chang et al (1994) suggested a measure of efficacy that takes into account both the incidence of disease and severity. A severity score is assigned to each incident case, with 0 assigned to noncases. Then the total is summed over all cases to have a burden of illness score. When the severity score for each case is one, the burden-of-illness score reduces to the vaccine efficacy based on the number of cases in the vaccinated compared with the unvaccinated group. When different cases have different severity scores, the burden-of-illness score for a group is a weighted sum of all of the cases in the group, where the severity scores serve as the weights. The burden-of-illness score divided by the number of subjects randomized to the group yields the burden-of-illness per randomized participant. The difference between the mean burden-of-illness in the two groups, or the relative difference is a measure of the net reduction in morbidity per participant. The reduction in burden of illness differs from the VE_P measures in that the denominator is still the susceptible people, and the first outcome post-randomization is illness, which is given a score. A number of vaccine studies have developed severity scores (Section 9.2.1). In a rotavirus vaccine study, the severity of each case of diarrhea was given a severity score between 0 and 20 (Ruuska and Vesikari 1990).

Let N_0 and N_1 be the number randomized to vaccine and control, and c_0 and c_1 the number of cases in the vaccine and control arms. The severity scores for the cases are $S_{01},\ldots,S_{0n_0}$ and $S_{11},\ldots,S_{1n_1}$ in the two groups with means μ_0, μ_1 and variances σ_0^2, σ_1^2. One design option is that the trial runs for a fixed time, after which it is stopped and analyzed. A second option is that the trial is stopped after a number of total cases c, where $c = c_0 + c_1$. If λ_0 and λ_1 are the hazards of disease in the two groups, then the expected number of cases in the two groups is $\lambda_0 N_0 t$ and $\lambda_1 N_1 t$, where t is the duration of follow-up. The number of cases in the control group, c_0, has a binomial distribution $\text{Binom}(c, p_0)$, where $p_0 = \lambda_0 N_0 t/(\lambda_0 N_0 t + \lambda_1 N_1 t)$, and $p_1 = 1 - p_0$. In the design with fixed time, the null hypothesis is that $\mu_0 = \mu_1$ and $p_0 = p_1$. In the design with fixed number of events, the null hypothesis is that $\mu_0 = \mu_1$ and $\lambda_0 = \lambda_1$. A test statistic T for both models is the difference in the mean burden of illness scores per participant:

$$T = \frac{1}{N_0}\sum_{i=1}^{n_0} S_{0i} - \frac{1}{N_1}\sum_{i=1}^{n_1} S_{1i}. \tag{6.16}$$

For both designs, under the null hypothesis, μ_0 and μ_1 are estimated by

$$\bar{x} = \left(\sum_{i=1}^{n_0} S_{0i} + \sum_{i=1}^{n_1} S_{1i} \right) / (n_0 + n_1) = (n_0 \bar{s}_0 + n_1 \bar{s}_1)/(n_0 + n_1). \tag{6.17}$$

The variances $j = 0, 1$ are estimated by

$$s_j^2 = \left(\sum_{i=1}^{n_j} (S_{ji} - \bar{S}_j)^2 \right) / (n_j - 1). \tag{6.18}$$

In the fixed time design, $\hat{p} = (n_0 + n_1)/(N_0 + N_1)$ estimates both p_0 and p_1. In the fixed number of events design, p_0 is estimated by $N_0/(N_0 + N_1)$, and p_1 by 1 minus the estimate of p_0. The observed standard test statistics are obtained from

$$\begin{aligned} \widehat{V}_H(T) &= [\bar{x}^2 \hat{p}(1-\hat{p})/(1/N_0 + 1/N_1) + \hat{p}(s_0^2/N_0 + s_1^2/N_1)] \\ \widehat{V}_H(T|n) &= c[\bar{x}^2/N_0 N_1 + (s_0^2/N_0 + s_1^2/N_1)/(N_0 + N_1)]. \end{aligned}$$

The two-sided rejection region of the null hypothesis for the fixed time design is $|T/\sqrt{\widehat{V}_H(T)}| > z_{\alpha/2}$ and for the fixed number of events design is $|T/\sqrt{\widehat{V}_H(T|n)}| > z_{\alpha/2}$. Chang et al (1994) also present a method to calculate sample size. Because the scores combine incidence with severity per case, one might think that the burden-of-illness scores can provide a more comprehensive measure of overall efficacy than would a separate analysis based simply on either incident cases, VE_S, or the per-case severity, VE_P with a continuous outcome (Chapter 9), alone. However, because there may be a large number of zeros in each group, the test can have poor power.

Mehrotra et al (2006) compared eight methods for a dual endpoint evaluation of efficacy in a proof-of-concept trial, including that of Chang et al (1994). The motivation for the comparison was the design of the first trial of an HIV vaccine based on cell-mediated immunity. The vaccine was expected to have very low efficacy against infection, but it was hoped that it would reduce viral load as a surrogate for progression to disease. The question was whether it was better to test the composite null hypothesis of no vaccine effect on either the incidence of HIV infection or the viral load setpoint among those who become infected relative to the placebo using just a single composite test or using two separate tests, one for the infection endpoint and one for viral load endpoint. They found that combining separate tests for the infection and viral load endpoints is generally more powerful than the unconditional burden-of-illness test of Chang et al (1994), especially at low or zero VE_S. At $VE_S = 0.60$ or higher, all methods and combinations of methods performed comparably. They recommended using either the unweighted Simes' or Fisher's combination test for the trial.

One of the problems in vaccine studies is that usually most of the participants do not become infected. Follmann et al (2009) took a different approach from that of Chang et al (1994) by introducing chop-lump Wilcoxon and t-tests. The approach again assigns a score S to each participant, 0 for uninfected participants, and a measure $S > 0$ of the post-infection outcome such as severity or parasite density in the infected participants. When the number of participants in each group is equal, the chop-lump test first removes an equal number of zeros from both groups, then performs the test on the remaining S scores, most of which are greater than 0. A permutation approach then provides a null distribution. The chop-lump Wilcoxon test is shown to be always more powerful than the usual Wilcoxon test when the true infection rates in the vaccine and the control group are the same. The R package `choplump` is available at http://cran.r-project.org/.

Problems

6.1. (a) Cholera study: compute one-sided and two-sided 95% confidence intervals for VE in Table 6.7. (b) Compare the results. (c) Why are two-sided confidence intervals generally recommended?

6.2. A randomized study of an influenza vaccine was conducted with 3000 children each in the vaccine arm and the control arm. There were 350 biologically confirmed cases in the control arm and 53 cases in the vaccine arm by the end of the influenza season. Compute the estimate of $\mathrm{VE}_{S,CI}(T)$ and the 95% confidence limits on the estimate.

6.3. (a) In an observational study in a cohort, some of whom are vaccinated and some not, how might the exposure to infection differ in the two groups?
(b) Would differing exposure to infection be a confounder in the study? How might it influence the vaccine efficacy estimates using $\mathrm{VE}_{S,CI}(T)$ or $\mathrm{VE}_{S,IR}$? Write out $\mathrm{VE}_{S,CI}(T)$ and $\mathrm{VE}_{S,IR}$ using the dependent happening expression (2.7) to explain your response.
(c) How might you ascertain differences in exposure to infection or control for it in the analysis?
(d) How would this vary for different infectious diseases?

6.4. Discuss how and why the vaccine efficacy estimates in Table 6.3 change with the changing case definition.

6.5. (a) Consider designing a relative efficacy trial of a live, attenuated influenza virus vaccine with a killed influenza virus vaccine. Assume a 5.0% attack rate in the children receiving killed vaccine and a 2.5% attack rate in the children receiving live, attenuated influenza virus vaccine. How large a sample size would be needed in each arm for 90% power with $\alpha = 0.5$ on a two-sided test? (b) Assume now attack rates of 1.0% and 0.05% in the two arms. What sample size would be needed in each arm to achieve the same power and α level?

6.6. (a) Explain the main difference between the approach of Chang et al (1994) in testing for differences in burden-of-illness in the vaccine and control groups and the chop-lump test of Follmann et al (2009).

Chapter 7
Modes of Action and Time-Varying VE_S

7.1 Mode of Action and Choice of Measures

Suppose you have just been vaccinated against an infectious agent. Your physician or health practitioner tells you that the protective efficacy of the vaccine is 90%. You might then wonder if that means that the vaccine reduces your probability of contracting the infection (or disease) by 0.90 at each exposure to infection. In other words, you still might have a finite probability of contracting the infection or disease each time you were exposed, but it would be much less than it would have been if you had not been vaccinated. Alternatively, you might think that it means that you have a 0.90 probability of being completely protected against the disease, but still a 0.10 probability that you received absolutely no protection against infection or disease compared to what it would have been had you not been vaccinated. That is, the vaccine fails to elicit a protective immune response in 10% of the vaccinated people. Would you behave differently if you knew which of these possibilities were actually true? Would it make a difference if the vaccine were against a disease with a high case fatality ratio? Would it make a difference if the efficacy were 60% rather than 90%?

In Chapter 6, vaccine efficacy results were reported simply based on relative cumulative incidence or rates without any further interpretation of the meaning of the efficacy estimate. In 1984, Smith et al published a paper that grew out of a student exercise that altered the discussion about interpreting and evaluating protective efficacy of vaccines. They considered two models of vaccine mechanism they called Type I and Type II. In the Type I mechanism, vaccination is assumed to reduce the instantaneous disease rate in all the vaccinated people by a constant proportion. That is, Type I assumes that protection is multiplicative on the baseline hazard of infection. The effect is homogeneous in the vaccinated population. In the Type II mechanism, vaccination is assumed to provide a constant proportion of individuals with complete immunity from the disease. That is, it completely protects a portion of the vaccinated people, but completely fails to protect in the other portion. Un-

M.E. Halloran et al., *Design and Analysis of Vaccine Studies*, Statistics for Biology and Health, DOI 10.1007/978-0-387-68636-3_7,

der the Type II mechanism, the distribution of protection is heterogeneous in the vaccinated population.

Smith et al (1984) considered how these assumed models affect the choice of analysis in cohort studies and sampling of controls in case-control studies. Their discussion considered two of the measures of vaccine efficacy that do not condition on exposure to infection, in particular, vaccine efficacy measures based on Level II and III information and vaccine efficacy based on Level IV information. The first, which they considered as one, was based on the hazard rate or cases per person-time at risk, $VE_{S,\lambda}$ or $VE_{S,IR}$. The second was based on the number of cases per person at risk, the cumulative incidence, or attack rate, $VE_{S,CI}$ or $VE_{S,AR}$. Their motivation was originally in the design of alternatives to randomized studies, but the results for the cohort studies apply as well to randomized controlled trials.

7.1.1 Leaky and all-or-none modes of action

Before continuing the discussion of the implications of the two models of vaccine action for choice of measures in vaccine studies, we divert to explain why we prefer the use of the term *leaky* for Type I and *all-or-none* for Type II models. In the early 1980s the possibility of developing effective malaria vaccines created a great deal of excitement. The malaria parasite has a complex life cycle with separate antigenic stages. Malaria sporozoites, the stage infective for humans, are injected by the mosquito into the human. Asexual blood stages, or merozoites, the stage responsible for malaria disease, subsequently develop. Sexual blood stage parasites, or gametocytes, the stage infective for mosquitoes, develop from the asexual blood stage parasites. Malaria vaccines were being developed against each of the three main stages, so vaccine candidates were directed at blocking infection, modifying disease once infected, and blocking transmission to the mosquito, corresponding to VE_S, VE_P, and VE_I. A sporozoite vaccine was expected to prevent infection either by inhibiting invasion of liver cells or by impairing effective reproduction once the parasite was in the liver. If the inhibition were not complete, then essentially the liver would let parasites through and be leaky. Struchiner et al (1989) and Halloran et al (1989) developed models of malaria vaccination that separately considered its effect on infection, disease, and transmission to mosquitoes. The mechanism of the vaccine model's effect on susceptibility to infection reduces the probability of infection given a bite by an infected mosquito, corresponding to the expected direct effects of a leaky sporozoite vaccine that does not provide sterile immunity. Thus the term "leaky" for a multiplicative effect on the transmission probability comes from the image of the malaria parasites getting through a leaky immunity in the liver. Halloran et al (1989) and Struchiner et al (1989) also considered waning of immunity and the role of natural boosting of infection in their dynamics models.

In a study of the use of case-control studies under complex disease transmission patterns, Struchiner et al (1990) adopted the term "leaky" rather than Model 1 as suggested by Smith et al (1984). The motivation was partly because it is more descriptive than the term Model 1, partly because it also was meant to take into account the effect on the transmission probability, and partly because the approach grew out of the malaria vaccine research. Smith et al (1984) did not discuss exposure to infection or any biological mechanism for the different models of vaccine action. There was considerable resistance in the early 1990s in parts of the vaccine community against the term "leaky" because of its potentially negative connotations. However, as recognition increased that vaccines often protect more against disease than infection, the term "leaky" has gained wide acceptance.

We also prefer the term "all-or-none" (Halloran et al 1991) to Model 2 for a vaccine that protects a portion of the vaccinated people completely and the rest of the vaccinated not at all because it is more descriptive. As early as 1915, Greenwood and Yule discussed possible heterogeneities in susceptibility in the vaccinated and unvaccinated groups. Correlation of the antibody response with the distribution of infection rates also suggests that there is heterogeneity in protective response. For example, in the first 17 months of follow-up in a hepatitis B vaccine trial, 10 of the 11 infections in vaccinees accrued in the hypo- or nonresponders (Francis et al 1982). In a live virus varicella vaccine trial, incidence in the 17% of vaccinees with low antibody titer was between 5 and 13% per year, whereas in vaccinees with high antibody titer, incidence averaged less than 2% per year (White et al 1992).

7.1.2 Implications for choice of efficacy measures

Consider a randomized controlled trial with equal numbers of individuals in the placebo and vaccinated groups with both groups followed for an equal period of time. In this simple example, assume there is no loss to follow-up or deaths, that all cases of disease are ascertained, and the time of onset of each case is known (Table 6.1). The measures of interest are based on the hazard rate or cases per person-time at risk, $VE_{S,\lambda}$ or $VE_{S,IR}$, and the cumulative incidence or attack rate, $VE_{S,CI}$ or $VE_{S,AR}$. If the incidence rates and the attack rates are low, then the two measures will be approximately equal, and it makes little difference which measure is used to compute vaccine efficacy, whereby the approach using the hazard rate or person-time at risk does allow for different follow-up times. However, in many cases the appropriate choice of vaccine efficacy measure may depend on whether the mode of action is leaky or all-or-none.

For the leaky model, Smith et al (1984) considered an essentially continuous-time model. Suppose that in a small interval of time $(t, t+\delta t)$ the probability of an unvaccinated person contracting disease is $\lambda_t \delta t$. Also, suppose that vaccination reduces the probability to $R\lambda_t \delta t$, with R assumed constant over time. Consider also that $\lambda_t = \lambda$ for all t, although this assumption is not necessary. Figure 7.1a shows the survival curves for the unvaccinated and vaccinated groups. The proportion of individuals in each group who would be expected to develop disease by time T would be $1 - e^{-\lambda T}$ and $1 - e^{-\lambda RT}$. Thus the calculated $VE_{S,CI}(T)$ given here as a function of T (Greenland and Frerichs 1988) is

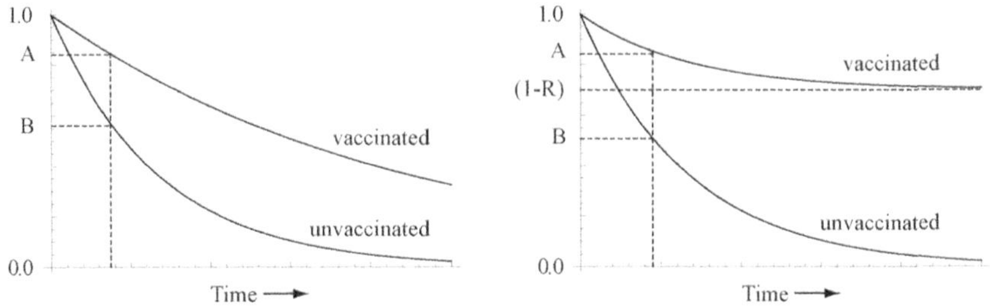

Fig. 7.1 Proportion of individuals without disease by time since start of trial under two models of vaccine action: (a) leaky, (b) all-or-none (adapted from Smith et al 1984).

$$\mathrm{VE}_{S,CI}(T) = 1 - \frac{1-e^{-\lambda RT}}{1-e^{-\lambda T}}. \tag{7.1}$$

$\mathrm{VE}_{S,CI}(T)$ in equation (7.1) decreases to zero as the follow-up time T increases. That is, this model allows everyone to get disease if the follow-up time is long enough. However, based on $\mathrm{VE}_{S,IR}(T) = 1-(c_1/Y_1)/(c_0/Y_0)$, or $\mathrm{VE}_{S,\lambda}$, it is easy to show (see Problem 7.1) that $\mathrm{VE}_{S,IR}(T)$ does not change with time, thus

$$\mathrm{VE}_{S,IR}(T) = 1-R. \tag{7.2}$$

Under the all-or-none model, the assumption is that vaccination provides a proportion $(1-R)$ of the vaccinated group with complete immunity from the disease. The probability of an unvaccinated person contracting disease in the small time interval $(t, t+\delta t)$ is still $\lambda_t \delta t$, and once again it is simple to assume that $\lambda_t = \lambda$ for all t. In the people who were vaccinated but in whom the vaccine provides no protection, the probability of contracting disease in a short interval is the same as in the unvaccinated people, $\lambda \delta t$. Figure 7.1b shows the survival curves for the vaccinated and unvaccinated groups under the all-or-none model. From the initiation of the trial up to time T, the proportions in each group expected to have developed disease would be $1-e^{-\lambda T}$ and $1-(1-R)-Re^{-\lambda T} = R(1-e^{-\lambda T})$. Thus the two expected efficacy measures would be

$$\mathrm{VE}_{S,CI}(T) = 1-R, \tag{7.3}$$

$$\mathrm{VE}_{S,IR}(T) = 1/[1+R(1-e^{\lambda T})/T\lambda(1-R)]. \tag{7.4}$$

Under the all-or-none model, the time-invariant measure of vaccine efficacy is $\mathrm{VE}_{S,CI}(T)$. The value of $\mathrm{VE}_{S,IR}(T)$ or $\mathrm{VE}_{S,\lambda}(T)$ will tend to increase to one as the people in the vaccinated group who are still susceptible to disease are depleted, leaving only those who are completely immune.

Smith et al (1984) showed that if in a randomized study, $\mathrm{VE}_{S,CI}(T)$ decreases with time, but $\mathrm{VE}_{S,IR}(T)$ ($\mathrm{VE}_{S,\lambda}(T)$) remains constant, the result would be suggestive of a leaky multiplicative mechanism. On the other hand, if $\mathrm{VE}_{S,CI}(T)$ is constant, but $\mathrm{VE}_{S,IR}(T)$ increases with time, the result would suggest an all-or-none mechanism. This result is the same for randomized prospective studies or observational cohort studies. Other mechanisms could explain time-varying efficacy estimates. In Section 7.3, we consider the situation that the efficacy within individuals actually does wane with time, which provides a biological mechanism for a time-varying vaccine efficacy. Also, heterogeneities in exposure to infection could play a role. In Chapter 8, we consider case-control studies, including the findings of Smith et al (1984). More general distributions of protection were developed (Halloran et al 1992). Brunet et al (1993) developed a method of estimation based on state space models.

7.1.3 Attack rates versus transmission probabilities

Suppose that the infection process occurs as discrete exposures to infection (Halloran et al 1991) rather than in continuous time models as in Smith et al (1984). The question then is to define a direct protective effect of vaccination given a specific amount of exposure to infection, not just comparable exposure to infection. To be biologically interpretable and to be robust to different transmission conditions, the parameters of interest might need to take account of the type and amount of exposure. The following argument shows how vaccine efficacy measured using the attack rate can depend on the number of exposures to infection, and thus could vary from population to population (Halloran et al 1991).

Let p_0 be the probability of transmission to an unvaccinated person after one exposure. Let $p_1 = \theta p_0$ be the probability of transmission to a vaccinated person after one exposure, where θ is the multiplicative leaky effect on the transmission probability in the vaccinated person. Let $\text{AR}_1(n)$, $\text{AR}_0(n)$ and $\text{VE}_{S,AR}(n)$ denote the attack rates and vaccine efficacy based on the cumulative incidence or attack rates that would be observed after everyone had n exposures to infection. Assume that everyone in the population receives one exposure to infection, and that there are N_0 and N_1 individuals in the unvaccinated and vaccinated groups. Then the attack rates in the vaccinated and unvaccinated groups are

$$AR_1(1) = \frac{p_1 N_1}{N_1} = p_1 = \theta p_0, \quad AR_0(1) = \frac{p_0 N_0}{N_0} = p_0 \, ,$$

so that the $\text{VE}_{S,AR}(1)$ and $\text{VE}_{S,p}$ are the same,

$$VE_{S,AR}(1) = 1 - \frac{AR_1(1)}{AR_0(1)} = 1 - \frac{p_1}{p_0} = VE_{S,p} = 1 - \theta. \qquad (7.5)$$

Now assume that everyone in the population is exposed to infection a second time. We assume a discrete model of infection and that each exposure is independent of the previous exposures. The attack rates in the unvaccinated would now be given by the probability of having been infected by the first infective plus the probability of being infected by the second infective given that a person was not infected by the first infective. Then

$$AR_1(2) = p_1 + (1-p_1)p_1 = p_1(2-p_1) = \theta p_0(2-\theta p_0) \quad (7.6)$$
$$AR_0(2) = p_0 + (1-p_0)p_0 = p_0(2-p_0) \quad (7.7)$$

Thus, after two exposures,

$$VE_{S,AR}(2) = 1 - \frac{p_1(2-p_1)}{p_0(2-p_0)} = 1 - \frac{\theta(2-\theta p_0)}{(2-p_0)}, \quad (7.8)$$

so that $\mathrm{VE}_{S,AR}(2) < \mathrm{VE}_{S,p}$. In general, for n exposures to infection,

$$VE_{S,AR}(n) = 1 - \frac{1-(1-p_1)^n}{1-(1-p_0)^n} = 1 - \frac{1-(1-\theta p_0)^n}{1-(1-p_0)^n}. \quad (7.9)$$

It can be shown by induction that for $n > 1$, $\mathrm{VE}_{S,AR}(n) < \mathrm{VE}_{S,p}$. Essentially, expression (7.9) is the vaccine efficacy for a leaky vaccine after n exposures using the binomial transmission model of Section 4.3.1.

7.1.3.1 Example

Suppose a vaccine has a multiplicative leaky effect that is the same in everyone and reduces the probability of transmission per potentially infective exposure by 80%, $\mathrm{VE}_{S,p} = 0.80$. Then the transmission probability in vaccinated people would be 20% of that in unvaccinated people, so that $p_1 = 0.20p_0$. Suppose we want to evaluate the efficacy of the vaccine in a study population of 2000, where 1000 individuals are vaccinated and 1000 are not. Assume for this disease that $p_0 = 0.25$, so that $p_1 = 0.20 \times 0.25 = 0.05$. At the end of one month, assume that every person in the study has had exactly five exposures to infection. What is the expected attack rate in each group and the $\mathrm{VE}_{S,AR}(5)$ after one month?

In the unvaccinated group, the probability of becoming infected is $1-(1-p)^5 = 1-0.75^5 = 0.76$, so the expected number of infections in the unvaccinated group is 1000 people $\times$ 0.76 = 760. In the vaccinated group, the probability of becoming infected after five exposures is $1-(1-0.05)^5 = 1-0.95^5 = 0.23$, so the expected number of infections in that group is 1000 people $\times$ 0.23 = 230. Then $\mathrm{VE}_{S,AR}(5) = 1-(230/1000)/(760/1000) = 1-0.30 = 0.70$, which is lower than the vaccine effect on the transmission probability, $\mathrm{VE}_{S,p} = 0.80$.

Suppose that after two months, each individual has had exactly 10 exposures. Now the expected number of infections in the unvaccinated group is $(1-0.75^{10}) \times 1000 = 943$, and in the vaccinated group, it is $(1-0.95^{10}) \times 1000 = 401$. After 10 exposures, the $\mathrm{VE}_{S,AR}(10) = 1-(401/1000)/(943/1000) = 0.57$. The vaccine seems less efficacious after two months even though the effect of vaccination on the transmission probability has not waned.

As the number of exposures in the two groups increases, the observed vaccine efficacy based on the attack rate will decrease to zero. Eventually everyone in both groups will become infected under the multiplicative assumption if they are exposed often enough, illustrating the meaning of a multiplicative or leaky model at the transmission probability level. In principle, people can still become infected if exposed often enough.

Suppose we use the model in continuous time (Section 4.3.3) similar to Smith et al (1984), but take into account the number of exposures to infection. Assume that c is the contact rate with infectives. Then $\lambda_0 = cp$ and $\lambda_1 = 0.20cp$. In continuous time, $\mathrm{VE}_{S,\lambda} = 1 - \lambda_1/\lambda_0 = 0.80$, giving the same answer as the multiplicative effect on the transmission probability. In the unvaccinated group, the probability of being infected after five exposures in the first month is $1 - \exp(-5 \times 0.25) = 0.713$ and in the vaccinated group is $1 - \exp(-5 \times 0.05) = 0.221$, so the expected number of infections is 713 in the unvaccinated group and 221 in the vaccinated group. The number of expected infections is different from that calculated above from the discrete model. The observed $\mathrm{VE}_{S,AR}(5) = 1 - 0.221/0.713 = 0.69$, similar but not identical to that calculated from the discrete model. After 10 exposures, the $\mathrm{VE}_{S,AR}(10) = 1 - 0.393/0.918 = 0.57$, the same as using the discrete model, though the expected number infected in the vaccinated and unvaccinated groups is different when calculated using the discrete model above.

7.2 Frailty Mixture Models for $\mathrm{VE}_{S,\lambda}$

In this section we consider estimation and interpretation of vaccine efficacy when the distribution of protection can include some people who are completely protected, some who have no protection, and the rest have a continuous distribution of protection (Longini and Halloran 1996; Halloran et al 1996). A frailty model is a survival analysis model that allows for unmeasured heterogeneity in the population. It is a special case of a random effects model. The frailty mixing model developed here falls into the general category of frailty models (Vaupel 1979) used in survival analysis, but like cure models (Farewell 1982), it allows for a point mass at 0.

7.2.1 Mixing models

In the following development it is important to distinguish between heterogeneity in the distributions of the hazard rates and heterogeneity in vaccine effects. Assume that the heterogeneity in susceptibility in the unvaccinated and vaccinated groups is described by the nonnegative mixing random variables Z_0 and Z_1. Assume that the distribution of susceptibility in each group is such that α_0 and α_1 are the proportion of people in each group that are highly protected, ie, not susceptible to infection such that Z_v, $v = 0, 1$ has point mass α_v at 0. The susceptibility in the susceptible proportion follows a continuous distribution $f_v(\cdot)$ with probability $1 - \alpha_v$. Thus,

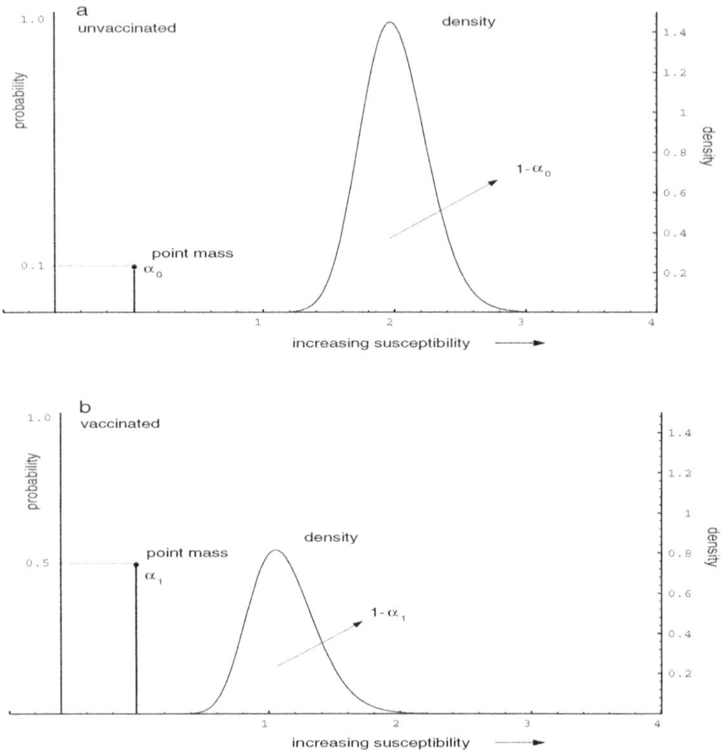

Fig. 7.2 Schematic distribution of susceptibility in the (a) unvaccinated and (b) vaccinated groups. The proportion highly protected is $\alpha_0 = 0.1$ in the unvaccinated and $\alpha_1 = 0.5$ in the vaccinated. The expectation of the random variable in the susceptible proportion of each group is equal to one. The area under each curve of susceptibles is $1 - \alpha_0$ and $1 - \alpha_1$ in the unvaccinated and vaccinated groups. In the vaccinated group the susceptibility is reduced by the factor $\theta = 0.5$ (from Halloran et al 1996, Am J Epidemiol, 144:83–97. Reprinted with permission).

$$\begin{aligned} P(Z_V = 0) &= \alpha_V, \\ Z_V | Z_V > 0 &\equiv X_V \sim f_V(\cdot), \text{ with probability } 1 - \alpha_V. \end{aligned} \tag{7.10}$$

The distribution f_V allows flexibility to model the shape and spread of the continuous part of the distribution of Z_V. However, in the estimation problem here the mean is not identifiable. Thus, let $f_V(\cdot)$ be from a two-parameter family, but with $E(X_V) = 1$. Furthermore, let $\text{var}(X_V) = \delta_V$. Then $E(Z_V = 1 - \alpha_V$, and $\text{var}(Z_V) = (1 - \alpha_V)(\delta_V + \alpha_V)$.

An example of the distribution of susceptibility in the vaccinated and unvaccinated groups if X_V follows a gamma distribution is shown in Figure 7.2. In this example, $\alpha_0 = 0.1$ and $\alpha_1 = 0.5$. The expectation of the random variable in the susceptible proportion of each group equals one. In the vaccinated group, the susceptibility is reduced by the factor $\theta = 0.5$ in the people still susceptible. The area under each curve of susceptibles is α_0 and α_1 in the unvaccinated and vaccinated groups. For a vaccine that highly protects some people while conferring partial protection on the rest, there are several measures of vaccine efficacy. The difference between the proportion highly protected in each group, $\mathrm{VE}_\alpha = \alpha_1 - \alpha_0$, measures the proportion of the population highly protected due to vaccination. The measure $\mathrm{VE}_\theta = 1 - \theta$ is the efficacy of the vaccine in conferring partial protection conditional both on a specified exposure to infection and on remaining to some degree susceptible.

The summary measure of protective vaccine efficacy is the expected relative reduction in susceptibility conferred by the vaccine at the beginning of observation,

$$\mathrm{VE}(0)_{S,SUM} = 1 - \frac{(1-\alpha_1)\theta}{1-\alpha_0}. \tag{7.11}$$

If the $\alpha_0 = 0$, ie, no one in the unvaccinated group is completely protected, then the summary measure of vaccine efficacy under heterogeneity is

$$\mathrm{VE}(0)_{S,SUM} = 1 - (1-\alpha)\theta. \tag{7.12}$$

7.2.2 *Frailty model*

Following the dependent happening expression (2.7), let $P(t)$ be the infection point prevalence at time t. Then the individual-level hazard rate to an unvaccinated and vaccinated person at time t is

$$\lambda_0(t) = Z_0 c p P(t) \text{ and } \lambda_1(t) = Z_1 c p P(t). \tag{7.13}$$

To derive the survival function, let $S_v(t)$ be the fraction of the stratum v that is considered to be at risk of infection at time t, $t \geq 0$. The assumption is made here that the population is closed to immigration, but open to emigration (ie, right censoring), so that $S_v(t)$ is a survival function. In addition, the assumption is made that vaccination takes place at or before time 0, and that the effects of vaccination do not wane over time. Then the population survival functions are

$$S_v(t) = E[\exp\{-Z_v\Lambda_v(t)\}] = L_{Z_v}\{\Lambda_v(t)\}, \tag{7.14}$$

where

$$\Lambda_0(t) = cp\int_0^t P(\tau)d\tau,$$

$\Lambda_1(t) = \theta\Lambda_0(t)$, and $L_Z(\,)$ is the Laplace transform (Aalen 1988, 1992). The Laplace transform of Z_v is

$$L_{Z_v}(s) = \alpha_v + (1 - \alpha v)L_{X_v}(s). \tag{7.15}$$

If X_v follows a gamma distribution with both scale and shape parameters equal to $1/\delta_v$, then from equations (7.14) and (7.15),

$$S_v(t) = \alpha_v + (1 - \alpha_v)\left\{\frac{1}{1 + \Lambda_v(t)\delta_v}\right\}^{1/\delta_v}. \tag{7.16}$$

When $\delta_v = 0$, then X_v is degenerate at 1, and

$$S_v(t) = \alpha_v + (1 - \alpha_v)\exp\{-\Lambda_v(t)\}. \tag{7.17}$$

7.2.2.1 Statistical inference

This approach is for data in grouped survival form with observations made at times $t_0(=0), t_1, \ldots, t_k$. Define the time intervals as $[t_{i-1}, t_i)$, $i = 1, \ldots, k$. Then let $P(t)$ be piecewise constant on these intervals, where $P(t) = P_i$ in interval i. Then from equation (7.14),

$$\Lambda_0(t) = cp\int_0^t P(\tau)d\tau = cp\kappa\left\{\sum_{j=1}^{i}(t_j - t_{j-1})P_j + (t - t_i)P_i\right\}, \quad t \in [t_i, t_{i+1}),$$

where κ is a proportionality constant related to the proportion of a time interval that infected individuals are infectious (Halloran et al 1996). Here the P_i are treated as observed and known quantitities and not as parameters to be estimated.

The parameters to be estimated are c, p, κ, α_0, α_1, δ_0, δ_1, and θ. Set $a = cp\kappa$, because c and p cannot be separately estimated from data with no contact information (Rhodes et al 1996), and κ is simply a proportionality constant. To formulate the likelihood function for observations from the population under study, let r_{iv} be the number of people at risk in group v at the beginning of interval i, minus half those who are lost to follow-up during the interval i, and let m_{iv} be the number infected during that interval. Then the likelihood function is

$$L(\text{data}|a, \alpha_0, \alpha_1, \delta_0, \delta_1, \theta) = \prod_{i=1}^{k}\prod_{v=0}^{1}\left\{\frac{S_v(t_i)}{S_v(t_{i-1})}\right\}^{r_{iv}-m_{iv}}\left\{\frac{S_v(t_i)}{1 - S_v(t_{i-1})}\right\}^{r_{iv}} \tag{7.18}$$

(see Aalen 1988). The likelihood function (7.18) can be maximized using standard methods.

Halloran et al (1996) explored the potential use of the frailty mixture model described above for the estimation of $\mathrm{VE}_{S,\lambda}$ over the parameter space that covers the possibilities of most vaccine studies. They showed that the parameters are identifiable under reasonable field conditions as long as there is not too much right-censoring. Most important they showed that the conventional VE_S estimators based

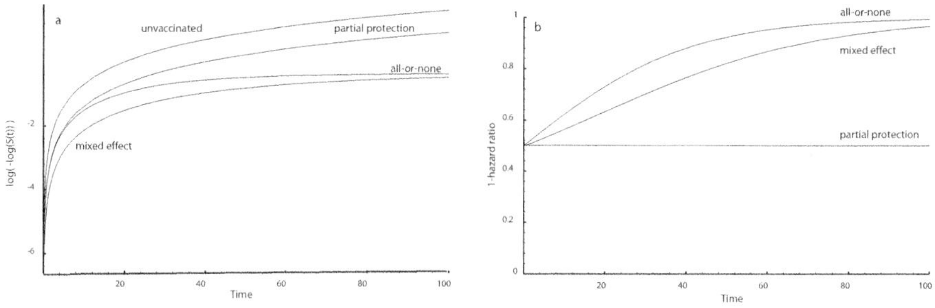

Fig. 7.3 (a) Diagnostic natural log minus log survival plots checking the proportional hazards assumption for vaccine conferring homogeneous partial protection, an all-or-none vaccine, and a mixed degenerate vaccine model compared with the unvaccinated group. (b) Plots of 1− hazard ratios for homogeneous partial protection ($\theta = 0.5$), the all-or-none vaccine ($\alpha_1 = 0.5$), and the mixed degenerate model ($\theta = 0.75, \alpha_1 = 0.33$). $VE_{SUM} = 0.5$ at time $t_0 = 0$ in these three cases (Halloran et al 1996, Am J Epidemiol, 144:83–97. Reprinted with permission).

on proportional hazards and cumulative incidence can be considerably biased when unmeasured heterogeneity is present. This bias is removed when the correct frailty mixture model is used. Violation of the proportional hazards assumption under frailty distributions is illustrated in Figure 7.3. The model is also applicable if there is heterogeneity in exposure to infection, although the interpretation of the estimates is different.

7.2.3 Measles outbreak in Burundi

A measles outbreak started in Muyinga, Burundi, in April 1988. The outbreak peaked in October 1988 and was over by December of that year (Chen et al 1994; Longini et al 1993). Measles illness histories were compiled after the outbreak for children aged 9 to 60 months. Only the month of onset of the measles illness was accurately recorded for most of the children (Table 7.1). Monthly measles incidence is given in the last column of Table 7.1. Initially 1436 children had no previous history of measles illness and known measles vaccination status, that is, they had childhood immunization cards. Of these 1436 children, 857 (60%) were vaccinated against measles before the outbreak. An additional 140 children were vaccinated during the outbreak. During the outbreak, 129 of the unvaccinated and 93 of the vaccinated children developed measles illness.

In the analysis of the data in Table 7.1, the vaccination times of the 140 children who were vaccinated during the outbreak were treated as right-censored times. The measles incidence in September was aberrantly high. There were only seven months, ($k = 7$), of measles incidence data, so δ_0 and δ_1 could not be estimated and were set to 0, so that the survival functions (7.17) were used in the likelihood function (7.18). In this case the summary vaccine efficacy is $VE_{SUM}(0) = 1 - (1 - \alpha_1)\theta$. The values calculated for $\{P_i\}$ were taken from the study population and are shown in Table 7.1.

Table 7.1 Numbers at risk, ill and monthly exposure for the measles epidemic Muyinga, Burundi, April–November 1998 (from Longini and Halloran 1996)

		Unvaccinated			Vaccinated			Exposure
i	Month	At Risk	Ill	%	At Risk	Ill	%	$p \times 100\%$
1	April	579	10	1.7	857	9	1.1	1.3
2	May	551	13	2.4	848	13	1.5	1.9
3	June	517	13	1.9	835	2	0.2	0.9
4	July	483	12	2.5	833	20	2.4	2.4
5	August	451	22	4.9	813	18	2.2	3.2
6	September	408	50	12.3	795	24	3.0	6.4
7	October	337	12	3.6	771	7	0.9	1.7
8	November	317	0	0.0	764	4	0.0	0.0
Total			129		93			

The maximum likelihood estimates and their standard errors are $\hat{a} = 1.66 \pm 0.14$, $\hat{\alpha}_1 = 0.805 \pm 0.060$, and $\hat{\theta} = 2.76 \pm 1.24$. The measles vaccine completely protected an estimated $\hat{\alpha}_1 = 0.805$, (95% CI, 0.687–0.924) of the vaccinated children. The estimate of θ is greater than 1, suggesting that, assuming equal exposure, the relative per-contact risk of contracting measles was higher in the vaccinated children who did not receive complete protection than it was in the unvaccinated children. The estimated summary measure of vaccine efficacy at time 0 is $\widehat{\text{VE}}_{SUM}(0) = 0.462$ (95% CI, 0.318–0671).

Table 7.2 gives the observed and expected (based on the fitted model) number of measles illness. The χ^2 goodness of fit statistic is 12.8 with 11 degrees of freedom. This yields a p-value of 0.3, so the model fits the data by this criterion. However, the distribution is not strictly χ^2 because of the correlation of the data over time. In future analyses, one might want to fit different models, such the leaky, all-or-none, and frailty mixture model, then use model selection tests such as likelihood ratio tests to choose among models (Hudgens and Gilbert 2009).

7.2.4 Model selection in low-dose challenge studies

In human field studies, we generally cannot observe the actual number of potentially infectious contacts that each person makes. However, in a challenge study in macaques with an HIV vaccine candidate, repeated, low-dose challenges were made and the infection status monitored (Ellenberger et al 2006). One of the 14 macaques in the control arm and four of the 16 in the vaccine arm were not infected when the study ended. Hudgens and Gilbert (2009) developed a clever method to distinguish using statistical methods whether the protective effect of the vaccine was leaky or all-or-none. The data are in the online supporting material of their paper. They used a discrete-time survival model similar to equation (7.9), but also including a term for complete protection, making it a discrete-time analogue of the summary measure of

Table 7.2 Observed and expected frequencies for the model fitted to the data from the measles epidemic Muyinga, Burundi, April–November 1998 (from Longini and Halloran 1996)

		Unvaccinated		Vaccinated	
i	Month	Observed	Expected	Observed	Expected
1	April	10	12.6	9	9.8
2	May	13	16.7	13	12.8
3	June	13	7.6	2	5.8
4	July	12	19.1	20	14.7
5	August	22	23.0	18	16.7
6	September	41.0	12.3	24	27.2
7	October	12	9.4	7	6.0
Total		129		93	

vaccine efficacy under heterogeneity in equation (7.12):

$$VE_S(n) = 1 - \frac{(1-\alpha)\{1-(1-\theta p)^n\}}{1-(1-p)^n}. \tag{7.19}$$

They developed maximum likelihood methods to estimate the transmission probability in the unvaccinated group, the proportion with complete protection, and the multiplicative effect on the transmission probability. They used a likelihood ratio test and the Akaike Information Criterion (AIC) to compare the leaky model, the all-or-none model, the summary model under heterogeneity, and the null model. They found that the statistical evidence suggested that the vaccine candidate had a significant leaky effect. These methods could be used for other repeated low-dose challenge studies or studies where the exposures to infection are known. The power for detecting an all-or-none effect was observed to be greater than the power to detect a leaky effect.

7.3 Estimating Waning Efficacy

Unmeasured heterogeneities in susceptibility, protection, and exposure to infection can produce time-varying estimates of $\text{VE}_{S,IR}(t)$ or $\text{VE}_{S,\lambda}(t)$ that are a result of the underlying heterogeneities, whereas true waning of protection or boosting of protection can lead to real time-varying effects. A traditional method to look for waning vaccine efficacy over time has been to partition the time axis into time intervals and to assume that the efficacy is constant within each interval. Then a separate constant $\text{VE}_{S,IR}(t)$ is estimated for each time interval. If the efficacy estimate depends on time, then the estimates will vary across the time intervals.

Table 7.3 Piecewise constant RR estimates, with approximate 95% confidence intervals for the oral whole cell and oral B-subunit whole cell vaccines, Matlab, Bangladesh, May 1, 1985 to November 30, 1989 (Durham et al 1999)

Year	Dates	Whole Cell Vaccine		BS Whole Cell Vaccine	
		RR	95% CI	RR	95% CI
1	May 1985–April 1986	0.44	[0.32–0.62]	0.33	[0.23–0.48]
2	May 1986–April 1987	0.45	[0.32–0.65]	0.47	[0.33–0.67]
3	May 1987–April 1988	0.55	[0.34–0.86]	0.86	[0.57–1.29]
4	May 1988–December 1989	1.21	[0.70–2.10]	0.83	[0.45–1.52]

7.3.1 Waning efficacy in the cholera vaccine trial

This method of partitioning the time axis was used to estimate $VE_{S,IR}(t)$ of oral killed whole cell (WC) and oral B subunit killed whole cell (BS-WC) oral cholera vaccines of a randomized, double-blinded vaccine trial in Matlab, Bangladesh (Clemens 1990) (Section 6.4.6). In a longer term follow-up from May 1, 1985 to November 30, 1989, 580 cases of cholera occurred, with 284, 150, and 146 in the placebo, WC vaccine, and BS-WC vaccine groups. The efficacy of both vaccines appeared to wane. The methods used to analyze waning vaccine efficacy from this trial involved partitioning the study duration into discrete time units and comparing piecewise constant incidence rate ratio estimates for successive time periods (Clemens et al 1990; van Loon et al 1996). For example, Table 7.3 gives the piecewise constant incidence rate ratio estimates for the whole cell and B-subunit whole cell vaccines. The incidence rate ratio for each year is calculated by using a ratio of incidence rates, where the incidence among those vaccinated is compared with the incidence among the unvaccinated. The time period called year 4 includes 19 months of follow-up, after which there were no observed cholera cases. The incidence rate ratio (RR) estimates appear to increase, so the efficacy estimates decrease across the time period.

Thus, we see a waning time trend in efficacy, with no significant protection by the fourth year. However, because the data have been grouped into years, it is difficult to be more precise about when and how these changes in efficacy occur. Because the partitioning boundaries are selected at one-year intervals, it is not clear if the waning protection is continuous or precisely at what point in time significant protection is lost. With use of a Poisson regression including covariates, the problem still remains of how to partition the time axis into piecewise constant components. The problem can be solved by the use of survival analysis methods.

Figure 7.4 shows plots of the log minus log Kaplan–Meier estimates of the survival curves for the placebo and two oral cholera vaccines. The good separation between the vaccine and placebo curves indicates that the vaccines give protection. The BS-WC vaccine provides better protection during the first year. The curves slowly approach one another indicating the waning of the protective effect, but this is difficult to see with plots based on cumulative incidence.

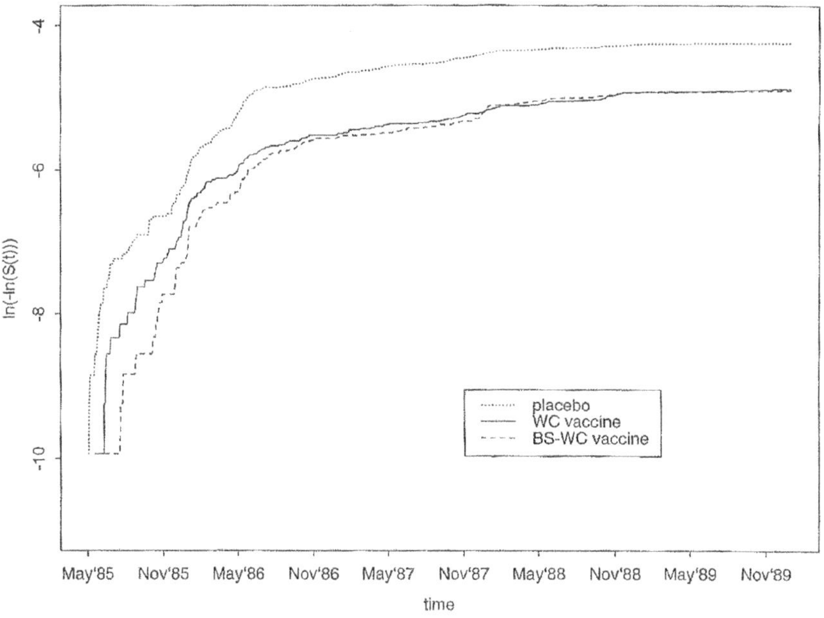

Fig. 7.4 Log-minus-log plots of the Kaplan–Meier estimates of the survival curves for the placebo and two cholera vaccines, Matlab, Bangladesh, May 1, 1985, through November 31, 1989. WC, killed whole cell; BS-WC, B subunit killed whole cell (Durham et al 1998, Am J Epidemiol, 147:948–959. Reprinted with permission).

7.3.2 Nonparametric estimation of time-varying vaccine effects

Durham et al (1999) adapted and compared two basic approaches for the nonparametric estimation of smoothed curves for $VE_{S,\lambda}(t) = 1 - RR(t) = 1 - \lambda_1(t)/\lambda_0(t)$. The first is a generalized additive models approach that involves using a time-varying coefficient, $VE_{S,\lambda}(t) = 1 - e^{\beta(t)}$ (Hastie and Tibshirani 1993), version of the proportional hazards model assuming a Poisson model (Whitehead 1980). This approach is useful for diagnostics to ascertain the shape of $\beta(t)$, but it cannot provide an estimator for $VE_{S,\lambda}(t)$.

The other method uses Schoenfeld residuals (Schoenfeld 1982; Grambsch and Therneau 1994). The general idea is to fit an ordinary proportional hazards model to the data, and then to compute the scaled differences between the actual and expected covariate values at each event time, called Schoenfeld residuals. The scaled residuals are added to the coefficient from the proportional hazards model. The time-varying regression coefficient $\beta(t)$ is recovered by smoothing the rescaled Schoenfeld residuals. Conceptually, we are nonparametrically estimating the instantaneous hazard rate ratio $e^{\beta(t)}$, thus $VE_{S,\lambda}(t)$. Both methods provide a hypothesis test for the null $H_0 : \beta(t) = \beta$ for all t, ie, for no time-varying effects. The method using the Schoenfeld residuals is easy to use, provides an estimate of $e^{\beta(t)}$ on the natural scale,

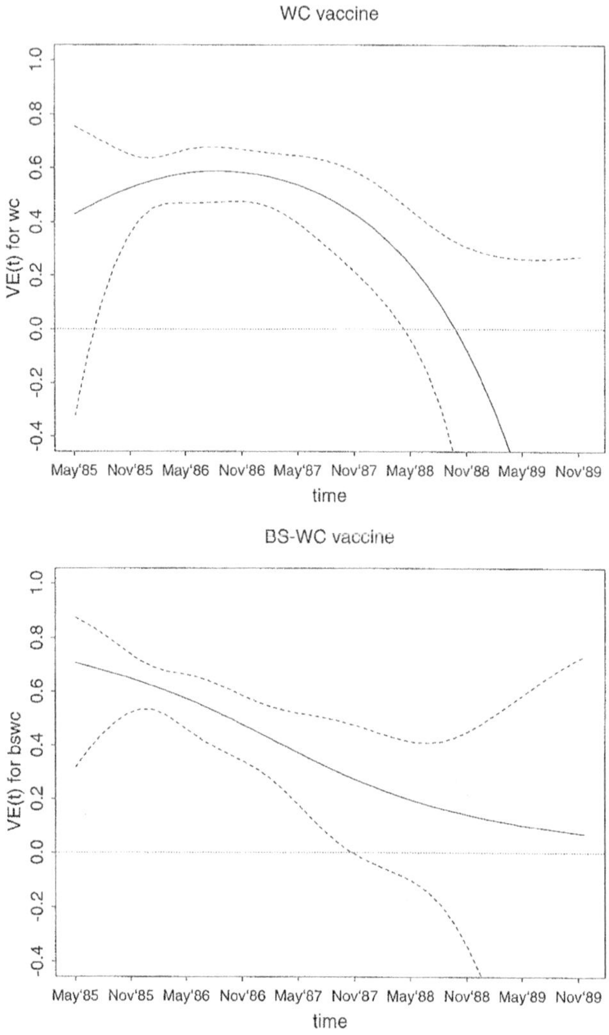

Fig. 7.5 Nonparametric smoothed plots of vaccine efficacy $\widehat{VE}_{S,\lambda}(t)$ versus time t, with 95% confidence intervals, for the killed whole cell (WC) and B subunit killed whole cell (BS-WC) vaccines, Matlab, Bangladesh, May 1, 1985, through November 31, 1989 (Durham et al 1998, Am J Epidemiol, 147:948–959. Reprinted with permission).

and allows easy incorporation of time-dependent covariates, so we recommend this approach in general.

Durham et al (1998) used the method involving Schoenfeld residuals to estimate smooth plots of the $\mathrm{VE}_{S,\lambda}(t)$ for the two oral cholera vaccines from the cholera vaccine trial described in Section 6.4.6. Figure 7.5 shows the plot of the $\mathrm{VE}_{S,\lambda}(t)$ estimates and the 95% CIs for the two vaccines. Table 7.4 gives the efficacy estimates

Table 7.4 Estimated vaccine efficacy over time, $VE_{S,\lambda}(t)$, with 95% confidence intervals for the the WC and BS-WC vaccines, Matlab, Bangladesh, May 1, 1985, through November 31, 1989 (Durham et al 1998)

Date	Day	Whole Cell Vaccine		BS Whole Cell Vaccine	
		VE(day)	95% CI	VE(day)	95% CI
May 1985	0	0.430	−0.342–0.758	0.713	0.320–0.879
November 1985	183	0.525	0.356–0.650	0.650	0.523 –0.743
May 1986	365	0.579	0.467–0.667	0.572	0.457–0.662
November 1986	548	0.583	0.478–0.667	0.476	0.344–0.582
May 1987	730	0.538	0.394–0.648	0.374	0.176–0.524
November 1987	913	0.433	0.220–0.588	0.280	0.006–0.478
May 1988	1095	0.245	−0.028–0.445	0.202	−0.089–0.416
November 1988	1278	−0.073	−0.664–0.308	0.141	−0.338–0.448
May 1989	1460	−0.590	−2.400–0.257	0.092	−0.955–0.578

and the approximate 95% confidence intervals for selected time points throughout the study. Age group (ages 2–5 years, >5 years) was included in the model as a covariate. The bending downward of the curves is indicative of waning. The *p*-values for the hypothesis test for departures from the proportional hazards assumption are 0.008 and 0.002 for the estimated model of the WC and BS-WC vaccines, respectively. The WC vaccine gives fairly constant and significant protection, with a $VE_{S,\lambda}(t)$ of about 0.50, for the first two and one-half years of the trial, but then protection appears to wane rapidly. After three years of the trial (May, 1988), the point estimate of the $VE_{S,\lambda}(t)$ is 0.245 and the 95% CI covers zero. Protection from the WC-BS vaccine starts out higher than that from WC vaccine, ie, 0.713 versus 0.430, but then gradually wanes at a fairly constant rate, about two to three percent per month. This analysis provides a more complete description of the $VE_S(t)$ than that based on yearly incidence ratios described above. Two further analyses studied the waning by age group and by biotype of the cases. The analysis was done using modifications of proportional hazards functions in available software. Details are in the appendix in Durham et al (1998).

The results of this method must be interpreted carefully. Smoothed values at the beginning and end of the observation period are uncertain, with large CIs. This typical effect of smoothing is exacerbated when the number of events decreases near the end of the observation period. For example, in the cholera vaccine trial, overall cholera incidence began to drop during the last year of the trial. Thus, the $VE_{S,\lambda}(t)$ estimates during the last year become unreliable. Nonetheless, a definite waning effect is apparent in Figure 7.5. This approach for estimating $VE_{S,\lambda}(t)$ provides a graphical interpretation of time-varying vaccine effects as well as a test for departure from the proportional hazards assumption.

Plots of $\ln(-\ln(S(t)))$ are frequently used to assess graphically whether the proportional hazards assumption holds for time-to-event data. Because these are cumulative hazard function plots, they can fail to give a clear picture of time-varying effects that occur later in the study after a substantial number of events have occurred (Figure 7.4). The estimated $\text{VE}_{S,\lambda}(t)$ (Figure 7.5) gives a clearer picture of the time-varying effects. If the proportional hazards assumption is valid, then these curves should be roughly straight lines, with zero slope rather than negative slope. In addition, the null hypothesis of a constant effect over time was rejected for both vaccines. This test, however, can be underpowered for small numbers of events.

7.3.3 Other approaches to estimate waning

Farrington (1992) reviewed some of the problems in estimating the occurrence and extent of waning vaccine protection. Kanaan and Farrington (2002) developed an approach to estimate vaccine efficacy in the presence of waning. The model is an extension of the all-or-none and leaky model in equation (7.12) to allow for waning. They also focus on observational data, allowing people to be vaccinated over time and also allowing for underreporting. First, assuming that the vaccine does not wane, they start from a version of the summary VE_S in equation (7.12),

$$\text{VE}_S = 1 - (1-\alpha)\theta, \tag{7.20}$$

where α is the proportion completely protected and θ is the leaky, or proportional hazards effect. Let a proportion π of the population be vaccinated, all at age τ. Then the model of waning for the all-or-none effect, assuming that $\theta = 1$, called a selection model, assumes that some people who were initially protected lose their protection. If the proportion initially protected when vaccinated is α_0, then one can model the proportion protected at time t after vaccination as

$$\alpha(t) = 1 - \alpha_0 \exp(-\alpha_1 t), \quad t \geq 0, \tag{7.21}$$

so that the age-specific vaccine efficacy at age x is

$$\text{VE}_S(x,\tau) = (1-\alpha_0)\exp(-\alpha_1(x-\tau)). \tag{7.22}$$

If $\alpha_1 = 0$, then the vaccine efficacy does not wane. In the deterioration model, the people who are initially completely protected are assumed to remain protected, but the leaky protection θ_0 in the initially partially protected people wanes with time. Under this model, age-specific vaccine efficacy is

$$\text{VE}_S(x,\tau) = 1 - (1-\alpha_0)\theta_0 \exp(-\theta_1(x-\tau)). \tag{7.23}$$

When $\theta_1 = 0$, the partial protection does not wane. The parameters α_0 and θ_0 represent the efficacy close to the age of vaccination τ. Kanaan and Farrington (2002) analyze two observational data sets of pertussis vaccination. The first is a cohort study of cases of pertussis in children born in 1970–1986 done by a general practitioner from 1977–1987 in children one to seven years old (Jenkinson 1988). The second was a case report study from the notifications of pertussis in the United

Kingdom in 1989–1990, divided into an epidemic and a nonepidemic period. The vaccine coverage for each age group was known (Ramsay et al 1993). The data for both studies are given in Kanaan and Farrington (2002).

Parametric survival analysis methods are used to estimate the parameters of interest. Calendar time effects are taken into account by allowing for epidemic and nonepidemic periods, E_k, and using a parametric approach to the baseline hazard. For the cohort data, the infection hazard is modeled both as an age-independent, time-dependent piecewise constant hazard $\lambda(a,t) = \rho_k, t \in E_k$, and as an age- and time-dependent gamma $\lambda(a,t) = \rho_k a \exp(-\beta a), t \in E_k$. For the case report data, the age and time effects are confounded, so the assumption is that $\rho_k = \rho$. Parameters are introduced that allow for complete ascertainment, equal and possibly incomplete ascertainment in the vaccinated and unvaccinated cases, incomplete ascertainment in the vaccinated cases only, and arbitrary differential ascertainment. The likelihood for the cohort model is an extension of equation (7.18) from Longini and Halloran (1996). The model for the case report data is an extension of the screening model (Section 8.1.4).

Not too surprisingly, with this number of parameters, estimating all of the parameters and choosing the model that fits best was somewhat difficult. It was not possible to differentiate between waning of the all-or-none protection or waning of partial protection, but there was strong evidence of waning in the cohort data. In the case report data, there was near-complete lack of identifiability of the vaccine efficacy because of the negative correlation between the proportion completely protected and the ascertainment proportions. The approach to modeling the waning is still valid, and could be used in future observational data sets where estimation of waning of vaccine efficacy was of interest.

7.4 Summary Strategy for Estimating Protective Effects

We present a general strategy for estimating $VE_{S,\lambda}(t)$ from time-to-event or incidence data (Halloran et al 1999). The first step is to conduct diagnostics. Then, with the help of the diagnostics, we find the best estimator of the VE_S. We begin by constructing log-minus-log plots of the Kaplan–Meier or actuarial estimates of the survival curves for the unvaccinated and vaccinated groups. These plots provide information about whether the vaccine effect is leaky, all-or-none, or a mixture. In addition, they provide some information about whether vaccine-induced protection is waning. If the curves are parallel, then the effect is mostly leaky (multiplicative), and we should model the vaccine effect with a proportional hazards model. Any divergence from parallelism indicates time-varying effects and the presence of some form of heterogeneity and/or waning protection. In this case, a model other than the proportional hazards model is needed. If the curves tend to diverge, then there is an all-or-none effect and if they tend to converge, then the model still may be leaky, but with an unmeasured random effect (heterogeneity). Convergence could also indicate waning protection. Although construction of log-minus-log plots is an important first diagnostic step, they are sometimes difficult to interpret. If there are a sufficient number of events, a more informative plot is a smoothed hazard ratio plot of $VE_{S,\lambda}(t) = 1 - \lambda_1(t)/\lambda_0(t)$ as described in Section 7.3.2. The possible patterns associated with different vaccine effects are shown in Figure 7.3. A line with zero slope indicates a purely leaky or multiplicative effect. The researcher can construct a formal hypothesis test for zero slope (Grambsch and Therneau 1994; Durham et al 1998).

If there is no evidence of time-varying effects from the diagnostics, then the $VE_{S,PH} = 1 - e^{\beta}$ can be estimated by fitting a proportional hazards model. If there is evidence of time-varying effects, then the investigator should fit the full family of frailty mixture models. If these models provide an adequate fit to the data, then the estimated parameters may be, but are not necessarily, the appropriate measures of the VE_S. Model selection methods can be used to choose among candidate models. If there is evidence of waning or other time-varying effects not attributable to unmeasured heterogeneity, then the nonparametric estimate of $VE_S(t)$ itself will provide the best estimate. In this case, it may be possible to construct a time-dependent parametric model of the $VE_S(t)$ that would provide tighter confidence intervals than the nonparametric approach.

7.4.1 Interpretation of measures

Which parameter to use to estimate VE_S in a particular study depends on the type and duration of the study, the infectious agent and its transmission mode, the resources available, and the assumptions of the distribution of protection within the vaccinated group. Even if time-dependent effects are detected, knowledge of the underlying biology will need to be used to interpret the effects and to help choose between actual waning, boosting, or heterogeneities. In many contemporary vaccine trials, immune response data are collected that can be used to help estimate and interpret vaccine effects. Also measuring actual or potential exposure to infection in individuals will help identify heterogeneities in exposure to infection. Some trials of vaccines for vector-borne diseases have entomological data. These help in quantifying potential exposure to infection.

Struchiner and Halloran (2007) show that randomization does not control for confounding in randomized vaccine trials, particularly when exposure to infection is an unmeasured confounder (Chapter 14). Differences in transmission intensity, previous exposure to infection, and pre-existing partial immunity and heterogeneities across communities result in different VE_S estimates, even when the actual biological action of the vaccine is the same conditional on these factors. Reviews of pertussis vaccine trials in different populations using different estimators consider some of these issues (Fine and Clarkson 1987; Fine et al 1988). Given the above discussion, there are clear limits on the interpretability and generalizability of estimates of VE_S.

Problems

7.1. (a) Show that under the leaky model (Smith et al 1984), $E(c) = N(1 - e^{-\lambda RT})$, $E(Y) = N(\int_0^T e^{-\lambda RT})dt = N(1 - e^{-\lambda RT})/\lambda R$.
(b) Show that under the all-or-none model, $E(c) = N(1 - e^{-\lambda RT})$, $E(Y) = N(\int_0^T [(1 - R) + Re^{-\lambda T}]dt) = N[T(1 - R) + R(1 - e^{-\lambda T})/\lambda]$.
(c) Derive the results in equations (7.1) to (7.4) from (a) and (b).

7.2. (a) Consider a cohort study with 2000 individuals each in the vaccinated and unvaccinated groups. Suppose that the hazard rate is 0.1/person/year in the unvaccinated group and that the protected efficacy VE*S* is 0.75. Under the leaky model $\text{VE}_S = 1 - \theta = 0.75$. Under the all-or-none model, $\text{VE}_S = \alpha = 0.75$. Compute the number of cases expected, the number at risk at the beginning of each year, and the person-years at risk each year, in the unvaccinated group for the first 8 years of follow-up.
(b) Compute the number of cases expected, the number at risk at the beginning of each year, and the person-years at risk during each year in the vaccinated group under the leaky model and then under the all-or-none model.
(c) Use the data so generated to compute $\text{VE}_{S,CI}(t)$ and $\text{VE}_{S,\lambda}(t)$ in each year for $t = 1,\ldots,8$ using the data generated under the two models. Discuss your results (Smith et al 1984, Tables A1 and A2).

7.3. What are the advantages of estimating waning vaccine effects in continuous time rather than estimating piecewise-constant vaccine efficacies?

7.4. Consider the summary vaccine efficacy measure $\text{VE}(0)_{S,SUM} = 1 - (1 - \alpha)\theta$ in (7.12). Would you prefer to learn about $\text{VE}(0)_{S,SUM}$ or the constituent values α and θ? What is the difference in the interpretations?

7.5. (a) Explain why the apparent efficacy would tend to increase if $\text{VE}_{S,\lambda}(t)$ were used to estimate efficacy with an all-or-none vaccine.
(b) How would you be able to distinguish such a situation from one in which the vaccine-induced protection were being boosted and enhanced by exposure to natural infection?

Chapter 8
Further Evaluation of Protective Effects

8.1 Case-Control Studies

Case-control studies can be used to estimate the relative risk measures in $VE_{S,CI}$ and $VE_{S,IR}$ ($VE_{S,\lambda}$). In a case-control study, cases of the disease are ascertained, and information on various covariates collected. A covariate of particular interest here is vaccination status. Then controls are selected in a manner discussed in more detail below, and the same covariates collected.

A case-control study can be thought of as a sample of data from a hypothetical cohort study. The cohort can also be thought of as a source population that gives rise to the cases. Ideally all cases from the underlying cohort or source population are ascertained. The controls are a sample of the underlying population drawn to give information about the distribution of vaccination and other covariates in the population. The ratio of the vaccinated cases (cases "exposed" to vaccine) to the unvaccinated cases (cases "unexposed" to vaccine) is divided by the ratio of vaccinated (exposed) controls to unvaccinated (unexposed) controls to give the exposure odds ratio (OR), or simply, odds ratio. A well-designed case-control study can provide good estimates of the relative risks of interest so that

$$VE_{S,CI,OR} = 1 - OR, \quad \text{or} \quad VE_{S,IR,OR} = 1 - OR. \tag{8.1}$$

In a case-control study, the number of individuals at risk for $VE_{S,CI}$ or the person-time at risk for $VE_{S,IR}$ ($VE_{S,\lambda}$) in the vaccinated and unvaccinated groups is not observed. Instead, the controls are used to estimate the distribution of vaccination in the population that is giving rise to the cases. Because controls are used to estimate the distribution of vaccination in the source population, controls should be chosen independent of their vaccination status.

In a seminal paper, Smith (1982) argued for the conduct of case-control studies to assess the effect on the incidence of tuberculosis of mass BCG campaigns that had been conducted in numerous countries in Asia and Africa beginning in the 1950s. Previous to that, case-control studies had not been widely used for evaluating vaccines. Case-control studies can be more feasible than the follow-up of large cohorts.

M.E. Halloran et al., *Design and Analysis of Vaccine Studies*, Statistics for Biology and Health, DOI 10.1007/978-0-387-68636-3_8,

Table 8.1 Number of cases and controls by vaccination status in a simple case-control study to evaluate a vaccine.

	Vaccinated	Unvaccinated	Total
Cases	c_1	c_0	c
Controls	d_1	d_0	d

They are less expensive than cohort studies. They can often be conducted in a relatively short period of time. Often a cohort study would be out of the question, so that case-control studies are the only feasible option. Orenstein et al (1988) argue that case-control studies allow large amounts of resources to be directed at a small number of cases and controls to assess vaccination status and history of disease most accurately, decreasing errors due to misclassification.

In a simple case-control study, suppose that c cases and d controls are ascertained, with c_1 vaccinated cases and c_0 unvaccinated cases, and d_1 vaccinated controls and d_0 unvaccinated controls. Then, vaccine efficacy estimated by the odds ratio is

$$\mathrm{VE}_{S,OR} = 1 - \text{exposure odds} = 1 - OR = 1 - \frac{c_1/c_0}{d_1/d_0} = 1 - \frac{c_1 d_0}{c_0 d_1}. \tag{8.2}$$

Under some circumstances the odds ratio will equal the cumulative incidence ratio or the incidence rate ratio, and $\mathrm{VE}_{S,OR}$ will equal either $\mathrm{VE}_{S,CI}$, $\mathrm{VE}_{S,IR}$, or $\mathrm{VE}_{S,\lambda}$.

Observational case-control studies suffer from the same potential biases that observational cohort studies do, and more. In particular, as in other observational studies, unmeasured confounders can bias the estimates of interest. Potential confounders that are measured can be adjusted for in the analyses. How similar estimates from a case-control study will be to estimates from a cohort study depends on the method of sampling the controls with respect to the cases and on the method of analysis. It is always important to be clear about what parameter one is estimating with an odds ratio and what the underlying assumptions are.

Practical aspects of case-control studies including how to define the source population for the cases, how to ascertain the cases, how to find the controls, and how to ascertain vaccination status or other covariates of the cases and controls will depend on the particular disease and population under study. Such issues are not covered here, but are discussed generally in Rothman et al (2008) and for vaccine studies in particular in Rodrigues and Smith (1999).

Here we focus on certain methodological considerations of sampling the controls. We begin with a discussion of estimating $\mathrm{VE}_{S,IR}$ ($\mathrm{VE}_{S,\lambda}$) from case-control studies. We then present the results of Smith et al (1984) about different sampling schemes for controls in a closed cohort when the vaccine has a leaky versus an all-or-none effect. None of the discussion up to that point requires the rare disease assumption. Finally, we present a commonly used approach to case-control studies that is a good approximation for the risk or rate ratio only if the proportion with the disease is relatively small.

8.1.1 Choosing controls to estimate $VE_{S,IR}$ ($VE_{S,\lambda}$)

Suppose that we are interested in conducting a case-control study to estimate $\mathrm{VE}_{S,IR} = \mathrm{VE}_{S,\lambda} = 1 - \theta$. The arguments also hold for $\mathrm{VE}_{S,PH}$. The goal of our case-control study is to estimate θ, the hazard ratio or incidence rate ratio. We assume that the vaccine efficacy does not wane with time and that the incidence rate ratio is constant, or equivalently, that the proportional hazards model holds.

The underlying cohort or source population can be a dynamic open cohort in which people can change their vaccination status over time. Controls should be chosen in a way that their probability of being chosen is proportional to the time they would contribute to the denominators of the incidence rate if a cohort study had been done. If θ is constant, the odds ratio yields a consistent and unbiased estimate of it under certain circumstances (Greenland and Thomas 1982). Three different odds ratios can be calculated, depending on the method of sampling person-time and the method of analysis. None of these odds ratios depends on the rare disease assumption to be a consistent estimator of a constant incidence rate ratio. Other assumptions, however, are important. Three key considerations are

1. Is the proportion vaccinated in the population changing over time?
2. Is the incidence rate ratio or hazard ratio constant?
3. Is the underlying incidence rate or hazard constant?

Risk set sampling, sometimes called matched density sampling, samples the relative distribution of person-time in the vaccinated and the unvaccinated groups matched on time by selecting controls from the population-at-risk at the time of onset of each case. The first odds ratio is the unmatched odds ratio based on risk set sampling, denoted ORU_{rs} and obtained using an unmatched analysis of the time-matched cases and controls. It is a consistent estimator of a constant incidence rate ratio if the proportion of the population at risk that is vaccinated is constant. The underlying incidence rate does not need to be constant. The second odds ratio, denoted ORM_{rs}, is also obtained using risk set sampling, but the time-matched controls are analyzed using a matched pair, or discordant pair, analysis. Risk set sampling with a time-matched analysis is equivalent to a failure time analysis if the incidence rate ratio is constant (Prentice and Breslow 1978). The matched odds ratio ORM_{rs} is a consistent estimator of a constant incidence rate ratio or hazard without further assumptions about the proportion vaccinated in the population or the baseline incidence.

In unmatched density sampling, controls are selected so that the expected ratio of the vaccinated controls to the unvaccinated controls equals the expected ratio of total person-time at risk in the vaccinated to the person-time at risk in the unvaccinated over the entire case ascertainment period. The third odds ratio, denoted ORU_{ds}, so obtained is a consistent estimator of a constant incidence rate ratio if either (1) the baseline incidence rate is constant or (2) the proportion of those at risk who are vaccinated is constant.

To show this, we follow the development in Greenland and Thomas (1982). Struchiner et al (1990) simulated case-control studies of malaria vaccines using the three different odds ratio estimators to estimate direct, indirect, and overall effects to illustrate the use of these methods under complex disease transmission patterns. Let $B_1(t)$ and $B_0(t)$ be the proportion vaccinated and unvaccinated in the underlying population at time t. Let the total number of people still at risk in the population at time t be $N(t)$. Then the numbers of vaccinated and unvaccinated people in the risk set at time t are $N_1(t) = N(t)B_1(t)$ and $N_0(t) = N(t)B_0(t)$. Let $\lambda(t)dt$ be the probability that an unvaccinated person still at risk becomes a case in small time interval dt, and $\theta\lambda(t)dt$ the corresponding probability in a vaccinated person. Then

$$\begin{aligned} N(t)B_1(t)\theta\lambda(t)dt &= \text{expected number of vaccinated cases in } dt, \\ N(t)B_0(t)\lambda(t)dt &= \text{expected number of unvaccinated cases in } dt, \end{aligned}$$

and $B_1(t)$ and $B_0(t)$ are the probabilities of choosing a vaccinated and unvaccinated control from the risk set at time t.

The expected number of discordant pairs of vaccinated cases and unvaccinated controls $m_{10}(t)$ and unvaccinated cases and vaccinated controls $m_{01}(t)$ in time interval dt are

$$\begin{aligned} m_{10}(t)dt &= [N(t)B_1(t)\theta\lambda(t)dt]B_0(t), \\ m_{01}(t)dt &= [N(t)B_0(t)\lambda(t)dt]B_1(t). \end{aligned} \tag{8.3}$$

Then

$$\begin{aligned} ORM_{rs} &= \frac{\text{discordant pairs (vaccinated case–unvaccinated control)}}{\text{discordant pairs (unvaccinated case–vaccinated control)}} \\ &= \frac{\int m_{10}(t)dt}{\int m_{01}(t)dt} \\ &= \frac{\int [N(t)B_1(t)\theta\lambda(t)dt]B_0(t)dt}{\int [N(t)B_0(t)\lambda(t)dt]B_1(t)dt} = \theta. \end{aligned} \tag{8.4}$$

Thus, $\mathrm{VE}_{S,IR} = \mathrm{VE}_{S,\lambda} = 1 - \mathrm{ORM}_{rs} = 1 - \theta$. This is similar to the discussion of Smith et al (1984) (Section 8.1.2) except that here it is shown that the baseline incidence or hazard can vary with time.

If the proportion in the risk set that was vaccinated were constant, it would not be necessary to do a matched analysis. In this case $B_1(t) = B_1$ and $B_0(t) = B_0$. Then

$$\begin{aligned} a_1(t)dt &= N(t)B_1\theta\lambda(t)dt = \text{expected number of vaccinated cases in } dt, \\ a_0(t)dt &= N(t)B_0\lambda(t)dt = \text{expected number of unvaccinated cases in } dt, \\ b_1(t)dt &= [a_1(t)dt + a_0(t)dt]B_1dt = \text{expected number of vaccinated controls in } dt, \\ b_0(t)dt &= [a_1(t)dt + a_0(t)dt]B_0dt = \text{expected number of unvaccinated controls in } dt. \end{aligned}$$

The odds ratio ORU_M not using a discordant pair analysis is

$$
\begin{aligned}
ORU_{rs} &= \frac{\text{no. vaccinated cases/no. vaccinated controls}}{\text{no. unvaccinated cases/no. unvaccinated controls}} \\
&= \frac{\int a_1(t)dt \int b_0(t)dt}{\int a_0(t)dt \int b_1(t)dt} \\
&= \frac{\int [N(t)B_1\theta\lambda(t)dt] \int [a_1(t)dt + a_0(t)dt]B_0 dt}{\int [N(t)B_0\lambda(t)dt] \int [a_1(t)dt + a_0(t)dt]B_1 dt} = \theta.
\end{aligned} \tag{8.5}
$$

The proportion vaccinated in the risk set will not be constant in a closed cohort if the vaccine protects against disease because there will be enrichment with time of vaccinated in the risk set. Thus, the matched analysis as in (8.4) would be necessary in a closed cohort.

If we believed that either the incidence rate or the proportion of the population that were vaccinated were constant, then we could use the third odds ratio ORU_{ds}.

$$
\begin{aligned}
ORU_{ds} &= \frac{\text{exposure odds in cases}}{\text{exposure odds in controls}} \\
&= \frac{\theta \int \lambda(t)B_1(t)N(t)dt / [\int \lambda(t)B_0(t)N(t)dt]}{\int B_1(t)N(t)dt / [\int B_0(t)N(t)dt]}.
\end{aligned} \tag{8.6}
$$

In general, expression (8.6) will not equal θ unless either $\lambda(t)$ or $B_1(t)$ (and $B_0(t)$) is constant. However, if the analysis is stratified finely on time, then it would be possible to estimate θ from the unmatched sampling design.

8.1.2 Choosing controls with leaky and all-or-none models

Now we return to consider case-control studies in a closed cohort where vaccination has a leaky or multiplicative effect on the hazard or an all-or-none effect. Smith et al (1984) consider designing a case-control study in a closed cohort in which all cases of disease are ascertained and the time of onset of each case is known. They assume that the study is randomized and that individuals are followed for an equal period of time. The hazard λ is assumed constant, but the argument holds for nonconstant hazard as well. Smith et al (1984) suggest that under a leaky model, controls should be chosen at the same time that cases occur from those individuals who had not yet developed the disease. This approach is the same as the risk set sampling in the previous section. Under risk set sampling, the controls can later become cases, and people can appear both in the case and control groups, but at different time points. In the closed cohort, the time-matched analysis is required. This approach gives a good estimate of the time-invariant $\mathrm{VE}_{S,IR} = \mathrm{VE}_{S,\lambda} = \theta$. This is the standard approach for sampling controls for a time-matched proportional hazards model. (Greenland and Thomas 1982; Prentice and Breslow 1978).

Smith et al (1984) point out that this approach would not give a good estimate of the proportion protected if the all-or-none model were in effect. Then one would want to estimate $\mathrm{VE}_{CI} = \alpha$, the proportion completely protected based on the rela-

Table 8.2 Vaccine efficacy under leaky and all-or-none models of vaccine action as measured in case-control studies. f_1: sampling fraction for cases; f_2: sampling fraction for controls; VE_k: vaccine efficacy calculated with "not yet cases" as controls; VE_r: vaccine efficacy calculated with "total population" as controls (Smith et al1984)

		Cases	Not Yet Cases	VE_k	Total Population	VE_r
Leaky model						
Year 3	Vaccinated	44 f_1	905 f_2	0.73	1000 f_2	0.64
	Unvaccinated	121 f_1	670 f_2		1000 f_2	
Year 6	Vaccinated	38 f_1	779 f_2	0.73	1000 f_2	0.43
	Unvaccinated	67 f_1	368 f_2		1000 f_2	
All-or-none model						
Year 3	Vaccinated	31 f_1	918 f_2	0.81	1000 f_2	0.74
	Unvaccinated	121 f_1	670 f_2		1000 f_2	
Year 6	Vaccinated	17 f_1	842 f_2	0.89	1000 f_2	0.75
	Unvaccinated	67 f_1	368 f_2		1000 f_2	

tive cumulative incidence or attack rates in the vaccinated and unvaccinated groups. Under the all-or-none model, the appropriate method of selecting controls would be to choose the controls for each case from among other individuals in the population whether or not they had already had the disease under study. Under the all-or-none model, the controls are used to estimate the proportion of the total population that had been vaccinated or unvaccinated, B_1 and B_0.

Table 8.2 has an illustrative example from Smith et al (1984). The results were generated assuming that the hazard of infection was 0.2 per person per year in the unvaccinated group. The vaccine efficacy was set to 75%, so $\theta = 0.25$ in the leaky model and $\alpha = 0.25$ in the all-or-none model. Under the leaky model, the hazard in the vaccinated group is 0.05 per person per year. Assume that the vaccinated and unvaccinated group each have 1000 persons and that the allocation is randomized. The results shown assume the controls were selected from among those who had not developed the disease at the start of the time interval under consideration. Greenland and Frerichs (1988) commented on a number of issues raised by Smith et al (1984).

8.1.3 Choosing controls from the nondiseased population

Case-control studies used to be commonly designed to choose controls only from the population that remained free of the disease of interest. Rothman et al (2008) call this design the cumulative or epidemic case-control design because it might be used to look for etiological factors after an outbreak. In this type of study, the rare disease assumption is needed if the odds ratio is assumed to be a close estimator for the relative risk of interest. A retrospective case-control study that only samples controls from the nondiseased population will yield a decent approximation of the incidence rate ratio only if less than about 20% of both the vaccinated and the unvaccinated groups have the disease and the proportion vaccinated does not change radically over the course of the outbreak.

8.1.4 Estimating VE_S using the screening method

Another approach related to a case-control approach is the screening method (Orenstein et al 1985). This approach expresses vaccine efficacy as a function of the proportion of the cases that are vaccinated and the proportion of the population that is vaccinated. If any two of the variables are known, the other can be estimated. Let PCV be the proportion of cases that are vaccinated and PPV be the proportion of the population that is vaccinated. Then vaccine efficacy can be estimated using the screening method by the following relation,

$$\mathrm{VE}_S = 1 - \frac{PCV(1-PPV)}{(1-PCV)PPV}. \tag{8.7}$$

Farrington (1993) discusses the screening method and its relation to case-control studies. An estimate of vaccine coverage in the population provides an estimate of the proportion vaccinated. Not all cases need to be ascertained, but the cases ascertained should be a random sample. Bias and precision of the method are considered. A method for computing a confidence interval allowing for extra variability and a method to determine sample size are provided. The screening method offers a simple, rapid, and inexpensive surveillance tool to get approximate estimates of vaccine effectiveness. It is called a screening method because it can be used to suggest when more accurate evaluation of a vaccine in the field might be needed.

8.2 Validation Sets for Outcomes

In vaccine field studies, often a nonspecific case definition rather than a more specific confirmatory diagnosis is used as the outcome. As seen in Chapter 6, estimates of VE_S will be lower when based on less specific case definitions, particularly when the diagnosis of the disease of interest is not biologically confirmed. Sometimes it would be prohibitively expensive or invasive to confirm each suspected case in a study biologically. However, if biological confirmation can be done in a small random sample of the suspected cases, this information can be used to estimate the expected number of cases of the true disease of interest among the suspected cases. The added uncertainty from not confirming all of the cases is taken into account with the statistical method, leading to a larger variance and wider confidence interval than would be obtained if all suspected cases were biologically confirmed.

In essence, this is a particular case of a missing data problem. The outcome of interest may be measured on some of the study participants in a subset called a validation sample, and the less specific outcome is measured on all participants. Then the result of the biological outcome is missing in those nonspecific cases that were not tested. Statistical missing data methods are available to use the outcomes of interest in the validation sample to correct the low estimates of VE_S based on the nonspecific case definition alone. Validation sets for exposure to infection can also improve joint estimation of VE_S and VE_I (Golm et al 1998, 1999). In the next sections, the use of validation sets and the improvements in estimation they can provide is illustrated by the analysis of an observational study of trivalent, live attenuated influenza vaccine in Central Texas.

8.2.1 Influenza vaccine field study in central Texas

A field study of trivalent, live attenuated, influenza virus vaccine (LAIV-T) was conducted in Temple-Belton, Texas, and surrounding areas during the 2000–2001 influenza season. The field study was part of a larger community-based, non-randomized, open-label field study conducted from 1998–2001 in Temple-Belton, Texas, as well as two other communities to evaluate the indirect effectiveness of LAIV-T vaccination of healthy children (Gaglani et al 2004; Piedra et al 2005, 2007). Temple-Belton was the intervention community. At that time, the Temple-Belton area had approximately 19,700 children from 18 months through 18 years of age. In Temple-Belton, eligible healthy children and adolescents aged 18 months through 18 years were offered LAIV-T vaccine through the Scott & White (S & W) Clinics from 1998–2001.

Halloran et al (2003a) evaluated the protection of LAIV-T against influenza during the influenza season of 2000–2001. They used surveillance cultures taken from a sample of the study participants to obtain more accurate estimates of protective efficacy against influenza than those obtained using the nonspecfic, clinical case definition. The analysis using validation set methods includes children who were S & W Health Plan (SWHP) members, and is concerned with the LAIV-T vaccinations administered in the influenza season 2000–01. Children received a single dose of LAIV-T each year they enrolled.

The primary clinical outcome was a non-specific case definition called medically attended acute respiratory infection (MAARI), which included all ICD-9-CM diagnoses codes (Codes 381–383, 460–487) for upper and lower respiratory tract infections, otitis media, and sinusitis. Any individual presenting with history of fever and any respiratory illness at S & W Clinics was eligible to have a throat swab (or nasal wash in young infants) for influenza virus culture. The decision to obtain specimens was made irrespective of whether a patient had received LAIV-T. The specific case definition is culture-confirmed influenza. Table 8.3 contains the number of children, the number of MAARIs, the number of cultures done, and the number of cultures positive for each group. The overall fraction of MAARI cases sampled was a little

Table 8.3 Study data for influenza epidemic season 2000–2001 (Halloran et al 2003a)

Age (Years)	Vaccine Status	Children	MAARI Cases	MAARI Proportion	MAARI Cases Cultured	Number Positive Cultures	Fraction Cultures Positive	Fraction Cultured
1.5-4	LAIV-T	537	389	0.72	16	0	0	0.041
	None	1844	1665	0.90	86	24	0.28	0.052
5-9	LAIV-T	807	316	0.39	17	2	0.12	0.054
	None	2232	1156	0.52	118	53	0.45	0.102
10-18	LAIV-T	937	219	0.23	19	3	0.16	0.087
	None	5249	1421	0.27	123	56	0.46	0.087
Total	LAIV-T	2281	924	0.41	52	5	0.10	0.056
	None	9325	4242	0.45	327	133	0.41	0.077

higher in the unvaccinated than in the vaccinated groups ($p = 0.03$). As expected, the proportion of cultures that were positive was consistently higher in the unvaccinated than in the vaccinated groups.

The risk of developing MAARI was compared in the children receiving LAIV-T with those children who had never received LAIV-T. The protective effectiveness of LAIV-T against MAARI was estimated as $VE_{S,CI,a} = 1 - RR$, where RR is the relative risk of MAARI in vaccinated children compared to unvaccinated children. The "a" stands for auxiliary outcome. Age-adjusted estimates were obtained using sample size weighted averages. Confidence intervals were based on the assumption of a normal approximation of the logarithm of the ratio of two independent binomial random variables (Katz 1978).

8.2.2 Analysis using surveillance samples

Estimates of the protective efficacy of LAIV-T against influenza using the surveillance samples, $VE_{S,CI,v}$, were obtained using the mean score method for auxiliary outcomes (Pepe et al 1994), an estimating equations approach for handling missing data. The "v" stands for validation sample. The method estimates the score contribution for main study members with only auxiliary outcome data from the mean of the score contributions of a sample of study subjects with the same observed covariate and auxiliary outcome values on whom the specific outcome has been measured. In this analysis, the clinical outcome MAARI was the nonspecific auxiliary outcome, and the actual influenza status was the specific outcome of interest. The confidence intervals take into account the uncertainty due to culturing only a sample of the MAARI cases.

The variable Y = outcome of interest (influenza status), A = auxiliary outcome (MAARI, yes or no), X = set of covariates (vaccination, age group), $P_\beta(Y|X)$ = binomial probability model, β = parameters to estimate in the probability model, S_β = score function, and $V, \overline{V}$ = in the validation set or not. The estimating equation

Table 8.4 Epidemic year 2000–2001: Vaccine effectiveness ($VE_{S,CI,a}$) against MAARI and efficacy ($VE_{S,CI,v}$) against combined influenza A (H1N1) and B taking missing influenza status into account (Halloran et al 2003a)

Age (Years)	$VE_{S,CI,a}$ MAARI	(95% CI)	$VE_{S,CI,v}$ Influenza	(95% CI)
1.5-4	0.20	(0.14,0.25)	0.91	(−0.34,0.99)
5-9	0.25	(0.15,0.34)	0.80	(0.26,0.95)
10-18	0.14	(0.01,0.26)	0.70	(0.13,0.90)
Total	0.18	(0.11,0.24)	0.79	(0.51,0.91)

is

$$\sum_{i \in V} S_\beta(Y_i|X_i) + \sum_{j \in \overline{V}} \hat{E}\{S_\beta(Y|X_j)|A_j, X_j\} = 0.$$

An unbiased estimator for a person who had no culture done is:

$$\hat{E}\{S_\beta(Y|X_j)|A_j, X_j\} = \sum_{i \in V(A_j, X_j)} S_\beta(Y_i|X_i)/n^V(A_j, X_j).$$

The variance was estimated on the adjusted log relative risk using the mean score and multivariate delta methods (Pepe et al 1994; Agresti 1990; Chu and Halloran 2004).

The analysis assumed that all children with negative MAARI were also negative for influenza disease. The mean score method produces valid estimates if the data are missing at random (MAR) (Pepe et al 1994) in the sense of Little and Rubin (2002). A continuity correction of 0.5 was added to the number of cultured samples and the number positive in the age group 1.5–4 years because there were no positive cultures in the vaccinated group.

The protective efficacy estimates against influenza taking missing influenza status into account are much higher than the estimates of the protective effects of LAIV-T against MAARI (Table 8.4). The overall vaccine effectiveness estimate based on the nonspecific case definition was 0.18 (95% CI, 0.11–0.24). The overall efficacy estimates incorporating the surveillance cultures using the mean score method was 0.79 (95% CI, 0.51–0.91), a fourfold increase in estimates, much closer to the efficacy estimate of 0.93 (95% CI, 0.88–0.97) obtained in a double-blind randomized controlled trial (Belshe et al 1998, Section 6.4.3). Although the point estimates are higher, the confidence intervals are wider due to the uncertainty resulting from not culturing all of the MAARI cases.

Table 8.4 contains the overall estimate obtained by pooling the data and avoiding the continuity correction. The age-adjusted $VE_{S,CI,v}$ obtained using sample size weighted averages, the continuity correction in the youngest age group, and the delta method for the variance estimate was $VE_{S,CI,v} = 0.77$ (95% CI, 0.48–0.90), similar to that in Table 8.4.

In this study, selection of children with MAARI for influenza cultures was not done randomly. Physicians might tend to choose MAARI cases that they believe to be influenza for culturing. If influenza disease is more moderate in the vaccinated group, then oversampling in the unvaccinated group might occur based on the influenza status, which is not measured on everybody. In this case, the MAR assumption is violated and the estimate assuming MAR could be biased.

If physicians know the vaccination status, they might oversample either the unvaccinated or the vaccinated children. They might tend to believe that vaccinated children would not have influenza, and therefore oversample the unvaccinated children. However, oversampling due to knowledge of the vaccination status alone would not bias the estimate, because the estimation procedure stratifies on the vaccination status of the child. The data are missing at random in this case (Little and Rubin 2002). In fact, in future studies, it would be desirable to oversample the vaccinated, non-specific cases for culturing. Oversampling in the vaccinated group would help avoid having zero positive cultures in the vaccinated groups.

The consistently higher proportion of cultures being positive in the unvaccinated groups could be partly due to vaccinated cases of influenza being less likely to be culture positive than unvaccinated cases. However, this would produce exactly the same bias that would be obtained if all of the MAARI cases had been cultured as in many randomized, double-blinded vaccine trials.

Future vaccine field studies that utilize validation samples could be intentionally designed so that the specific outcome would be missing at random within any given observed stratum of the study subjects. The sample size needed in the validation sample to correct the bias from using the nonspecific outcome is not necessarily large. In this case the overall sampling fraction was well below 10%.

8.3 Sensitivity Analysis for Selection Bias

The analysis in Section 8.2 relies on the nonidentifiable assumption that the outcome of interest is missing at random (MAR) (Little and Rubin 2002). If the outcome is not MAR, the vaccine efficacy estimates could be subject to selection bias. Rotnitzky et al (1998, 2001), Scharfstein et al (1999), and Robins et al (2000b) developed a frequentist selection model that displays the sensitivity analysis over a plausible range of selection parameters. Scharfstein et al (2003) developed a Bayesian approach that allows the formal incorporation of prior beliefs about the degree of the selection bias on the odds ratio scale to obtain the full posterior distribution, a single summary of the sensitivity analysis. Scharfstein et al (2006) extended this work to the relative risk parametrization of selection bias, discrete covariates, and dependence of the priors for the relative risk parameters across treatment groups. They reanalyzed the data from the Texas influenza study (Section 8.2.1) with the methods. They relied on an influenza expert to provide informative priors for the Bayesian analysis.

8.3.1 Sensitivity analysis in the vaccine study

In the vaccine field study, let n be the total number of participants, and n_0 and n_1 the number of unvaccinated and vaccinated participants. Let Z denote the vaccination indicator, taking on the value 1 if a participant is vaccinated and 0 if not vaccinated. Let $A(0)$ and $A(1)$ denote the indicator of MAARI (1: yes; 0: no), for a participant if she had been, possibly contrary to fact, unvaccinated or vaccinated, respectively. The observed MAARI outcome $A = A(Z)$ is observed for every participant. Let $Y(0)$ and $Y(1)$ denote influenza status (1: positive; 0: negative) for a participant if she had been, possibly contrary to fact, unvaccinated and vaccinated, respectively. Only one of these outcomes can be potentially observed. In this study, influenza status is biologically confirmed by a culture. In the validation substudy, a possibly nonrandom sample of the participants is biologically confirmed, so that influenza status, $Y = Y(Z)$ is known for a subset of the participants. Let R be the validation indicator, where $R = 1$ if sampled for validation and $R = 0$, otherwise. Sampling for validation only occurs for those with $A = 1$. Let X denote age category (0: 1.5–4 years; 1: 5–9 years; 2: 10–18 years) measured at the time of study entry.

The observed data for an individual are $O = (Z,X,A,R,Y : A = R = 1)$. We assume we observe n i.i.d. copies, $\mathcal{O} = \{O_i : i = 1,\ldots,n\}$. Throughout, probabilities P, indexed by subgroup subscripts indicate restriction to the associated subpopulation. For example, for events A and B, $P_{z,x}[A] = P[A|Z = z, Z = x]$ and $P_{z,x}[A|B] = P[A|B, Z = z, X = x]$.

8.3.1.1 Vaccine Efficacy

The scientific goal is to use the observed data to estimate the causal effect of vaccination on the outcome Y, within age levels as well as overall. Specifically, the goal is to estimate age-specific vaccine efficacy

$$VE_{S,CI,x} = 1 - \frac{P_x[Y(1) = 1]}{P_x[Y(0) = 1]} \tag{8.8}$$

and overall vaccine efficacy

$$VE_{S,CI} = 1 - \frac{\sum_{x=0}^{2} P_x[Y(1) = 1]P[X = x]}{\sum_{x=0}^{2} P_x[Y(0) = 1]P[X = x]}. \tag{8.9}$$

To identify $VE_{S,CI,x}$, it is sufficient to identify $P_x[Y(z) = 1]$ for $z = 0,1$. For $VE_{S,CI}$, we must identify $P_x[Y(z) = 1]$ for all z and x, and the marginal distribution of X. Although the marginal distribution is identified from the observed data without additional assumptions, the conditional probabilites $P_x[Y(z) = 1]$ will require nonidentifiable assumptions.

Two structural assumptions facilitate identification of $P_x[Y(z) = 1]$. The first assumption is that vaccination status is independent of the potential outcomes

$\{A(0), A(1), Y(0), Y(1)\}$, given age ($X$). Although the Texas influenza study was not randomized, the expert had no information to conclude that one group differed substantially from another. The second assumption is that if a participant, under vaccination status z, does not have MAARI, then she does not have medically attended influenza. The interest is in efficacy against medically attended, culture-confirmed influenza, not influenza infection.

8.3.1.2 Identification of $P_x[Y(z) = 1]$

With these assumptions, we can write

$$P_x[Y(z) = 1] = P_{z,x}[Y(z) = 1] = P_{z,x}[Y = 1]$$
$$= \sum_{r=0}^{1} P_{z,x}[Y = 1|A = 1, R = r] P_{z,x}[A = 1, R = r]. \qquad (8.10)$$

For all z, x, r, $P_{z,x}[Y = 1|A = 1, R = 1]$ and $P_{z,x}[A = 1, R = r]$, are identifiable but $P_{z,x}[Y = 1|A = 1, R = 0]$ are not. Thus, identification of $P_x[Y(z) = 1]$ will require identification of these latter probabilities.

The most common assumption used to identify these probabilities is that of missing at random (MAR) (Little and Rubin 2002). MAR states that R is independent of Y given (Z, A, X). This implies that, for all z, x, $P_{z,x}[Y = 1|A = 1, R = 0] = P_{z,x}[Y = 1|A = 1, R = 1]$. As a result, $P_x[Y(z) = 1]$ becomes identifiable. Because the assumption of MAR is untestable and was considered questionable by the scientific expert, it is useful to perform a sensitivity analysis to outcomes that are missing not at random (MNAR).

8.3.2 Frequentist sensitivity analysis

Scharfstein et al (1999, 2003) and Robins et al (2000b) introduced a sensitivity analysis methodology in which the estimands of interest are presented over a range of posited models (including MAR), each yielding identification of $P_{z,x}[Y = 1|A = 1, R = 0]$. Scharfstein et al (2006) developed a selection model approach to sensitivity analysis. In the selection model, for subjects with $Z = z, X = x$ and MAARI, the selection bias parameter $\alpha_{z,x}$ is interpreted as the log odds ratio of being unvalidated for diseased versus undiseased subjects. So, $\alpha_{z,x}$ positive or negative indicates that diseased subjects have lower or higher odds of being validated, respectively.

When eliciting plausible ranges for $\alpha_{z,x}$, the expert found it easier to think about selection bias on a relative risk as opposed to an odds ratio scale. Specifically, he felt more comfortable expressing opinions about the relative risk of being validated given that a MAARI participant has influenza compared with the MAARI participant having another influenza-like illness. As a result, the selection models were reformulated in terms of the relative risk selection bias parameters

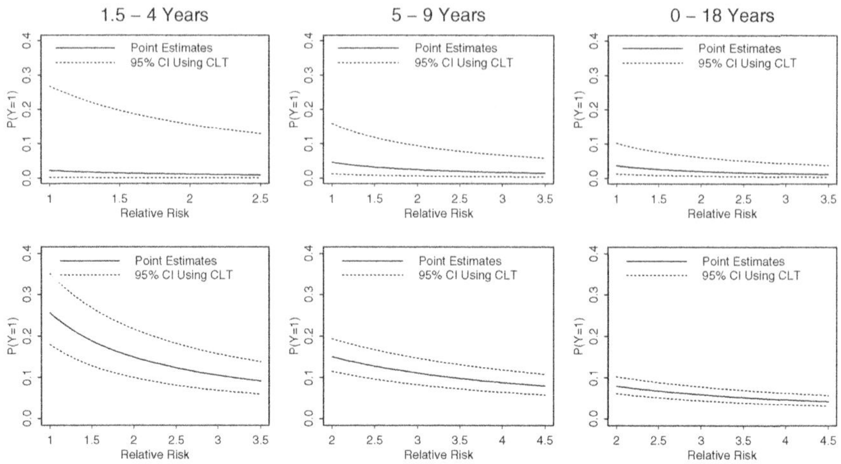

Fig. 8.1 Frequentist sensitivity analysis of $P_{z,x}[Y=1]$. Shown are the estimated probabilities and 95% confidence intervals for influenza in the vaccinated and unvaccinated groups, for each age stratum, as a function of the relative risk selection bias parameter $\beta_{z,x}$, varied over the 90% ranges elicited from the expert (Scharfstein et al 2006, , Biostatistics 7:615–629, reprinted with permission).

$$\beta_{z,x} = \frac{P_{z,x}[R=1|A=1,Y=1]}{P_{z,x}[R=1|A=1,Y=0]}. \tag{8.11}$$

Then specification of $\beta_{z,x}$ leads to identification of $P_x[Y(z)=1]$ via the following formula,

$$P_x[Y(z)=1] = \frac{P_{z,x}[Y=1|A=1,R=1]P_{z,x}[A=1]}{\beta_{z,x}P_{z,x}[Y=0|A=1,R=1]+P_{z,x}[Y=1|A=1,R=1]}$$
$$= \frac{P[Z=z,X=x,A=1,R=1,Y=1]P[Z=z,X=x,A=1]/P[Z=z,X=x]}{\beta_{z,x}P[Z=z,X=x,A=1,R=1,Y=0]+P[Z=z,X=x,A=1,R=1,Y=1]}. \tag{8.12}$$

The frequentist nonparametric estimator of $P_x[Y(z)=1]$ can be found by replacing the probabilities P in (8.12) by their empiricals $\tilde{P}$. Plugging the estimates $\widehat{P}_x[Y(z)=1]$ into equations (8.8) and (8.9) yields the estimates $\widehat{VE}_{S,CI,x}$ and $\widehat{VE}_{S,CI}$. The right-hand side of estimated equation (8.12) reduces to the results with the mean score method when $\beta_{z,x}=1$, for all z and x. Supplementary material for Scharfstein et al (2006) give the derivation of the large sample-based confidence intervals for $VE_{S,CI,x}$ and $VE_{S,CI}$. The frequentist sensitivity analysis proceeds by varying the $\beta_{z,x}$ over plausible ranges.

Figure 8.1 shows the estimated probabilities and 95% confidence intervals for influenza in the vaccinated and unvaccinated groups, for each age stratum, as a function of $\beta_{z,x}$. Figure 8.2 shows the point estimates and lower 95% confidence bounds

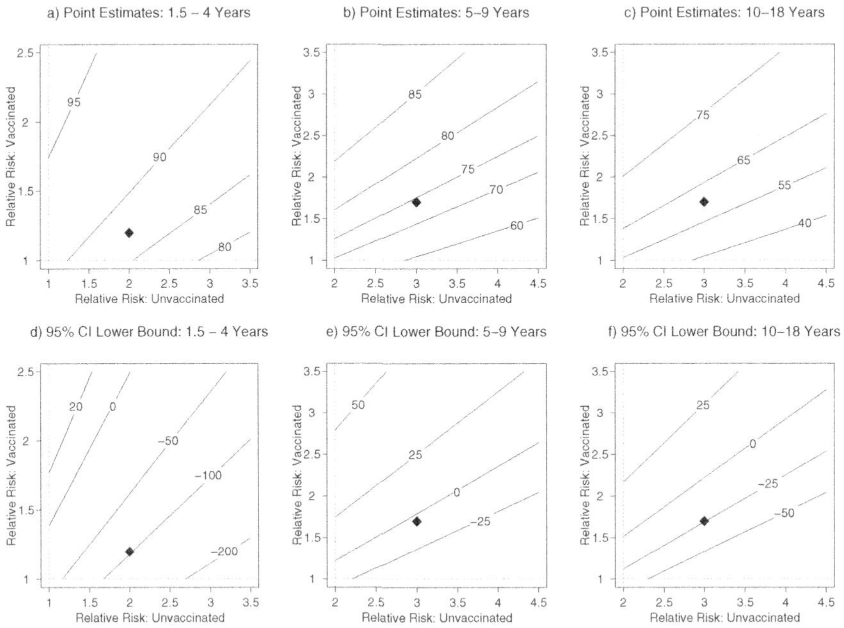

Fig. 8.2 Frequentist sensitivity analysis of point estimates and lower 95% confidence bounds for the age-group-specific vaccine efficacy as a function of the relative risk selection bias parameters $\beta_{1,x}$ (vaccinated) and $\beta_{0,x}$ (unvaccinated) varied over the 90% ranges elicited from the expert. Black diamonds indicate the results at the best guess of the expert. Black lines with numbers indicate the contours (Scharfstein et al 2006, Biostatistics 7:615–629, reprinted with permission).

for the age-group-specific efficacy. The selection bias parameters were varied over the 90% ranges elicited from the expert. Within these ranges and within each age group, the vaccine efficacy estimates based on the validation sets are higher than the point estimates based on the nonspecific definition, which were 0.2, 0.25, and 0.14 for the age groups 1.5–4, 5–9, and 10–18 years, respectively. The lower confidence bounds indicate the degree of variability. A key drawback of the frequentist sensitivity analysis methodology is that it is not feasible to present parsimoniously the overall results. This is a motivation for the Bayesian sensitivity analysis.

8.3.3 *Bayesian inference*

In the Bayesian analysis, we can specify prior distributions on the relative risk selection bias parameters $\beta_z = (\beta_{z,0}, \beta_{z,1}, \beta_{z,2})'$, $\beta = (\beta_0', \beta_1')$. Models for $\text{VE}_{S,CI,x}$ and $\text{VE}_{S,CI}$ are developed analogously to (8.8) and (8.9), whereby prior distributions are required for all model parameters.

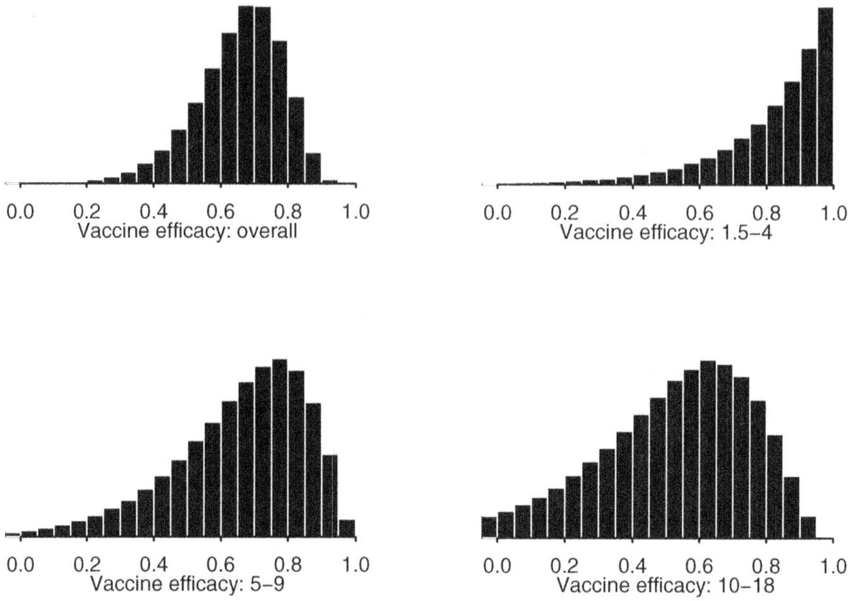

Fig. 8.3 Posterior distributions of the overall vaccine efficacy and by age group using the informative prior distributions (Scharfstein et al 2006, , Biostatistics 7:615–629, reprinted with permission).

In the prior specification for β, Scharfstein et al (2006) provided two options: (1) Bayesian analogue of the frequentist sensitivity analysis and (2) fully Bayesian analysis. For option (1), point-mass priors were specified on β and the posterior distributions of the estimands of interest were estimated over a range of β. This approach is comparable to the frequentist sensitivity analysis described above, but does not rely on large sample approximations. For option (2), a nondegenerate prior distribution on β was specified as elicited from a subject-matter expert. This approach has the advantage of providing a single summary of the posterior inference about the estimands, which naturally incorporates the uncertainty due to selection bias. Details are in Scharfstein et al (2006). To sample from the posterior, they constructed a Gibbs sampling algorithm with data augmentation (Tanner and Wong 1987) and slice sampling (Damien et al 1999).

8.3.3.1 Informative priors

For Bayesian inference, informative priors are specified for the selection bias relative risk parameters, β, by age group and vaccination status. An influenza expert was asked the following question: *If a physician were doing surveillance cultures during an influenza season, what is the probability that he would select the chil-*

Table 8.5 Best guess and 90% range for the informative prior distributions on the selection bias parameter β and log β (Scharfstein et al 2006)

Age Group (Years)		β (Relative Risk) Scale				Log β Scale			
		Unvaccinated		Vaccinated		Unvaccinated		Vaccinated	
		Best Guess	90% Range	Best Guess	90% Range	Best Guess	90% Range	Best Guess	90% Range
1.5–4	Elicited	2.00	1.00, 3.50	1.20	1.00, 2.50	0.69	0.00, 1.25	0.18	0.00, 0.92
	Used	2.00	1.00, 4.00	1.20	0.58, 2.50	0.69	0.00, 1.39	0.18	−0.55, 0.92
5–18	Elicited	3.00	2.00, 4.50	1.60	1.00, 3.50	1.10	0.69, 1.50	0.47	0.00, 1.25
	Used	3.00	2.00, 4.50	1.70	1.00, 2.89	1.10	0.69, 1.50	0.53	0.00, 1.06

dren who actually had true influenza over the children who just had nonspecific respiratory symptoms to culture? He responded that this was very hard to answer. One "would be more likely to be correct in the unvaccinated," because unvaccinated children presenting with true influenza would have more typical, severe disease than the vaccinated children. One would be "less likely to be correct in young children under five years," because children under five years experience many other severe respiratory diseases that could be mistaken for influenza, whereas older children are already immune to such diseases. He added that the degree of selection bias would also "depend on the rules for collection, for example, a certain number per week or with specific symptoms."

Another influenza expert had similar views. He provided his best guess for each of the univariate relative risk selection bias parameters $\beta_{z,x}$ defined in (8.11) and his belief about the interval that would likely contain 90% of the prior distribution for each $\beta_{z,x}$. He also provided the degree of correlation of the selection bias by age group and vaccine status. The expert did not have different prior beliefs about the selection bias in the 5–9 and 10–18 year age groups. Thus the prior distributions for these two age groups are presented as one group in Table 8.5.

For the analysis, the elicitations were plugged into a multivariate Normal prior on the log β scale as follows. The elicited best guesses for each $\beta_{z,x}$ and 90% range were transformed to the log $\beta_{z,x}$ scale. In the unvaccinated 5–18 year olds, the elicitation was quite consistent with a Normal distribution. In the other three groups, adjustments were necessary as shown in Table 8.5. The expert felt comfortable with the changes in elicited and proposed priors in light of the uncertainty about the selection bias. The expert believed that the correlation in selection bias among the strata would be quite high, even as high as 0.90. The corresponding covariance matrices for $\pi(\beta)$ were constructed from the marginal univariate Normal distributions and the correlations.

Figure 8.3 shows the Bayesian posterior distribution of the age-group-specific efficacy and overall efficacy using the informative prior distributions from Table 8.5, assuming a correlation of 0.9. The mode is 1.00 in the age group 1.5–4 years, because there are no positive cultures in the vaccinated group in that age group. The results assuming a zero correlation were nearly identical (not shown).

Table 8.6 Results of Bayesian and frequentist sensitivity analyses using surveillance cultures assuming NMAR and MAR. For the Bayesian analyses, the posterior means (95% credible intervals) for vaccine efficacy are reported, for the frequentist analyses, the point estimates (95% confidence intervals). The estimates using just the nonspecific MAARI case definition are included for comparison (Scharfstein et al 2006)

	Age Group			
Analysis	1.5–4 Years	5–9 Years	10–18 Years	Overall
Bayesian:				
Informative $\pi(\beta)$	0.80 (0.23,1.00)	0.65 (0.13,0.93)	0.51 (−0.12,0.88)	0.65 (0.35,0.86)
$\pi(\beta)$ fixed at best guess	0.77 (0.11,0.99)	0.63 (0.10,0.93)	0.50 (−0.12,0.86)	0.64 (0.32,0.85)
$\pi(\beta)$ fixed at 1 (MAR)	0.84 (0.41,0.90)	0.73 (0.40,0.94)	0.64 (0.26,0.89)	0.73 (0.53,0.88)
Frequentist:				
β fixed at best guess	0.88 (−0.97,0.99)	0.74 (−0.05,0.88)	0.61 (−0.25,0.88)	0.73 (0.34,0.89)
β fixed at 1 (MAR)	0.91 (−0.34,0.99)	0.80 (0.26,0.95)	0.70 (0.13,0.90)	0.79 (0.52,0.91)
MAARI alone:	0.20 (0.14,0.25)	0.25 (0.15,0.34)	0.14 (0.01,0.26)	0.18 (0.11,0.24)

Table 8.6 compares the summaries of the Bayesian posterior distributions and of the frequentist estimates and 95% confidence intervals. The assumption of MAR results in an overestimate of the vaccine efficacy compared with the selection bias relative risk assumptions elicited from the expert. The frequentist result with β fixed at 1 (MAR) is identical to the result in Table 8.4. The Bayesian posterior means are somewhat lower than the frequentist estimates.

8.4 Validation Sets with Time-to-Event Data

The Texas field study (Section 8.2.1) continued in the fall of 2003 (Halloran et al 2007b). Children were not vaccinated in the 2002–2003 season. In the meantime the vaccine was licensed but not approved for children under 5 years old. In the 2003–2004 season, healthy children and adolescents aged 5–18 years were eligible to enroll and were offered LAIV-T vaccination at public schools, the Temple Mall, churches, and Scott & White (S & W) Clinics. In the 2003–2004 influenza season, the predominant circulating influenza A (H3N2) virus in the United States was similar antigenically to A/Fujian/411/2002 (H3N2), a drift variant of A/Panama/2007/99 (H3N2), the vaccine strain. Comparison of the vaccinated with the unvaccinated children within Temple-Belton allows prospective evaluation of the direct protective effects of LAIV-T against the drift variant during the 2003–2004 influenza season. Children who were contraindicated to receive LAIV-T, such as history of asthma, were offered trivalent inactivated vaccine (TIV). Thus, there were three main vaccinated groups of interest: 1) those receiving LAIV-T in 2003, whether or not they had received LAIV-T before, 2) those having received LAIV-T in the seasons 1998–1999 through 2001–2002, but not in 2002–2003 or in the fall of 2003, and 3) those receiving TIV in the fall of 2003. The distributions of chronic obstructive pulmonary diseases and other similar potential confounders were similar in the LAIV-T, the previously vaccinated, and the unvaccinated groups. The TIV group had a much higher percentage of COPD and other diseases than the other groups, so that comparison of the TIV group with the unvaccinated group is not valid. Age-eligible members of the SWHP on October 10, 2003 were considered for inclusion in the analysis. The final inclusion was restricted to children living within zip codes in the Temple-Belton area. The definition of a case of medically attended acute respiratory illness (MAARI) is the same as in Section 8.2.1.

Some of the children who had surveillance cultures done were in the SWHP, and others were not. Those in the SWHP were included in the SWHP administrative database. The non-SWHP children were not in the SWHP database, although their culture results, age, and vaccination status were available. The primary influenza season was defined as the weeks with the most intense influenza activity accounting for 80–85% of all positive influenza cultures (Nichol et al 1999; Piedra et al 2005). The primary influenza season occurred during the 10-week period from October 10 to December 20, 2003. The MAARI cases and cultures occurring within this 10-week period were included in the analysis. The influenza season started early in Texas, so vaccination occurred during the influenza season.

A total of 6403 age-eligible children in the SWHP database living in the zip codes in the Temple-Belton are included in the analysis, of whom 1706 received LAIV-T and 548 received TIV in 2003 before the end of the study period. Of the remaining children, 983 had been previously vaccinated in 1998–2001 and 3166 had never been vaccinated by the end of the study period. About four weeks into the period, by November 8, 2003, 50% of the vaccinees had been vaccinated with either LAIV-T or TIV. Table 8.7 contains the number of MAARI events, child-days at risk, and rate per 1000 by age and vaccine status used in the analysis. Table 8.8 shows the influenza surveillance data and proportion of cultures positive by age and vaccine status at the time of culture.

8.4.1 Time-to-event analysis

The effectiveness of protection against MAARI and the efficacy of protection against culture-confirmed influenza were computed using the basic equation $VE_{S,IR} = 1 - RR$, where RR is the ratio of the number of MAARI (estimated influenza) cases/ child-days in the vaccinated compared to the unvaccinated group. In this section, we denote it simply as VE. The main interest was in the efficacy of LAIV-T, but estimates were also obtained for the previously vaccinated in 1998–2001 (PREV), both being compared to the unvaccinated group. Age-group specific values were computed for the two age groups 5–9 years and 10–18 years. Overall efficacy was computed by weighting the contributions of the age groups by the combined number of child-days at risk in the vaccinated and unvaccinated groups in each age group.

A child who began the season as either unvaccinated or previously vaccinated could be switched to the LAIV-T group or the TIV group once they got vacci-

Table 8.7 MAARI events, child-days at risk, and rate per 1000 child-days at risk by age group and vaccine status (Halloran et al 2007b)

Age (Years)	Vaccination Status	MAARI Events	Child-Days at Risk	Rate/1000 Child-Days at Risk
5–9				
	LAIV-T	105	35,886	2.93
	TIV	80	10,598	7.55
	PREV	143	26,902	5.32
	UNVAC	261	61,522	4.24
10–18				
	LAIV-T	117	42,991	2.72
	TIV	82	13,741	5.97
	PREV	273	71,424	3.82
	UNVAC	641	179,828	3.56
Combined				
	LAIV-T	222	78,883	2.81
	TIV	162	24,383	6.64
	PREV	416	98,297	4.23
	UNVAC	902	241,331	3.74
Totals				
5–9		589	134,908	4.37
10–18		1113	307,984	3.61
Combined		1702	442,896	3.84

nated in 2003. To take the changing vaccine status into account and to integrate the surveillance cultures into the analysis, we grouped the data by week over the 10-week period. If vaccination occurred before the day of MAARI, the child was counted as a vaccinated MAARI case. Otherwise, the child was counted as a previously vaccinated or unvaccinated MAARI case. We assumed that multiple visits in a week were not independent. Only the first MAARI case in the week was included if a child had more than one MAARI presentation in that week. Vaccine effectiveness against MAARI was denoted as VE^a.

To estimate the efficacy against culture-confirmed influenza illness, the expected number of influenza cases in each week for each age and vaccine group was estimated by multiplying the proportion of positive surveillance cultures in each age and vaccine group by the number of MAARI cases in that group (Halloran and Longini 2001; Halloran et al 2007b). Children who had positive cultures were considered to be no longer at risk for influenza and did not contribute further child-days at risk for the rest of the 10-week period.

The data are grouped within one-week time intervals τ, $(t_{\tau-1}, t_\tau]$, $\tau = 1, \ldots, T$, $T = 10$. Let k, $k = 1, \ldots, K$, indicate the relevant strata, in our case age groups, and $K = 2$. Let $n_{\nu\tau}$, $\nu = 0, 1$, be the number of participants in the unvaccinated and vaccinated group at risk of influenza at the beginning of each time interval, with $n_{k\nu\tau}$, $\nu = 0, 1$, $k = 1, \ldots, K$, the corresponding number in each stratum. For each stratum k, $k = 1, \ldots, K$, and vaccine status ν, $\nu = 0, 1$, let the number of MAARI cases ascertained in each time interval be $w_{k\nu\tau}$, the number of surveillance cultures be $r_{k\nu\tau}$,

Table 8.8 Influenza surveillance data (number positive/number cultured (proportion)), Temple-Belton, Texas, 2003–2004 (Halloran et al 2007b)

Age Group	SWHP		Non-SWHP		Combined	
(Years)	Unvaccinated	LAIV-T	Unvaccinated	LAIV-T	Unvaccinated	LAIV-T
5–9	8/20 (0.40)	3/15 (0.20)	19/34 (0.56)	4/9 (0.44)	27/54 (0.50)	7/24 (0.29)
10–18	35/56 (0.63)	5/13 (0.38)	30/49 (0.61)	4/11 (0.36)	65/105 (0.62)	9/24 (0.38)
Total	43/76 (0.57)	8/28 (0.29)	49/83 (0.59)	8/20 (0.40)	92/159 (0.58)	16/48 (0.33)
	TIV	PREV	TIV	PREV	TIV	PREV
5–9	2/5 (0.40)	3/9 (0.33)	0/3 (0.33)	7/21 (0.33)	2/8 (0.25)	10/30 (0.33)
10–18	3/3 (1.0)	15/29 (0.52)	5/6 (0.83)	8/15 (0.53)	8/9 (0.89)	23/44 (0.52)
Total	5/8 (0.63)	18/38 (0.47)	5/9 (0.56)	15/36 (0.42)	10/17 (0.59)	33/74 (0.44)

and the number of positive cultures be $c_{kv\tau}$. For each τ, estimate the proportion $\rho_{kv\tau}$ of true influenza cases among the MAARI cases in each age and vaccine group by $\hat{\rho}_{kv\tau} = c_{kv\tau}/r_{kv\tau}$. Multiply $w_{kv\tau}$ by $\{\hat{\rho}_{kv\tau}\}$ to obtain an estimate of the number of influenza cases in each interval. Summing over the weekly estimates of the number of true influenza cases, the total expected number of influenza cases in each age and vaccine group during the study is estimated. The outcome of interest, the result of a culture, is assumed to be missing at random (Little and Rubin 2002).

To compute child-days at risk, everyone is assumed to be at risk for influenza at the beginning of the study period. For each time interval τ, the child-days at risk in each stratum, $d_{kv\tau}$, were computed as $7 \times (n_{kv\tau} - 0.5\hat{\rho}_{kv\tau}w_{kv\tau})$, $v = 0, 1$, $k = 1, \ldots, K$. That is, the expected number of influenza cases times half the time interval was subtracted from the number at risk at the beginning of the interval to adjust the child-days at risk. Children who had positive cultures were considered to be no longer at risk for influenza and did not contribute further child-days at risk for the rest of the 10-week period. The incidence rate of true influenza in each vaccine and age group was estimated based on the above, and from that, the stratum specific vaccine efficacy, $\mathrm{VE}_{k,v}$, based on the validation set as

$$\widehat{\mathrm{VE}}_{k,v} = 1 - \frac{[\sum_{\tau=1}^{T} \hat{\rho}_{k1\tau} w_{k1\tau}]/[\sum_{\tau=1}^{T} d_{k1\tau}]}{[\sum_{\tau=1}^{T} \hat{\rho}_{k0\tau} w_{k0\tau}]/[\sum_{\tau=1}^{T} d_{k0\tau}]} . \tag{8.13}$$

Overall VE_v is computed by weighting the contributions of the age groups by the combined number of child-days at risk in the vaccinated and unvaccinated groups in each age group.

Two different estimates using the surveillance cultures can be computed. The first, denoted VE^{in}, uses just the surveillance cultures from the SWHP members in the database. The second, denoted VE^{ex}, uses the surveillance cultures from both the SWHP members and the non-SWHP children. Confidence intervals were obtained using 2000 bootstrap samples (Efron and Tibshirani 1993). When spread over a 10-week period, the culture data were too sparse to obtain a separate weekly estimate of

Table 8.9 Vaccine effectiveness of LAIV-T: VE^a against MAARI (95% CI), against culture-confirmed influenza using just SWHP surveillance cultures VE^{in} (95% CI), and against culture-confirmed influenza using surveillance cultures from the children in the SWHP database and children not in the SWHP database, VE^{ex} (95% CI) (Halloran et al 2007b)

Vaccine Status	Age Group (Years)	VE^a (95% CI)‡ MAARI	VE^{in} (95% CI) Influenza	VE^{ex} (95% CI) Influenza
LAIV-T*	5–9	0.31 (0.11,0.47)	0.66 (−0.03,1.0)	0.60 (0.25,0.84)
	10–18	0.24 (0.03,0.40)	0.53 (0.12,0.86)	0.54 (0.23,0.78)
	All	0.26 (0.11,0.39)	0.56 (0.24,0.84)	0.56 (0.32,0.75)
PREV†	5–9	−0.25 (−0.61,0.05)	−0.04 (−1.9,1.0)	0.17 (−0.50,0.61)
	10–18	−0.07 (−0.28,0.10)	0.11 (−0.37,0.46)	0.09 (−0.28,0.39)
	All	−0.13 (−0.30,0.03)	0.08 (−0.38,0.44)	0.11 (−0.19,0.37)

∗ Vaccinated with LAIV-T in 2003, regardless whether previously vaccinated.
† Previously vaccinated in 1998-2001, but not in the 2002–2003 season or in 2003.
‡ Percentile bootstrap confidence intervals based on 2000 bootstrap samples.

$\rho_{kv\tau}$ for use in equation (8.13). So the overall estimated proportion positive in Table 8.8 in each group was used as the estimate for the proportion positive in equation (8.13).

The estimates of VE^a, VE^{in}, and VE^{ex} are given in Table 8.9. Overall effectiveness of LAIV-T against MAARI VE^a is 0.26 (95% CI 0.11–0.39). Overall efficacy against culture-confirmed influenza using just surveillance cultures from children in the SWHP database, VE^{in}, is 0.56 (95% CI 0.24–0.84). The point estimates for VE^{in} and VE^{ex} are quite similar, but the confidence intervals using all of the surveillance cultures are narrower than those using just the surveillance cultures from SWHP, reflecting the higher precision conferred by the larger number of cultures.

8.5 Assessing Differential Protection Against Variants

In a series of papers, Gilbert et al (1998), Gilbert (2000), and Gilbert et al (1999) described statistical procedures for hypothesis testing, estimation, and confidence intervals for assessing strain variations in vaccine efficacy, called *sieve analysis*. Gilbert et al (2001) demonstrated use of these methods on examples of cholera, HIV, and hepatitis, rotavirus, and pneumococcal vaccines. Sun et al (2009) extended these methods to a continuous competing risk model to assess efficacy based on the distance of genetic divergence of the infecting strain and the vaccine strain.

Problems

8.1. What is the purpose of matching on time when selecting controls in the closed cohort?

8.2. Suppose that we do a BCG efficacy study and we choose our matched controls from within the same household (in a similar age group). What is the purpose of this matching?

8.3. Consider a study using a random sample of surveillance cultures for influenza as a validation set for a nonspecific outcome influenza-like illness. The purpose is to estimate vaccine efficacy for influenza illness. The design called for cases vaccinated for influenza to have a sampling fraction twice that of cases not vaccinated. Would this result in selection bias in the estimate of vaccine efficacy using the surveillance cultures as a validation set?

Chapter 9
Vaccine Effects on Post-Infection Outcomes

9.1 Scientific Questions of Interest

A common question of interest is whether clinical cases in infected vaccinated people are less severe than clinical cases in infected unvaccinated people. As early as 1939, Kendrick and Eldering described less severe disease in children with pertussis who had been inoculated with pertussis vaccine compared to children with pertussis who had not been inoculated. Children vaccinated against chickenpox who develop clinical symptoms have less severe disease than unvaccinated children (Vazquez et al 2001). In evaluating malaria vaccine candidates, a question of interest might be whether the density of malaria blood-stage parasites is lower in infected vaccinated children than in infected unvaccinated children. In assessing an HIV vaccine, a scientific question of interest might be whether infected vaccinated people have a slower progression to clinical AIDS disease than infected unvaccinated people. In such a study, because the clinical endpoint of AIDS could take years to develop, the post-infection outcomes viral load and CD4 count could be used as surrogates for the clinical endpoint of interest.

Common to all of these questions is that the comparison is not between outcomes in uninfected vaccinated and unvaccinated individuals, but in people who have either become infected or developed clinical symptoms. We denote the vaccine effects on post-infection or post-clinical symptom outcomes broadly as VE_P.

9.1.1 Different measures of VE_P

If the interest is in an outcome in infected people, then VE_P is defined as one minus the ratio of a summary measure, such as the mean, of the post-infection outcome in the infected vaccinated people and a summary measure of the post-infection outcome in the infected unvaccinated people:

M.E. Halloran et al., *Design and Analysis of Vaccine Studies*, Statistics for Biology and Health, DOI 10.1007/978-0-387-68636-3_9,

$$\mathrm{VE}_P = 1 - \frac{\dfrac{\text{vaccinated post-infection outcome}}{\text{infected vaccinated people}}}{\dfrac{\text{unvaccinated post-infection outcome}}{\text{infected unvaccinated people}}}. \tag{9.1}$$

Similarly, if a post-clinical outcome in the clinical cases is of interest, then VE_P is defined as one minus the ratio of a summary measure of the post-clinical outcome in the vaccinated cases and a summary measure of the post-clinical outcome in the unvaccinated cases:

$$\mathrm{VE}_P = 1 - \frac{\dfrac{\text{vaccinated post-clinical outcome}}{\text{vaccinated clinical cases}}}{\dfrac{\text{unvaccinated post-clinical outcome}}{\text{unvaccinated clinical cases}}}. \tag{9.2}$$

Throughout this chapter, the methods are applicable to post-infection outcomes given infection as well as to post-clinical outcomes given a clinical case. We do not repeat everywhere the result for both situations. In this chapter, if the interest is on post-infection outcomes, then VE_S, VE_{SP}, and VE_P denote vaccine efficacy for susceptibility to infection, vaccine efficacy for susceptibility to the post-infection outcome not conditional on infection, and vaccine efficacy for the post-infection outcome conditional on being infected. If the interest is in some post-clinical outcome in clinical cases, the vaccine efficacies are defined analogously. For example, we use the notation VE_S, VE_{SP}, and VE_P to denote vaccine efficacy against a clinical case, vaccine efficacy against a further outcome, such as severe disease, not conditional on being a case, and vaccine efficacy against severe disease conditional on being a clinical case.

Just as with VE_S, different post-infection or post-clinical outcomes can be used to measure VE_P. Some options for outcomes in VE_P are summarized in Table 9.1. In the table, the occurrence of the infection or clinical outcome on which the post-infection or post-clinical outcome is conditioned is assumed to be dichotomous (0,1), but more complex forms or assumptions are possible. Depending on the scientific question of interest, the post-infection outcome could be dichotomous (0,1), continuous, as with parasite density, or time-to-event, such as the time between ascertaining infection and developing a clinical outcome of interest. Thus, we could differentiate VE_P measures based on different outcomes by the notation as in Table 2.2, such as $\mathrm{VE}_{P,\lambda}$ analogous to $\mathrm{VE}_{S,\lambda}$ if based on the time-to-event. If the outcome is the time to an event after infection, an incidence rate or survival analysis that begins with the observation at the time of infection might be appropriate. For continuous or time-to-event post-infection outcomes, the mean, median, or some other summary measure in the two groups could be used. The exact form of the VE_P estimator depends on the choice of outcome.

Transmissibility for others is also a post-infection outcome. Thus, vaccine efficacy for infectiousness, VE_I, is a special case of a vaccine effect on a post-infection outcome. If measured by level of viral shedding or some other laboratory measure, then VE_I is similar to a VE_P measure, or at least a surrogate measure. If VE_I is measured epidemiologically based on the transmission probability or secondary attack

Table 9.1 Different types of post-infection and post-clinical outcomes, VE_P. Ascertainment can be on infection or on clinical disease, which determines the VE_S (VE_{SP})

VE_S Outcome	Postinfection VE_P Outcome	Examples
Infection 0,1	Dichotomous	Clinical case (0,1) Clinical case within time interval (0,1) Transmission to other (0,1)
	Continuous	Malaria parasite density HIV viral load
	Time-to-event	Time to developing symptoms
Clinical case 0,1	Dichotomous	Severe disease (0,1) Death Transmission to other (0,1)
	Continuous	Malaria parasite density Chickenpox: number of lesions
	Time-to-event	Time to clearing infection Time to death

rate in others, it is more complex than simple VE_P measures (Chapters 10 through 12).

9.1.2 Vaccine effects on dichotomous post-infection outcomes

If the post-infection outcome is dichotomous, we can define the post-infection attack rate (PAR) as the number with the post-infection outcome of interest divided by the number of infections:

$$\text{PAR} = \frac{\text{number with post-infection outcome}}{\text{number infected}}. \tag{9.3}$$

Letting p denote the control group and v denote the vaccinated group, then VE_P using a dichotomous outcome can be defined as

$$VE_P = 1 - \frac{PAR(v)}{PAR(p)}. \tag{9.4}$$

As an example of VE_P based on a dichotomous outcome in people with clinical disease, Préziosi and Halloran (2003a) proposed a method to estimate the efficacy of vaccine in reducing the probability of developing severe disease in clinical cases:

$$\text{VE}_P = 1 - \frac{\frac{\text{severe vaccinated cases}}{\text{all vaccinated cases}}}{\frac{\text{severe unvaccinated cases}}{\text{all unvaccinated cases}}}. \tag{9.5}$$

Pathogenicity is a measure of the ability of an infectious agent to cause disease in an infected person. A measure of pathogenicity is the probability of developing clinical disease if infected. If a vaccine decreases the probability of infected people developing clinical disease, it decreases pathogenicity. An example of VE_P based on a dichotomous outcome in infected people is the vaccine effect on the probability that an infected person will develop clinical symptoms, the vaccine efficacy for pathogenicity. Asymptomatic infections have not traditionally been ascertained in most vaccine studies, because ascertainment was generally by clinical case. However, asymptomatic infections could still be infectious. Thus for understanding the overall public health effects of vaccination programs and for dynamic models, ascertaining people with asymptomatic infections and estimating the effect of vaccination on the probability of developing symptoms is important.

9.1.2.1 Relation of VE_P, VE_S, and VE_{SP}

For dichotomous infection outcomes and dichotomous post-infection outcomes, a simple relation exists among VE_P, VE_S, and VE_{SP}. Let ψ denote the relative risk of the post-infection outcome in the infected vaccinated people compared with the infected unvaccinated people, and θ be the relative risk of infection in the vaccinated compared with the unvaccinated people. Then VE_P is

$$\mathrm{VE}_P = 1 - \frac{\frac{\text{vaccinated cases}}{\text{vaccinated infections}}}{\frac{\text{unvaccinated cases}}{\text{unvaccinated infections}}} = 1 - \psi. \tag{9.6}$$

Letting

$$VE_{S,CI} = 1 - \frac{\frac{\text{vaccinated infectious}}{\text{vaccinated people}}}{\frac{\text{unvaccinated infections}}{\text{unvaccinated people}}} = 1 - \theta, \tag{9.7}$$

then

$$\begin{aligned} VE_{SP,CI} &= 1 - \frac{\frac{\text{vaccinated cases}}{\text{vaccinated people}}}{\frac{\text{unvaccinated cases}}{\text{unvaccinated people}}} \\ &= 1 - \frac{\frac{\text{vaccinated infections}}{\text{vaccinated people}}}{\frac{\text{unvaccinated infections}}{\text{unvaccinated people}}} \times \frac{\frac{\text{vaccinated cases}}{\text{vaccinated infections}}}{\frac{\text{unvaccinated cases}}{\text{unvaccinated infections}}} \\ &= 1 - (1 - VE_S)(1 - VE_P) = 1 - \theta\psi. \end{aligned} \tag{9.8}$$

These relations hold under the assumption that the infected people in the control arm are comparable to the infected people in the vaccine arm. If any two of the three are estimated, the other can be derived from equation (9.8). In general, to use (9.8), asymptomatic infections need to be determined. A similar relation as that in equation (9.8) holds for $VE_{SP,CI}$, when the post-clinical outcome is severe cases of the disease of interest, and VE_S is based on clinical cases.

9.1.3 *Statistical validity and VE_P*

In randomized studies, approaches that use the originally randomized populations in the denominators, such as VE_S and VE_{SP}, enjoy the statistical validity associated with an intent-to-treat analysis. One can think of the events after randomization of uninfected individuals as occurring on a continuous time line. Perhaps first is infection, followed by symptoms or not, followed by severe symptoms or not, followed by death or not. An analysis that uses any of these outcomes, as long as it is the first outcome post-randomization used in the analysis, enjoys the statistical validity associated with an intent-to-treat analysis. In any particular study, vaccine efficacy against differing definitions or severity of the symptomatic disease can be estimated, yielding more than one estimate of VE_{SP}. The efficacy estimate may be higher for more stringent case definitions (Chapter 6), but the statistical validity of the comparison is not compromised.

However, VE_P conditions on infection or clinical disease to estimate a net effect of the vaccine on the post-infection or post-disease endpoint in just those people who become infected or have clinical disease. The infected vaccinated group and the infected control group may not be comparable, so the comparison may not be statistically valid, and the VE_P estimate may not have a causal interpretation. In the first sections in this chapter, we assume that the comparison is valid. In Sections 9.3 and 9.4, we relax this assumption and show the implications.

9.2 Effect of Vaccination on Disease Severity

Préziosi and Halloran (2003a) analyzed a study of pertussis vaccination in the Niakhar study area of Senegal to estimate the effect of vaccination on reducing the severity of clinical pertussis cases. The study population and surveillance for pertussis in the Niakhar study area are described in Section 10.2.3. Briefly, the Niakhar study area is 150 km southeast of Dakar, Senegal, and includes 30 villages. Surveillance began in March 1983 with annual, and after 1987, weekly visits to residential compounds. Pertussis was endemic, with epidemics every 3–4 years, and 1993 was a pertussis epidemic year. Active surveillance was conducted in children <15 years of age by weekly visits to the compounds by trained field workers. They reported cases in children <15 years old who had potential pertussis (cough of >7 days duration). A physician then visited to confirm clinically and collect laboratory samples.

Table 9.2 Scale used to assess the severity of illness among children with symptoms of pertussis (Préziosi and Halloran 2003a)

Variable	No. of Points
Severity of cough	
Typical paroxysms with whoops	4
Typical paroxysms without whoops	3
Atypical paroxysms only	1
Apnea	6
Pulmonary sign[a]	3
Mechanical complication[b]	3
Facial swelling	3
Conjunctival injection	3
Post-tussive vomiting	2
Total score (severity)[c]	
Mild disease	≤ 6
Severe disease	>6

[a] Bronchitis or bronchopneumonia.
[b] Subjunctival hemorrhage or umbilical or inguinal hernia.
[c] The overall median total score was 6 in this study.

A case of pertussis was defined by confirmation of pertussis infection by presence of at least one of three laboratory criteria: (1) isolation of *B. pertussis* from a nasopharyngeal aspirate (culture positive), (2) significant increase or decrease in pertussis toxin or filamentous hemagglutinin antibodies (serology positive), or (3) signs and symptoms of disease in an individual who lived in the same compound as a child who had onset of culture-positive disease within 28 days (epilink).

9.2.1 Global score of disease severity

Estimating VE_P requires defining the disease outcomes of interest carefully. To compare the severe to nonsevere cases, definitions of a severe case and a nonsevere case, or other levels of severity, such as moderate severity, are needed. Préziosi and Halloran (2003a) proposed a scale to assess the global clinical severity of pertussis cases, rather than analyzing each individual symptom. Severity of illness was assessed according to the scale in Table 9.2. Death is not included, because there was only one death due to pertussis in the study period. Each relevant symptom was given a score based on the judged severity of the symptom. The global symptom score for each child was obtained by the simple sum of the child's scores for individual clinical signs and symptoms. Severe disease was defined by a score greater than a particular threshold value. The main outcome measure was defined using the overall severity median score in the confirmed clinical cases.

Sex, age, and type of case (primary or post-infection) were included in a multivariate analysis using logistic regression and then backtransformed to the relative

Table 9.3 Number of cases of severe pertussis, among 834 children who had or had not received pertussis vaccine, and efficacy of the vaccine in reducing severity, according to severity score (Préziosi and Halloran 2003a).

	No. (%) of cases			
Score[a]	All ($n = 837$)	In unvaccinated children ($n = 243$)	In vaccinated children ($n = 594$)	Vaccine efficacy, % VE_P (95% CI)
>0	738 (88)	233 (96)	505 (85)	11 (8–15)
>1	728 (87)	231 (95)	497 (84)	12 (8–16)
>2	677 (81)	227 (93)	450 (76)	19 (14–23)
>3	559 (67)	205 (84)	354 (60)	29 (23–35)
>4	529 (63)	194 (80)	335 (56)	29 (22–36)
>5	443 (53)	178 (73)	265 (45)	39 (32–46)
>6	339 (41)	149 (61)	190 (32)	48 (39–55)
>7	315 (38)	139 (57)	176 (30)	48 (39–56)
>8	268 (32)	119 (49)	149 (25)	49 (38–58)
>9	151 (18)	76 (31)	75 (13)	60 (47–70)
>10	147 (18)	75 (31)	72 (12)	61 (48–71)
>11	130 (16)	67 (28)	63 (11)	62 (48–72)
>12	31 (4)	20 (8)	11 (2)	78 (54–89)
>13	30 (4)	19 (8)	11 (2)	76 (51–89)
>14	24 (3)	17 (7)	7 (1)	83 (60–93)

[a] The scale used to assign the severity score is shown in Table 9.2. The overall median score was 6. A score ≤6 indicates mild disease; a score >6 indicates severe disease.

risk scale (Halloran et al 2003b) (Chapter 12.3.2). Confidence intervals were obtained using the bootstrap (Efron and Tibshirani 1993).

In 1993, 2123 individuals with potential cases of pertussis were identified in 518 of 1800 residential compounds, 98% under 15 years of age. Nearly all children under 6 months or 9 years and older were unvaccinated, so these age groups could not be included in the comparison. Cultures were done on 99% of all suspected cases, and serological testing in 69% of unvaccinated and 83% of vaccinated suspected cases. In all, 834 children with 837 cases of laboratory-confirmed pertussis were identified. Details of confirmation criteria and clinical signs and symptoms are in Préziosi and Halloran (2003a).

9.2.2 VE_P for severity of pertussis disease

Based on the median threshold global severity score of 6 for mild versus severe disease, there were 190 severe vaccinated cases in 594 vaccinated cases, and 149 severe unvaccinated cases in 243 vaccinated cases. Thus, 61% of cases in unvaccinated children and 32% of cases in vaccinated children had severe disease. Based on this threshold, using equation (9.5), the estimated VE_P is

$$\widehat{\mathrm{VE}}_P = 1 - \frac{190/594}{149/243} = 0.48 \quad (95\%\ \mathrm{CI}\ 0.39,\ 0.55). \tag{9.9}$$

Thus, clinical cases in unvaccinated children were twice as likely as clinical cases in vaccinated children to have severe disease. Table 9.3 presents a sensitivity analysis of the estimate of VE_P to the choice of threshold for defining a severe case. The threshold varies from 1 to >14. The estimated VE_P varies from 11% to 83%, becoming higher as the threshold for defining a severe case gets higher. The lower limit of the 95% CI was greater than 0 for all thresholds. The results indicate that pertussis vaccination substantially decreases the severity of breakthrough disease in children who receive three doses of vaccine, compared with that in unvaccinated children. The majority of vaccinated children who developed pertussis had mild disease.

Because this is an observational study, there is a potential for selection bias, particularly in (1) ascertainment and (2) laboratory confirmation. Both are minimal in this case because (1) surveillance was active, and (2) most children with suspected cases had laboratory tests done. To assess potential bias in the selection of the confirmed cases, Préziosi and Halloran (2003a) examined clinical illnesses among children with a potential case of pertussis whose biological tests were negative and among children for whom no laboratory samples were available. A comparison of the vaccinated and unvaccinated children who had no biological test done or whose tests were all negative yielded no appreciable vaccine effect in these groups.

In a secondary analysis, VE_{SP} was also estimated, first using all cases, and then using just severe cases. Child-years at risk were computed for 1993 among susceptible children six months up to eight years old. Standard CIs were computed assuming log-normality of relative risks. In the secondary analysis, the estimate of VE_{SP} for all cases was 0.29 (95% CI, 0.19–0.39), and the estimate of VE_{SP} for severe cases was 0.64 (95% CI, 0.55–0.71). It is typical that the estimated VE_{SP} is higher for more severe or stringent case definitions.

9.2.3 Rotavirus vaccine in Finland

Vesikari et al (1990) analyzed a randomized, double-blinded, placebo controlled trial of a *Rhesus* rotavirus candidate vaccine. The trial was conducted in children two to five months of age from 1985–1987 in Finland with 100 children randomized to each arm. The effect of the vaccine on the clinical course of infection was considered by comparing severity (mild, moderate, or severe) between vaccinees and control individuals with confirmed *Rotavirus* diarrhea using Fisher's exact test. Combining the severe and moderately severe cases, 5 of 10 cases in the vaccinated group were severe or moderately severe, and 13 of 16 cases in the placebo group were severe or moderately severe. Using equation (9.5) yields $\widehat{\mathrm{VE}}_P = 0.38$, (95% CI, −0.11–0.74).

9.3 Causal Effects on Post-Infection Outcomes

In Sections 9.1 and 9.2 the assumption was made that the infected vaccinated group and the infected unvaccinated group were comparable. However, conditioning on an event, such as infection, that occurs subsequent to receipt of vaccine or control could result in selection bias, even if the study were randomized (Struchiner et al 1994; Halloran and Struchiner 1995). Issues related to interpreting malaria vaccine trials motivated Struchiner et al (1994) to consider the problem of vaccinated and unvaccinated groups not being comparable after being infected even in randomized trials. With the development of HIV vaccine candidates, the assumption about the comparability of the infected vaccinated and infected unvaccinated groups gained considerable attention (Hudgens et al 2003; Gilbert et al 2003a). The initial HIV vaccine candidates were hoped to protect against infection and also slow progression to AIDS post-infection. The HIV vaccine trials were designed to draw blood from all the participants to ascertain infection at three-month intervals. Because the incubation period to the development of AIDS after HIV infection is usually several years, post-infection measures in the blood such as viral load and CD4 cell count are used as surrogates of potential future development of AIDS. Concern grew that the infected people in the vaccinated group and infected people in the unvaccinated group might not be comparable, leading to biased estimates of the effect of vaccination on post-infection outcomes.

9.3.1 Post-infection selection bias

For example, assume that the potential immune response to HIV has a distribution in the population before individuals are randomized to vaccine or control. Randomization would assure that in large samples, the potential distribution of the immune response to HIV would be the same in the vaccine and the control groups. It could be that the vaccine enhances protection only in people who have the stronger immune system, conferring some level of protection against infection if exposed. Then the people in the vaccinated group who become infected would be the ones with weaker immune systems, whereas the infected people in the unvaccinated group would be those with a weaker immune system as well as those with the stronger immune system. In this situation, if we compare a post-infection outcome in the vaccinated group with that in the unvaccinated group, it could appear that the vaccine makes things worse, even if vaccination has absolutely no effect on anything after infection.

For example, if people with a weaker immune system tend to have a higher viral load after being infected than those with a stronger immune system, then the mean viral load in the infected vaccinated group would be higher than the mean viral load in the infected unvaccinated group (Figure 9.1). The resulting VE_P estimate would be negative. This observation could lead to the false conclusion that the vaccine made the post-infection outcome worse, possibly resulting in rejection of a potentially useful vaccine candidate (Hudgens et al 2003; Gilbert et al 2003a). However,

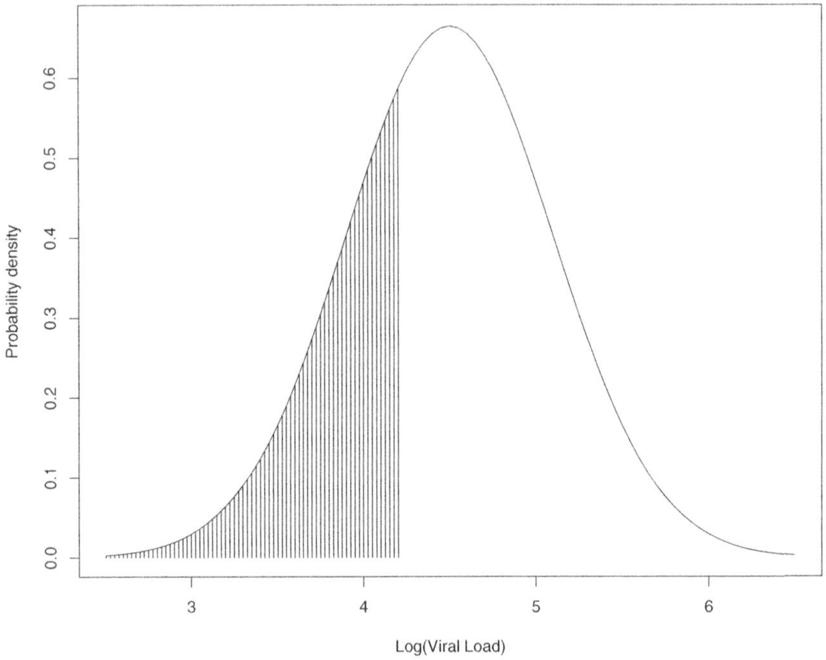

Fig. 9.1 Viral load distribution for infected participants under a selection model. The normal distribution represents the viral loads of the infected controls. The shaded area represents the potential viral loads of the vaccine efficacy $\times$ 100% that are protected by the vaccine. The unshaded area (after appropriate scaling) represents the viral load distribution of the infected vaccinees (adapted from Hudgens et al 2003).

the vaccine in this case actually does not make anything worse. The problem is that the infected vaccinated group and infected control group are no longer comparable because of selection bias.

Struchiner et al (1994) examined the post-infection selection bias from the point of view of a lack of exchangeability (Greenland and Robins 1986) of the vaccinated and unvaccinated groups, motivated by malaria vaccine trials. A similar problem exists in principle for diseases and vaccines other than HIV and malaria, but it has received considerably less attention. When the benefits of vaccination are clearly positive, selection bias might not lead to discarding the vaccine, but to either an over- or an underestimate of the public health benefits. Thus, it is important both scientifically and for public health purposes to be able to differentiate the effects of vaccines on infection from their effects on post-infection outcomes, and to account for potential selection bias.

9.3.2 Defining causal estimands for post-infection outcomes

How do we account for possible selection bias in estimating VE_P if we do not know whether it is present? Different methods have been used to adjust analyses for post-treatment variables such as infection (Robins and Greenland 1992, 1994; Rosenbaum 1984). The method presented here is based on the potential outcomes approach to causal inference introduced in Section 1.4. In Table 1.1, four types of people are defined based on their joint potential outcome under vaccine and control, namely immune, harmed, protected, and doomed. If infection is the potential outcome of interest, then the four types of people are defined by their joint potential infection outcomes under vaccine and control. Because the set of individuals who would become infected if vaccinated is likely not identical to the set of those who would become infected if given control, comparisons that condition on infection do not have a causal interpretation (Rosenbaum 1984; Frangakis and Rubin 2002).

Frangakis and Rubin (2002) propose a method to adjust for post-treatment variables, called *principal stratification*, that stratifies on the joint potential post-treatment variables under each of the treatments being considered. The causal effects of one treatment compared to the other on a main outcome of interest are defined within each of these principal strata and are called principal effects. If infection is considered as a post-treatment variable, then the post-infection outcome is defined under both vaccine and placebo only in the doomed stratum, in which people would be infected under both vaccine and placebo. The post-infection outcome is not defined for anyone in the immune stratum. It is defined only under placebo in the protected stratum, and only under vaccine for the harmed stratum. The importance of estimating quantities defined only in a subpopulation in which the outcomes are defined was presented in the context of outcomes censored by death (Kalbfleisch and Prentice 1980). Robins (1986, Remark 12.2,) considered inference about causal effects in the stratum that would survive under either treatment.

Several papers have been published using this approach to assess vaccine effects on post-infection outcomes. In studying HIV vaccines, Hudgens et al (2003) and Gilbert et al (2003a) adopted the principal stratification approach to assess HIV vaccine effects on the continuous post-infection outcome viral load. Hudgens et al (2003) developed bounds. Gilbert et al (2003a) adapted methods for sensitivity similar to that of Scharfstein et al (1999) and Robins et al (2000b). Shepherd et al (2006a) considered sensitivity analyses comparing outcomes only existing in a subset selected post-randomization, conditional on covariates, with application to HIV. Jemiai et al (2007) developed extensions of Gilbert et al (2003a) that allow the estimation of treatment effects conditional on covariates. Shepherd et al (2007) developed the methods for a time-to-event post-infection outcome, also with application to HIV vaccine. The time-to-event postinfection outcome was the time from infection diagnosis to initiation of antiretroviral therapy. Hudgens and Halloran (2006) developed methods for the causal vaccine effects on binary post-infection outcomes with applications to pertussis and rotavirus vaccines. Table 9.4 summarizes literature on bounds and sensitivity analyses of causal vaccine effects for different types of post-infection outcomes.

Table 9.4 Bounds and sensitivity analyses of causal vaccine effects, VE_P, for different types of post-infection outcomes assuming SUTVA, randomization, and monotonocity

Infection Outcome VE_S	Postinfection Outcome VE_P	Analysis	Reference
0, 1	Continuous	Bounds	Hudgens et al 2003
		Sensitivity analysis	Gilbert et al 2003a
		Covariates	Shepherd et al 2006a Jemiai et al 2007
	Binary	Bounds and sensitivity analysis	Hudgens and Halloran 2006
	Ttime-to-event	Bounds and sensitivity analysis	Shepherd et al 2007

Because the development for continuous and time-to-event post-infection outcomes involves complex integral equations, we focus on the development of methods for binary post-infection outcomes by Hudgens and Halloran (2006). The approach for continuous and time-to-event outcomes is similar. The common steps in developing the methods regardless of the type of post-infection outcome are as follows.

1. Assume (i) the stable unit treatment value assumption (SUTVA) and (ii) an assignment mechanism independent of the potential outcomes, for example, randomization.
2. Define the causal VE_P in the doomed (always-infected) basic principal stratum, which is not identifiable from the observed data without further assumptions.
3. Assume that the harmed principal stratum is empty, called the monotonicity assumption.
4. The monotonicity assumption implies that all infected vaccine recipients are in the doomed stratum, so the numerator of the causal VE_P is identifiable. However, the infected placebo recipients could be in either the protected or the doomed stratum, so the denominator of the causal VE_P is not identifiable.
5. Bounds can be set on the estimates of the causal VE_P by extreme assumptions about the distribution of the post-infection outcome in the infected placebo recipients in the protected stratum compared with the distribution of the post-infection outcome in the infected placebo recipients in the the doomed stratum.
6. Sensitivity analyses can be done by varying a selection bias parameter over reasonable ranges of selection bias, with the assumption of no selection bias being a special case.

To formalize these concepts, we use an extension of the causal model introduced in Section 1.4 and Table 1.1. Let $Z_i = v$ if the ith individual is assigned vaccine, and $Z_i = p$ if assigned control. Denote the potential infection outcome of the ith individual if assigned Z_i as $S_i(Z_i)$, where $S_i(Z_i) = 0$ if uninfected and $S_i(Z_i) = 1$ if infected. The focus is on evaluating the causal effect of vaccine on the outcome Y that occurs after an individual becomes infected. Y could be a continuous random variable, a time-to-event variable, or a binary outcome. Here we develop the notation for a binary outcome. If $S_i(Z_i) = 1$, then $Y_i(Z_i) = 1$ if the ith individual has the worse, or more severe post-infection outcome, and $Y_i(Z_i) = 0$ otherwise. If an individual's potential infection outcome for an assignment is uninfected, that is, $S_i(Z_i) = 0$, then $Y_i(Z_i)$ is undefined and denoted by $*$. Let S_i^{obs} denote the observed infection outcome $S_i(v)$ or $S_i(p)$, depending on treatment assignment, and analogously Y_i^{obs} for the observed post-infection outcome.

In the following, we assume the potential outcomes for each individual are independent of the treatment assignment of other individuals. That is, we assume there is no interference between individuals (SUTVA). We further assume that the assignment to vaccine or control is independent of the potential infection outcomes and the potential post-infection outcomes. Randomization is one assignment mechanism where the treatment assignment is independent of the potential outcomes.

A *basic principal stratification* P_0 is defined according to the joint potential infection outcomes $S^{P_0} = (S(v), S(p))$ (Frangakis and Rubin 2002). Table 9.5 summarizes the four basic principal strata defined by the joint potential infection outcomes, $(S(v), S(p))$, and the strata defined by the joint potential post-infection outcomes, $(Y(v), Y(p))$, within each principal stratum. The four basic principal strata are composed of immune (not infected under both vaccine and placebo), harmed (infected under vaccine but not placebo), protected (infected under placebo but not vaccine), and doomed individuals (infected under both vaccine and placebo). Because membership in a basic principal stratum is not affected by whether an individual is actually assigned vaccine or placebo, the strata can be used in the same way as pre-treatment covariates, with causal post-infection vaccine effects defined within a basic principal stratum S^{P_0}.

In general, causal effects are defined in terms of potential outcomes. From Table 9.5, we see the doomed basic principal stratum, $S^{P_0} = (1,1)$, is the only stratum in which both potential post-infection endpoints, and thus their joint distribution, are defined. For this reason, defining individual post-infection causal vaccine effects makes sense only in the doomed basic principal stratum, $S^{P_0} = (1,1)$. In other words, we can speak of a vaccine causing an improvement or worsening of a post-infection outcome only for an individual who would become infected whether vaccinated or not. Thus, two population-level causal estimands can be validly defined: (1) the effect of vaccine on infection (S) for all participants, and (2) the effect of vaccine on the post-infection outcome (Y) for those participants who would be infected under both treatment assignments.

Regardless of the type of post-infection outcome, the population causal vaccine efficacy to prevent infection $S = 1$ can be defined as

$$\mathrm{VE}_S = 1 - \frac{\Pr(S(1) = 1)}{\Pr(S(0) = 1)}, \tag{9.10}$$

Table 9.5 Basic principal stratification P_0 based on the potential infection outcomes $(S(v),S(p))$ with potential post-infection strata based on $(Y(v),Y(p))$ (Hudgens and Halloran 2006)

Potential Infection Strata		Potential Post-infection Strata	
Basic Principal Stratum, S^{P_0}	Potential Infection Outcomes $(S(v),S(p))$	Potential Post-Infection Outcomes $(Y(v),Y(p))$	Post-Infection Interpretation
Immune	(0,0)	(∗,∗)	Always undefined
Harmed	(1,0)	(0,∗)	Not severe vaccine, undefined placebo
		(1,∗)	Severe vaccine, undefined placebo
Protected	(0,1)	(∗,0)	Undefined vaccine, not severe placebo
		(∗,1)	Undefined vaccine, severe placebo
Doomed	(1,1)	(0,0)	Never severe
		(1,0)	Harmed by vaccine
		(0,1)	Helped by vaccine
		(1,1)	Always severe

the relative average causal effect (RACE) of vaccination on infection (Hudgens and Halloran 2006). Under randomization, it follows that

$$\mathrm{VE}_S = 1 - \frac{E\{S(v)|Z=v\}}{E\{S(p)|Z=p\}} = 1 - \frac{E\{S^{obs}|Z=v\}}{E\{S^{obs}|Z=p\}}.$$

Using the basic principal stratification shown in Table 9.5, Hudgens and Halloran (2006) propose an estimand for the causal effect of vaccination on a binary post-infection outcome. In particular, the individual causal vaccine effect on the post-infection outcomes is defined as

$$\mathrm{VE}_{Pi} = 1 - \frac{Y_i(v)}{Y_i(p)},$$

for individuals within the doomed principal stratum only. Assuming SUTVA and randomization, define the population post-infection causal vaccine effect VE_P within the doomed principal stratum as

$$\mathrm{VE}_P = 1 - \frac{E\{Y(v)|S^{P_0}=(1,1)\}}{E\{Y(p)|S^{P_0}=(1,1)\}}. \tag{9.11}$$

All of the papers listed in Table 9.4 define an analogous causal estimand for post-infection outcomes based on the individuals within the doomed principal stratum only. The form is different for continuous and time-to-event outcomes. Like VE_S, (9.11) could equivalently be given in terms of probabilities because the post-infection random variables $Y(v)$ and $Y(p)$ are assumed to be binary such that VE_P

can be interpreted as the causal estimand measuring the relative reduction in the probability of the worse post-infection outcome given vaccine compared to placebo in those individuals who would be infected under either treatment assignment.

The problem with this approach is that it is not possible to tell to which stratum any individual belongs, at least without further assumptions. For example, a person who is vaccinated and becomes infected could belong to either the doomed or the harmed stratum. A person who receives control and is infected could belong to either the doomed or the protected stratum. Thus it is not possible to estimate the causal VE_P from the observed data without further assumptions.

One assumption that is plausible for most vaccines is helpful in this situation. If we assume that the vaccine does not harm people with respect to infection, then we can claim that the harmed stratum is empty. This assumption is called the monotonicity assumption. Under the monotonicity assumption, a vaccinated person who becomes infected must be in the doomed stratum. The monotonicity assumption does not help with the people who receive control and become infected. Infected people in the control arm can still be in either the protected or the doomed stratum.

Although it is not possible to identify who of the infected control group is in the protected or doomed stratum, it is possible to set upper and lower bounds on the vaccine effect on the post-infection outcome, $\widehat{VE}_P^{upper}$ and $\widehat{VE}_P^{lower}$. Estimating the causal vaccine effect under an extreme degree of selection bias is useful in bounding the estimate of the post-infection effect above and beyond any possible selective effects. However, the true degree of selection bias is likely less than the extreme models, such that using $\widehat{VE}_P^{upper}$ or $\widehat{VE}_P^{lower}$ may be too conservative. Therefore, it is useful to do sensitivity analyses by varying the amount of selection bias, in which the case of no selection and extreme bounds are included as special cases.

Gilbert et al (2003a), Shepherd et al (2006a), and Shepherd et al (2007) adapted methods for sensitivity similar to those of Scharfstein, et al (1999) and Robins et al (2000b) for continuous outcomes. In this approach, the sensitivity analysis is performed by varying a selection bias parameter β over a range. In particular the odds ratio, $OR = \exp(\beta)$, is varied from 0 to $+\infty$, with no selection bias being at $OR = 1$. The odds ratio is interpreted as given infection in the placebo arm, for a one-unit increase in the Y outcome, the odds of being infected if randomized to the vaccine arm multiplicatively increases by $OR = \exp(\beta)$.

Figure 9.2 illustrates different degrees of selection bias associated with varying the odds ratio, showing the distributions of the potential continuous Y outcome in the infected control group in the protected stratum and the infected control group in the doomed stratum. The shaded area represents the distribution of the potential Y outcome in the infected control group in the doomed stratum. The area under the clear distribution is that in the protected stratum. When the odds ratio equals 1, there is no selection bias, and the distributions in the two strata are the same. As the odds ratio tends to 0, the distribution of the Y outcome in the doomed stratum tends to be lower than the Y outcome in the protected stratum. As the odds ratio tends to ∞, the distribution of the Y outcome in the doomed stratum tends to be higher than the Y outcome distribution in the protected stratum. The data do not provide information

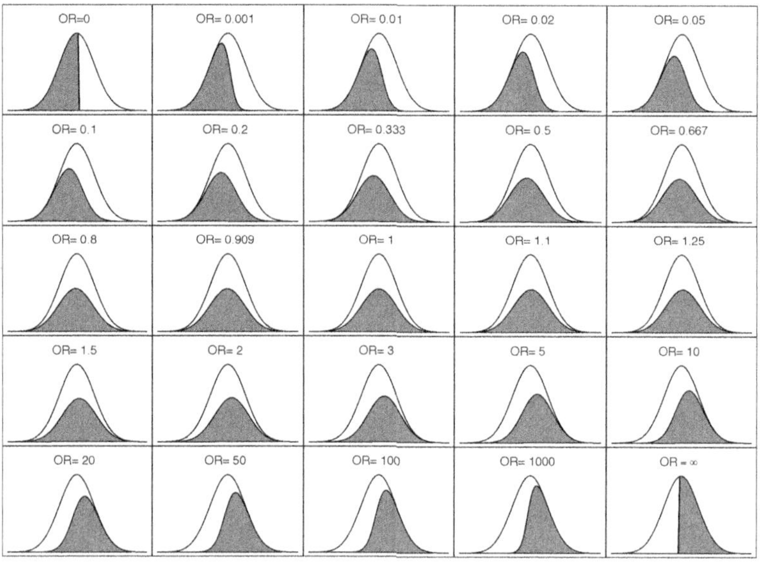

Fig. 9.2 Distribution of the potential post-infection outcome Y in the infected control group in the protected stratum and the infected control group in the doomed stratum for different values of the selection bias odds ratio $\exp(\beta)$. The shaded area represents the distribution of the potential Y outcome in the infected control group in the doomed stratum. The area under the clear distribution is that in the protected stratum (courtesy of B. Shepherd).

about the degree of selection bias. Then outside knowledge or expert opinion can be used to choose a plausible range for the selection bias (Shepherd et al 2006b).

9.4 Causal Effects for Binary Post-Infection Outcomes

The causal vaccine efficacy for a binary post-infection outcome for those participants who would be infected under both treatment assignments, VE_P, is defined in equation (9.11). Two further estimands regarding the effect of vaccination on the binary post-infection outcome Y can be formally defined (Hudgens and Halloran 2006).

The approach to assessing vaccine effects on post-infection endpoints based on the observed data in Section 9.1.2 is the *net* vaccine effect estimand that conditions on infection, ie,

$$\text{VE}_P^{net} = 1 - \frac{E\{Y^{obs}|S^{obs} = 1, Z = v\}}{E\{Y^{obs}|S^{obs} = 1, Z = p\}} = 1 - \frac{E\{Y(v)|S(v) = 1\}}{E\{Y(p)|S(p) = 1\}},$$

with the second equality following from the independence, eg, randomization assumption. As discussed in Section 9.3.1, in general, VE_P^{net} does not have a causal interpretation since the set of individuals with $S(v) = 1$ is not necessarily identical to the set of individuals with $S(p) = 1$.

An estimand that defines the effect of vaccination on disease rather than infection, or severe disease rather than disease, as in Chapter 6, might be considered intent-to-treat (ITT) because it does not condition on the post-treatment variable S^{obs}. It incorporates all individuals according to their treatment assignment. $\text{VE}_{SP,CI}$ in equation (9.8) is an example of an ITT estimand. Formally,

$$\text{VE}_{SP,CI} = \text{VE}_P^{ITT} = 1 - \frac{E\{Y(v) \times S(v)\}}{E\{Y(p) \times S(p)\}},$$

where the convention sets $Y(z) \times S(z) = 0$ if $S(z) = 0$, $z = v, p$. This is a general form for what Préziosi and Halloran (2003a) called "VE_{SP} for severity." The VE_P^{ITT} estimand has a causal interpretation, but it combines vaccine effects on susceptibility and the post-infection outcome. Formally, equation (9.8), and equivalently equation (2.12), can be written as

$$\text{VE}_P^{ITT} = 1 - (1 - \text{VE}_S)(1 - \text{VE}_P^{net}).$$

9.4.1 Parameterization

Let the parameters θ govern the probabilities associated with the basic principal strata (Hudgens and Halloran 2006). By the monotonicity assumption, the harmed stratum $S^{P_0} = (1,0)$ is empty, so let $\theta = (\theta_{00}, \theta_{01}, \theta_{11})$ where

$$\Pr\{S^{P_0} = (i,j); \theta\} = \theta_{ij} \text{ for } i,j = 0,1; i \leq j. \tag{9.12}$$

Next let the parameters $\phi = (\phi_{00}, \phi_{01}, \phi_{10}, \phi_{11})$ govern the probabilities associated with the joint potential post-infection outcomes in the doomed basic principal stratum $S^{P_0} = (1,1)$, where

$$\Pr\{(Y(v), Y(p)) = (k,m) | S^{P_0} = (1,1); \phi\} = \phi_{km} \text{ for } k,m = 0,1. \tag{9.13}$$

Let the parameters $\gamma = (\gamma_0, \gamma_1)$ govern the probabilities associated with the two possible potential post-infection outcomes under placebo in the protected basic principal stratum, $S^{P_0} = (0,1)$, where

$$\Pr\{Y(p) = i | S^{P_0} = (0,1); \gamma\} = \gamma_l \text{ for } l = 0,1. \tag{9.14}$$

Finally, let the law of Z be given by $\Pr\{Z = z; \varphi\} = \varphi_z$ for $z = v, p$.

Under this parameterization, the causal estimand of vaccine efficacy for susceptibility is

$$\mathrm{VE}_S = 1 - \frac{\theta_{11}}{\theta_{01} + \theta_{11}}.$$

Based on the definition of the causal estimand VE_P given in (9.11), we are not interested in the joint probabilities ϕ_{km} $(k,m = 0,1)$, but rather just two of the marginal probabilities. In particular, let

$$\begin{aligned}\Pr\{Y(v) = 1|S^{P_0} = (1,1)\} &= \phi_{10} + \phi_{11} = \phi_{1\cdot}\,,\\ \Pr\{Y(p) = 1|S^{P_0} = (1,1)\} &= \phi_{01} + \phi_{11} = \phi_{\cdot 1}\,.\end{aligned}$$

Then

$$\mathrm{VE}_P = 1 - \frac{\phi_{1\cdot}}{\phi_{\cdot 1}}, \tag{9.15}$$

Under this parameterization,

$$\mathrm{VE}_P^{net} = 1 - \frac{\phi_{1\cdot}}{\gamma_1 \mathrm{VE}_S + \phi_{\cdot 1}(1-\mathrm{VE}_S)}, \quad \text{and} \quad \mathrm{VE}_P^{ITT} = 1 - \frac{\phi_{1\cdot}(1-\mathrm{VE}_S)}{\gamma_1 \mathrm{VE}_S + \phi_{\cdot 1}(1-\mathrm{VE}_S)}.$$

9.4.2 Estimation

Suppose we observe n i.i.d. realizations of (Z, S^{obs}, Y^{obs}), where Y^{obs} is undefined or does not exist if $S^{obs} = 0$. There are six possible observed combinations of (Z, S^{obs}, Y^{obs}). Let $n_{sy}(z)$ be the number of each combination observed in the study population where $s = 0,1$ is the observed infection outcome S^{obs}; $y = 0,1,*$ is the observed post-infection outcome Y^{obs}; and $z = v,p$. That is,

$$\begin{aligned}n_{0*}(p) &= \textstyle\sum_i I(Z_i = p, S_i^{obs} = 0, Y_i^{obs} \text{ does not exist})\\ n_{10}(p) &= \textstyle\sum_i I(Z_i = p, S_i^{obs} = 1, Y_i^{obs} = 0)\\ n_{11}(p) &= \textstyle\sum_i I(Z_i = p, S_i^{obs} = 1, Y_i^{obs} = 1)\end{aligned}$$

$$\begin{aligned}n_{0*}(v) &= \textstyle\sum_i I(Z_i = v, S_i^{obs} = 0, Y_i^{obs} \text{ does not exist})\\ n_{10}(v) &= \textstyle\sum_i I(Z_i = v, S_i^{obs} = 1, Y_i^{obs} = 0)\\ n_{11}(v) &= \textstyle\sum_i I(Z_i = v, S_i^{obs} = 1, Y_i^{obs} = 1)\end{aligned}$$

where the summations are over $i = 1,\ldots,n$. The double subscripts for the ns do not have the same meaning as for the ϕs and θs. Assume that each of the six combinations is observed at least once. Let $n(p) = n_{0*}(p) + n_{10}(p) + n_{11}(p)$ and $n(v) = n_{0*}(v) + n_{10}(v) + n_{11}(v)$ denote the number of individuals assigned to placebo and vaccine. Let $n_{1\cdot}(p) = n_{10}(p) + n_{11}(p)$ and $n_{1\cdot}(v) = n_{10}(v) + n_{11}(v)$ denote the number of infected individuals assigned placebo and vaccine. Let

$$AR_z = \frac{n_{1\cdot}(z)}{n(z)} \text{ for } z = v,p,$$

ie, AR_z is the observed attack rate in the group assigned treatment z. Finally, let

$$PAR_z = \frac{n_{11}(z)}{n_{1\cdot}(z)} \text{ for } z = v, p,$$

ie, PAR_z is the observed post-infection attack rate in the group infected given treatment z.

Maximum likelihood estimators (MLEs) of the identifiable vaccine efficacy estimands can be found by maximizing the likelihood

$$L(\theta, \gamma, \phi) \propto \prod_{i=1}^{n} \Pr[Y_i^{obs} = y_i, S_i^{obs} = s_i | Z_i = z_i; \theta, \gamma, \phi],$$

subject to constraints on θ, γ, ϕ that ensure (9.12–9.14) are probability functions. Hudgens and Halloran (2006) show that the MLE of VE_S is given by

$$\widehat{\text{VE}}_S = \begin{cases} 1 - \frac{AR_v}{AR_p} & \text{if } AR_v \leq AR_p, \\ 0 & \text{otherwise.} \end{cases} \tag{9.16}$$

This is the usual estimator of VE_S based on the attack rates, or cumulative incidence. Furthermore, the MLE of VE_P^{net} is

$$\widehat{\text{VE}}_P^{net} = 1 - \frac{PAR_v}{PAR_p}, \tag{9.17}$$

the same as in equations (9.1), (9.2), and (9.6). The MLE of VE_I^{ITT} is

$$\widehat{\text{VE}}_P^{ITT} = 1 - (1 - \widehat{\text{VE}}_S) \frac{PAR_v}{PAR_p}, \tag{9.18}$$

or equivalently

$$\widehat{\text{VE}}_P^{ITT} = \begin{cases} \widehat{\text{VE}}_P^{net} & \text{if } \widehat{\text{VE}}_S = 0, \\ 1 - \frac{n_{11}(v)/n(v)}{n_{11}(p)/n(p)} & \text{if } \widehat{\text{VE}}_S > 0, \end{cases} \tag{9.19}$$

analogous to equation (9.8). In summary, the three MLEs $\widehat{\text{VE}}_S$, $\widehat{\text{VE}}_P^{net}$, and $\widehat{\text{VE}}_P^{ITT}$ derived formally by the methods of causal inference correspond to the usual estimators associated with these measures as in equation (9.8).

The causal estimand VE_P is not identifiable because $\phi_{\cdot 1}$, the denominator of the right side of (9.15), is not identifiable. On the other hand, $\phi_{1\cdot}$, the numerator of the right side of (9.15), can be identified by the observable random variables. The corresponding MLE is given by

$$\widehat{\phi}_{1\cdot} = PAR_v, \tag{9.20}$$

ie, the observed post-infection attack rate in the vaccine arm. Finally, although $\phi_{.1}$ is not identifiable, we can identify

$$\Pr[Y(p)=1|S(p)=1;\theta,\gamma,\phi]=\gamma_1\mathrm{VE}_S+\phi_{.1}(1-\mathrm{VE}_S). \tag{9.21}$$

The MLE of (9.21) is PAR_p such that any feasible pair $(\widehat{\gamma}_1,\widehat{\phi}_{.1})$ satisfying

$$PAR_p=\widehat{\gamma}_1\widehat{\mathrm{VE}}_S+\widehat{\phi}_{.1}(1-\widehat{\mathrm{VE}}_S), \tag{9.22}$$

is an MLE of $(\gamma_1,\phi_{.1})$.

9.4.3 Applications

9.4.3.1 Rotavirus candidate vaccine

In the rotavirus candidate vaccine study (Vesikari et al 1990), the observed data were

$$\begin{array}{ll} n_{0*}(p)=84 & n_{0*}(v)=90 \\ n_{10}(p)=3 & n_{10}(v)=5 \\ n_{11}(p)=13 & n_{11}(v)=5. \end{array}$$

From (9.16), $\widehat{\mathrm{VE}}_S=1-(10/100)/(16/100)=0.375$. It then follows from (9.19) that $\widehat{\mathrm{VE}}_P^{ITT}=1-(5/100)/(13/100)=0.62$. The post-infection attack rates are $\mathrm{PAR}_v=\widehat{\phi}^{1\cdot}=5/10=0.50$ and $\mathrm{PAR}_p=13/16=0.81$ such that $\widehat{\mathrm{VE}}_P^{net}=1-(5/10)/(13/16)=0.385$, as in Section 9.2.3.

To consider estimation of the causal VE_P, we examine the relation of the observed data to the basic principal strata and the strata of joint potential post-infection outcomes within each basic principal stratum. By the assumptions of SUTVA, independence, and monotonicity, we know the following:

- All $n_{10}(v)+n_{11}(v)=10$ belong to the doomed stratum $S^{P_0}=(1,1)$.
- All $n_{0*}(p)=84$ belong to the immune stratum $S^{P_0}=(0,0)$.
- The $n_{0*}(v)=90$ could belong to the immune stratum $S^{P_0}=(0,0)$ or the protected stratum $S^{P_0}=(0,1)$.
- The $n_{10}(p)+n_{11}(p)=16$ could belong to the protected $S^{P_0}=(0,1)$ or the doomed $S^{P_0}=(1,1)$.

Ignoring statistical variability, by the independence assumption, because there are 10 vaccine recipients in the doomed stratum, there are 10 placebo recipients in the doomed stratum. Because there are 84 placebo recipients in the immune stratum, there are 84 vaccine recipients in the immune stratum. So there must be 6 from each of the vaccinated and unvaccinated groups in the protected stratum. Thus, we can estimate the size of the unobserved principal stratum $S^{P_0}=(0,1)$. However, we do not know which 6 of the 16 infected placebo recipients are in protected stratum $S^{P_0}=(0,1)$ or which 10 of the 16 are in the doomed stratum $S^{P_0}=(1,1)$. Why do we care?

Because to estimate the causal VE_P, we need to know the post-infection outcomes of those in the doomed stratum. This illustrates the need for further assumptions to identify VE_P.

9.4.3.2 Pertussis vaccine

The pertussis vaccine analysis presented in Section 9.2 included exactly one year of follow-up, the calendar year 1993, so the person-years at risk are a close approximation to the number of persons at risk. Thus, we use the person-years at risk for $n(v)$ and $n(p)$. During that one calendar year, there were 3845 and 1020 person-years at risk in the vaccinated and unvaccinated children. Using slightly different inclusion criteria for cases than in Section 9.2, of 548 cases in the vaccinated group, 176 were severe, and of 206 cases in the unvaccinated group, 129 were severe. Based on equation (9.5), $\widehat{\mathrm{VE}}_P = 0.49$ (95% CI, 0.40–0.56). Although vaccine status was not randomized, there was no evidence of systematic differences between the vaccinated and unvaccinated groups, so that the independence assumption might be reasonable. The observed data are

$$\begin{array}{ll} n_{0*}(p) = 814 & n_{0*}(v) = 3297 \\ n_{10}(p) = 77 & n_{10}(v) = 372 \\ n_{11}(p) = 129 & n_{11}(v) = 176. \end{array}$$

From (9.16), $\widehat{\mathrm{VE}}_S = 1 - (548/3845)/(206/1020) = 0.29$. The post-infection attack rates are $\mathrm{PAR}_v = \widehat{\phi^{1\cdot}} = 176/548 = 0.32$ and $\mathrm{PAR}_p = 129/206 = 0.63$ such that $\widehat{\mathrm{VE}_P^{net}} = 1 - (176/548)/(129/206) = 0.49$, which is the same as $\widehat{\mathrm{VE}}_P$ yielded by using (9.5). Finally $\widehat{\mathrm{VE}_P^{ITT}} = 1 - (176/3845)/(129/1020) = 0.64$, which in Préziosi and Halloran (2003a) was $\widehat{\mathrm{VE}}_{SP}$ for severity.

9.4.4 Selection bias models

The inability to identify the causal VE_P is due to $\phi_{\cdot 1}$ and γ_1 not being separated in the term

$$\theta_{01}\gamma_1 + \theta_{11}\phi_{\cdot 1} = \Pr[Y^{obs} = 1, S^{obs} = 1 | Z^{obs} = p]. \tag{9.23}$$

For any fixed values of θ_{01}, θ_{11}, and $\Pr[Y^{obs} = 1, S^{obs} = 1 | Z^{obs} = p]$ all pairs of parameters

$$\{(\gamma_1, \phi_{\cdot 1}) : 0 \le \gamma_1 \le 1, 0 \le \phi_{\cdot 1} \le 1, \text{ and (9.23) holds}\}, \tag{9.24}$$

will yield the same distribution of (Z, S^{obs}, Y^{obs}). The selection models presented in this section place additional constraints on the parameter space such that only one pair of parameters satisfies (9.24).

9.4.4.1 No selection bias

The assumption of no selection implies that the probability of the post-infection outcome conditional on infection under placebo is independent of infection status under vaccine:

$$\Pr\{Y(p) = y|S^{P_0} = (1,1);\phi\} = \Pr\{Y(p) = y|S^{P_0} = (0,1);\gamma\} \quad \text{for } y = 0,1, \tag{9.25}$$

which implies $\phi_{\cdot 1} = \gamma_1$. Under assumption (9.25), from (9.22), the resulting MLE is

$$\widehat{\phi}_{\cdot 1} = \mathrm{PAR}_p. \tag{9.26}$$

From (9.20), (9.26), and the definition of VE_P given by (9.15), it follows that the MLE of the causal VE_P equals $\widehat{\mathrm{VE}}_P^{net}$ as given in (9.17). In other words, under the additional assumption of no selection bias as specified by (9.25), the MLE of the causal vaccine effect is the usual post-infection attack rate ratio estimator one obtains when conditioning on infection as in equations (9.1) and (9.2).

9.4.4.2 Upper and lower bounds

The upper bound selection model yields the parameter pair $(\gamma_1, \phi_{\cdot 1})$ consistent with the observed data that has the largest $\phi_{\cdot 1}$, thus largest VE_P. Because (9.24) is simply the intersection of the unit square and a line with negative slope, it follows that the pair with maximal $\phi_{\cdot 1}$ must be on the edge of the square, ie, when either of the following conditions holds:

$$\Pr[Y(p) = 1|S^{P_0} = (1,1)] = \phi_{\cdot 1} = 1, \tag{9.27}$$

$$\Pr[Y(p) = 1|S^{P_0} = (0,1)] = \gamma_1 = 0. \tag{9.28}$$

In words, the upper bound selection bias model assumes either (i) all placebo recipients in the doomed principal stratum have the worse post-infection outcome or (ii) all placebo recipients in the protected principal stratum have the better post-infection outcome. From (9.22) it follows that the unique MLE of VE_P assuming either (9.27) or (9.28) is given by:

$$\widehat{\mathrm{VE}}_P^{upper} = \begin{cases} 1 - PAR_v & \text{if } \widehat{\mathrm{VE}}_S > 1 - PAR_p, \\ \widehat{\mathrm{VE}}_P^{ITT} & \text{if } 0 < \widehat{\mathrm{VE}}_S \le 1 - PAR_p, \\ \widehat{\mathrm{VE}}_P^{net} & \text{if } \widehat{\mathrm{VE}}_S = 0. \end{cases} \tag{9.29}$$

All MLEs obtained under the three key assumptions must be less than or equal to $\widehat{\mathrm{VE}}_P^{upper}$.

Similarly, the lower bound selection bias model assumes that under assignment to placebo, the worse post-infection outcome occurs either with probability zero in the doomed principal stratum,

$$\Pr[Y(p)=1|S^{P_0}=(1,1)]=\phi_{\cdot 1}=0, \tag{9.30}$$

or with probability one in the protected principal stratum,

$$\Pr[Y(p)=1|S^{P_0}=(0,1)]=\gamma_1=1. \tag{9.31}$$

The resulting unique MLE of VE_P is

$$\widehat{\text{VE}}_P^{lower} = \begin{cases} -\infty & \text{if } \widehat{\text{VE}}_S > PAR_p, \\ 1-PAR_v/\left\{\frac{PAR_p-\widehat{\text{VE}}_S}{1-\widehat{\text{VE}}_S}\right\} & \text{if } 0<\widehat{\text{VE}}_S \le PAR_p, \\ \widehat{\text{VE}}_P^{net} & \text{if } \widehat{\text{VE}}_S = 0. \end{cases} \tag{9.32}$$

Hudgens and Halloran (2006) derived the circumstances when the upper bound will be negative (suggesting harm) and when the lower bound will be positive (suggesting benefit). For example, $\widehat{\text{VE}}_P^{upper}$ will be negative if and only if $\widehat{\text{VE}}_S \le 1-PAR_p$ and $\widehat{\text{VE}}_P^{ITT} < 0$. Similarly, $\widehat{\text{VE}}_P^{lower}$ will be positive if and only if $\widehat{\text{VE}}_S \le PAR_p$ and $PAR_v < (PAR_p-\widehat{\text{VE}}_S)/(1-\widehat{\text{VE}}_S)$. On the other hand, for $\widehat{\text{VE}}_S > \max\{PAR_p, 1-PAR_p\}$, $\widehat{\text{VE}}_P^{upper}$ will be always positive and $\widehat{\text{VE}}_P^{lower}$ will be always negative. In other words, for large enough $\widehat{\text{VE}}_S$ the sign of VE_P cannot be determined unless further assumptions are made beyond SUTVA, independence, and monotonicity.

9.4.4.3 Sensitivity analysis for selection bias

Hudgens and Halloran (2006) present three approaches to sensitivity analysis that allow selection models to range from no selection to the extreme maximum possible levels.

9.4.4.4 Log odds ratio of infection

The first approach is similar to that of Scharfstein et al (1999) and Robins et al (2000b). The sensitivity model is defined in terms of the log odds ratio of having the severe post-infection endpoint under placebo in the doomed versus protected principal strata:

$$\exp(\beta)=\frac{\Pr[Y(p)=1|S^{P_0}=(1,1)]/\Pr[Y(p)=0|S^{P_0}=(1,1)]}{\Pr[Y(p)=1|S^{P_0}=(0,1)]/\Pr[Y(p)=0|S^{P_0}=(0,1)]}. \tag{9.33}$$

For example, if $\exp(\beta) = 2$, then doomed individuals have twice the odds of having the worse post-infection outcome under placebo compared to protected individuals. In terms of this parameterization, this implies

$$\phi_{\cdot 1} = \frac{\gamma_1 \exp(\beta)}{\gamma_0 + \gamma_1 \exp(\beta)}. \tag{9.34}$$

For fixed β, one can solve equations (9.22) and (9.34) for $\phi_{\cdot 1}$ and, in turn, VE_P. The sensitivity analysis is done by repeating this process over a range of different βs. The bounds are given above.

9.4.4.5 Conditioning on γ_1 as the sensitivity analysis parameter

The second approach to a sensitivity analysis conditions on the nuisance parameter γ_1 which governs the post-infection endpoint distribution in the protected stratum. If γ_1 is assumed known, from (9.22), the resulting MLE of VE_P is

$$\widehat{\mathrm{VE}}_P = 1 - PAR_v / \left\{ \frac{PAR_p - \gamma_1 \widehat{\mathrm{VE}}_S}{1 - \widehat{\mathrm{VE}}_S} \right\}, \tag{9.35}$$

where γ_1 varies between

$$\max\left\{0, \frac{PAR_p - (1 - \widehat{\mathrm{VE}}_S)}{\widehat{\mathrm{VE}}_S}\right\} \le \gamma_1 \le \min\left\{1, \frac{PAR_p}{\widehat{\mathrm{VE}}_S}\right\}, \tag{9.36}$$

with the left side of (9.36) giving rise to $\widehat{\mathrm{VE}}_P^{upper}$ and the right side of (9.36) giving rise to $\widehat{\mathrm{VE}}_P^{lower}$.

9.4.4.6 Complete data model

The third approach to sensitivity analysis regards the unknown basic principal stratum membership of the infected placebo recipients as missing data and formulates the sensitivity analysis in terms of the complete data likelihood. The observed data are $n_{10}(p)$ and $n_{11}(p)$. If we could know the basic principal stratum membership, the complete data would be $n^d_{10}(p)$ and $n^d_{11}(p)$, the number of infected placebo recipients in the doomed stratum with $Y(p) = 0$ and $Y(p) = 1$, and $n^p_{10}(p)$ and $n^p_{11}(p)$, the corresponding number in the protected stratum. Given the complete data, $\phi_{\cdot 1}$ becomes identifiable. Maximizing the complete data log-likelihood for (θ, ϕ, γ) yields the MLE

$$\widehat{\phi_{\cdot 1}} = \frac{n^d_{11}(p)}{n^d_{10}(p) + n^d_{11}(p)}, \tag{9.37}$$

the post-infection attack rate under placebo in the doomed stratum. The sensitivity analysis involves estimating VE_P using (9.37) for all possible complete data configurations consistent with the assumptions and the constraints implied by the observed data. Molenberghs et al (2001) call this set of point estimates the *region of ignorance*. They call the collection of confidence intervals (CIs) or other measures of precision together with the region of ignorance the *region of uncertainty*.

9.4.4.7 Statistical variability

Once a particular selection model has been assumed, it becomes a finite-dimensional parametric inference problem with a unique MLE. Conditional on a selection model, standard methods can be used to obtain CI estimates for VE_P. For example, CIs can be computed assuming the usual χ^2 limiting distribution of the profile likelihood ratio (Barndorff-Nielsen and Cox, 1994). Alternatively, using the observed information and the delta method, Wald-type CIs for VE_P can be determined. The resulting CIs can then be used to determine a region of uncertainty for any of the sensitivity analyses described above. A region of uncertainty that excludes zero implies a statistically significant post-infection causal effect of the vaccine.

9.4.4.8 Applications, continued

9.4.4.9 Rotavirus candidate vaccine

For these data, $\widehat{\mathrm{VE}}_S > 1 - PAR_p$, so from (9.29), $\widehat{\mathrm{VE}}_P^{upper} = 1 - PAR_v = 0.50$. On the other hand, $0 < \widehat{\mathrm{VE}}_S \leq PAR_p$, so from (9.32),

$$\widehat{\mathrm{VE}}_P^{lower} = 1 - \frac{5/10}{\frac{\{13/16-(1-(10/100)(16/100))\}}{(10/100)/(16/100)}} = 0.29.$$

Figure 9.3a shows the sensitivity analysis of $\widehat{\mathrm{VE}}_P$ as a function of the odds ratio e^{β}. For this figure, profile likelihood-based CIs are presented. Wald-type CIs give qualitatively similar results. The vertical dotted line in Figure 9.3 corresponds to the assumption of no selection bias. The lack of statistical significance in this example may be due simply to small sample size. If the study had had 1000 participants in each arm with the same observed marginal distributions, then the 95% CI for VE_P under the lower bound model would have been [0.09, 0.46], indicating a significant causal vaccine effect on rotavirus disease severity in individuals who would have been infected under assignment to either vaccine or control.

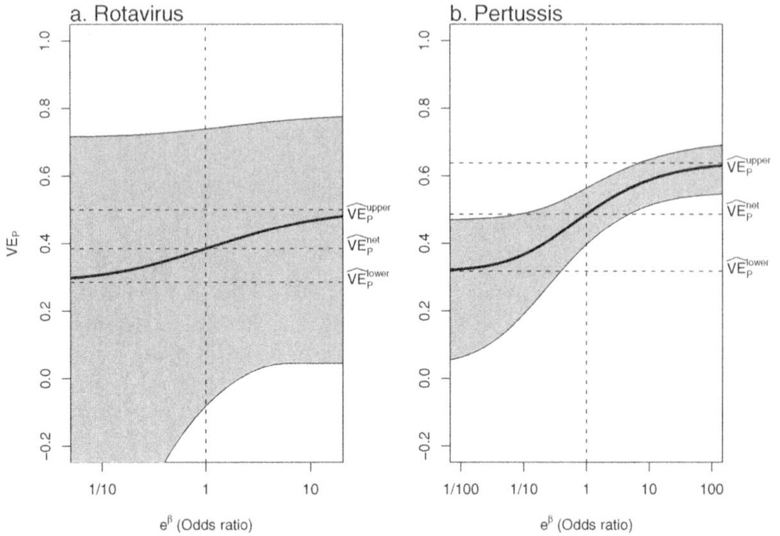

Fig. 9.3 Sensitivity analysis using the odds ratio of having the severe post-infection endpoint under placebo in the doomed versus protected principal strata: (a) rotavirus; (b) pertussis. The vertical dotted line corresponds to the assumption of no selection bias (from Hudgens and Halloran 2006, Journal of the American Statistical Association, 101:51-64. Reprinted with permission).

9.4.4.10 Pertussis vaccine

For the pertussis vaccine data, $0 \leq \widehat{\text{VE}}_S \leq 1 - PAR_p$, so from (9.29), $\widehat{\text{VE}}_P^{upper} = \widehat{\text{VE}}_P^{ITT} = 0.64$. On the other hand, $0 \leq \widehat{\text{VE}}_S \leq PAR_p$, so from (9.32), $\widehat{\text{VE}}_P^{lower} = 0.32$. Figure 9.3b shows the sensitivity analysis of $\widehat{\text{VE}}_P$ as a function of the odds ratio e^β. The lower limit of the 95% CIs are well above zero over the range of the selection model, suggesting pertussis vaccination causes significant protection against severe disease in children who would develop pertussis regardless of vaccination status.

Problems

9.1. In a study of the effect of varicella vaccine (Vazquez et al 2001), of the 56 vaccinated children with chickenpox, 48 had mild disease. Of the 187 unvaccinated children with chickenpox, 89 had mild disease. A case-control study conducted concurrently estimated VE_S against clinical chickenpox to be 0.85 (95% CI 0.78 to 0.90). Compute the VE_P^{net}, VE_P^{ITT}, and the upper and lower bounds on the MLE of the causal VE_P of the varicella vaccine against combined moderate and severe chickenpox.

9.2. In two studies of the influenza antiviral agent oseltamivir (Hayden et al 2004; Welliver et al 2001), because asymptomatic infections, as well as symptomatic disease (Section 10.3.5), had been ascertained in all household contacts of index cases, it was possible to estimate the influenza pathogenicity and the antiviral efficacy in reducing pathogenicity, AVE_P. In the contacts receiving prophylaxis, 10 symptomatic cases occurred in 46 infected people. In the contacts not receiving prophylaxis, 33 symptomatic cases occurred in 75 infected people (Halloran et al 2007a). Compute the pathogenicity of the influenza virus in the two groups and the efficacy of post-exposure prophylaxis against pathogenicity, AVE_P.

9.3. (a) Write out the complete data log-likehood discussed in the third approach to sensitivity analysis in Section 9.4.4.6.
(b) How many complete-data configurations are there for the rotavirus example?
(c) What are the different values of $\widehat{VE}_P$ corresponding to those configurations?
(d) The sensitivity analysis for the pertussis vaccine data using the complete data likelihood would proceed similarly as for the rotavirus vaccine candidate. However, there are many more possible data configurations and the unequal sizes of the vaccinated and unvaccinated arms need to be taken into account. Sketch out the sensitivity analysis using the complete data approach for the pertussis vaccine example.

9.4. (a) What is the range for γ_1 in the rotavirus vaccine example? in the pertussis vaccine example?
(b) Produce a graph of VE_P over the range of γ_1 for the rotavirus vaccine example and for the pertussis vaccine example. Mark VE^{upper}, VE^{lower}, and VE^{net}, and the γ_1 corresponding to the assumption of no selection bias.

Chapter 10
Household-Based Studies

10.1 Concepts of Household Studies

In Chapter 2 we introduced vaccine efficacy parameters that require conditioning on exposure to infection. Household studies were used as the basis for defining exposure to infection in vaccine studies as early as the 1930s in evaluating the efficacy of pertussis vaccines (Kendrick and Eldering 1939). In addition to evaluating vaccine efficacy, household studies have been used to learn about transmission and natural history of many infections. Aspects of the natural history studied in households include the transmissibility, the incubation and latent periods, the duration of infectiousness, and the serial interval between cases (Hope-Simpson 1952; Bailey 1957). Household studies have also been used to evaluate other interventions, such as post-exposure prophylaxis with influenza antiviral agents (Welliver et al 2001; Hayden et al 2004). Exposure to an infectious case within a household can be used as a natural challenge study, for example, when studying immunological correlates of protection (Storsaeter et al 1998). Longitudinal studies of pneumococcal carriage in households and schools have been used to estimate the acquisition and clearance rates for asymptomatic pneumococcal carriage.

The general idea of a transmission unit is that individuals make contact sufficient for transmission within it. Households are the most common form of transmission unit used in studies. It allows easy identification of contacts between a case and susceptibles, and families are convenient units of study. Many other settings are also used as transmission units in studies and analyses that condition on exposure to infection. These include sexual partnerships, classrooms, schools, school buses, airplanes, day care centers, and workplaces, among others. Here we talk mostly about household studies, but many of the study designs and analyses are applicable with possibly slight modification to other transmission units as well. The term household is much easier for exposition than is "transmission unit".

Historically the use of household studies to evaluate vaccine effects focused on evaluating the protective effects of vaccination. The relative risk of developing illness in vaccinated compared to unvaccinated susceptibles exposed to cases in their

M.E. Halloran et al., *Design and Analysis of Vaccine Studies*, Statistics for Biology and Health, DOI 10.1007/978-0-387-68636-3_10,

household was the basis of estimating the protective effects. In recent years, the vaccine effect on the ability to transmit the infection in vaccinated infected people compared to unvaccinated infected people, VE_I, has gained attention. In contrast to protective effects, VE_I generally needs contact and exposure to infection information for its evaluation. An additional measure of interest is the overall reduction in transmission if both the infective person and the susceptible person who make contact are vaccinated compared to if neither is vaccinated, VE_T. The analysis is often based on the relative secondary attack rate (SAR), between the vaccinated and unvaccinated individuals of interest. The SAR is a special case of the transmission probability. The secondary attack rate is the probability that an individual infects another person during some period of time. The secondary attack rate can be estimated from the proportion of susceptibles who become infected when exposed to an infectious person. In the secondary attack rate, the contact between the infectious susceptible persons may be defined as occurring over some time period, such as the duration of infectiousness, or over the period of the study. For example, the *household SAR* is the probability that a susceptible individual living in the same household with an infectious person during his or her period of infectiousness will become infected (Fine et al 1988; Orenstein et al 1988).

Considering the estimates of VE based on the relative secondary attack rates, there are three main unstratified vaccine effects:

$$\begin{aligned} VE_{S.1/.0} &= 1 - \frac{SAR_{.1}}{SAR_{.0}}, \qquad VE_{I1./0.} = 1 - \frac{SAR_{1.}}{SAR_{0.}}, \\ VE_T &= 1 - \frac{SAR_{11}}{SAR_{00}}. \end{aligned} \tag{10.1}$$

If one stratifies on the vaccine status of the infective person or the susceptible person, then there are four further stratified measures of VE_S and VE_I:

$$\begin{aligned} VE_{S01/00} &= 1 - \frac{SAR_{01}}{SAR_{00}}, \qquad VE_{S11/10} = 1 - \frac{SAR_{11}}{SAR_{10}}, \\ VE_{I10/00} &= 1 - \frac{SAR_{10}}{SAR_{00}}, \qquad VE_{I11/01} = 1 - \frac{SAR_{11}}{SAR_{01}}. \end{aligned} \tag{10.2}$$

Equations (10.1) and (10.2) give the three main unstratified and three stratified vaccine effects conditional on exposure to infection data, conditional on exposure to infection. The vaccine efficacies in (10.1) and (10.2) could also be defined in terms of the relative transmission probabilities or transmission rates.

Despite being widespread for some infections such as pertussis, household studies of vaccine effects have not generally been used for primary licensure efficacy trials. Household studies are sometimes nested within randomized controlled studies and provide secondary analyses. The primary analysis is generally based on one of the unconditional measures of vaccine efficacy, such as $VE_{S,IR}$ or $VE_{S,CI}$. When an exposure is determined to have occurred, for instance, when a sibling of a vaccine study participant has a case of pertussis, then the outcomes are evaluated in a secondary analysis. Household studies are also used in observational evaluation of vaccines. In observational studies, evaluating vaccine efficacy under conditions of household exposure can help reduce bias generated by unequal exposure in vaccinated and unvaccinated people.

In this and the following two chapters, we consider household studies not only for evaluating vaccine effects, but in a broader context. Some of these concepts may be useful for future vaccine studies. The household- and school-based pneumococcal carriage studies were conducted as a prelude to the introduction of pneumococcal vaccines. Similar studies are now being prepared by the MenAfriCar Consortium to anticipation of introducing the meningococcal A vaccine in the meningitis belt in Africa. This chapter provides several examples of household studies and discusses general design considerations. Design considerations include how the households are ascertained, whether the cases are ascertained on infection status or symptomatic cases, and whether the studies are randomized or observational. The data structure and follow-up period can depend on whether the infection results in immunity that lasts at least as long as the study period, such as in influenza, colds, or measles, or whether a person can experience repeated episodes of infection, carriage or disease during the study, such as pneumococcal nasopharyngeal carriage. In many analyses of household studies, the households are assumed to be independent of one another, so that susceptible contacts are assumed exposed only by the first case within the household. When the statistical model assumes that the households are embedded within a community, the analysis allows estimation of the risk of being infected in the community as well as the risk of infection by exposure to a case within the household and the vaccine effects at both levels. Chapters 11 and 12 cover methods of analysis in more detail. Chapter 11 presents several methods for analyzing data assuming that households are embedded in communities. Chapter 12 presents methods of analysis assuming that households are independent.

We introduce a few terms that are used. The *index case* in a household is the case that draws attention to the household and leads to ascertainment of the household. The index case is often, but not necessarily, temporally the first, that is, the *primary case* in the household. A case that occurs too soon after the primary case to have resulted from infection by the primary case is called a *co-primary case*.

10.2 Pertussis Vaccination

10.2.1 History

Household exposure studies have long been used to evaluate pertussis vaccination. Pertussis vaccines were developed in the 1920s and the first hopeful results were observed in the Faroe Islands in the early 1920s (Madsen 1933; Medical Research Council 1951). Most pertussis vaccines were based on killed whole cells until the 1980s. Concern about efficacy and adverse effects of whole cell pertussis vaccines resulted in some countries stopping to recommend their use. For example, Sweden completely discontinued pertussis vaccination in 1979 because the efficacy seemed to be negligible (Trollfors and Rabo 1981). A new generation of acellular vaccines was developed as an alternative to the killed whole cell ones. In the 1980s and early 1990s, considerable interest in evaluating the relative efficacy of the two types generated a number of papers on how methodological compared to biological effects of vaccines affected the efficacy estimates. Fine and Clarkson (1987) and Fine et al (1988) give a thoughtful review of sources of variability in pertussis vaccine efficacy estimates. They compare estimates based on controlled trials, cohort studies, case-control studies, and secondary attack rate studies. Efficacy estimates were often lower in household studies, possibly due to more intense and prolonged exposure.

In countries that did not recommend pertussis vaccination, trials of the efficacy of the new vaccines could be conducted with a placebo arm. In countries that recommended use of the whole cell pertussis vaccines, it was unethical to have a placebo arm, and the whole cell and acellular vaccines had to be compared head to head. Children not in the study who were not vaccinated could be followed and provide an unvaccinated study arm as part of an observational study. Pertussis vaccine is generally combined with the diphtheria and tetanus toxoids and given three to four times early in the first year of life. The vaccine combination without the pertussis component is denoted DT, and with it is denoted DTP. We present several examples of pertussis vaccine studies in households.

10.2.2 Michigan, USA

Kendrick and Eldering (1939) report on a study of pertussis immunization in children between 8 months and <5 years (<6 years for a short time at the beginning) in Grand Rapids, Michigan, USA, and surrounding areas from March 1, 1934 to November 1, 1937. Although the study was not randomized, efforts were made to create a control group comparable to the test group. Children receiving the vaccine were self-selecting. They obtained the vaccine by presenting themselves at the city immunization clinics. As children were immunized, comparable children were selected at random from a population-based roster to match the vaccinated children on age and district. House visits were made by nurses to all participants initially at three- to four-month intervals, but after November 1935 at two-month intervals. Public health and other sources of reports of whooping cough cases were followed up as well.

The diagnoses in the study were primarily based on detailed clinical histories. Kendrick and Eldering discuss the difficulties associated with diagnosing an attack of pertussis with certainty, particularly one in which the usually accepted clinical criteria are lacking or at least not prominent. The difficulty of choosing the best case definition for pertussis persists even today.

The main analysis was based on the relative number of cases per person-years at risk in the vaccinated group compared with the control group (Figure 1.2 and equation (2.3)). However "from the beginning, one important objective in the study was to obtain as exact information as possible with regard to exposures to pertussis and subsequent related attacks" (Kendrick and Eldering 1939, page 146). They had clearly established definitions of exposures. To be considered an exposure, the source case of the exposure had to have a written case history with diagnosis made on the same basis as the study participants. The contact had to be recorded. Different levels of exposure were defined. The levels of exposure were (1) definite in their own household, (2) definite in other households, (3) indefinite, and (4) no exposure history. To be considered definite, an exposure had to occur within 21 days of onset of the source case. A maximum incubation period of 30 days was assumed. Definite exposures in other households had to be of at least 30 minutes duration. Indefinite exposures could occur under less intimate conditions, such as outdoors or after the 21st day, but no later than the 35th day of onset of the source case. The data are shown in Figure 1.3 and the vaccine efficacy estimate based on definite household exposure is in equation (2.4).

10.2.3 Niakhar, Senegal

Active population surveillance has been conducted since 1983 in Niakhar, Senegal, a sub-Saharan rural community of 30 villages. The community is very homogeneous, composed of Sereer peasant families, living in compounds, the residential unit for extended families. As part of many research components (Garenne and Cantrelle 1998), pertussis was under prospective and active surveillance (Préziosi et al 2002). As a result, information for each child was available not only on pertussis illnesses and vaccination but also on contacts. Extended families were under longitudinal observation beginning in March 1983, based on annual visits, and from 1987 to 1996, based on weekly visits to each compound. In addition, during pertussis vaccine trials 1990–1996 comparing whole cell to acellular vaccine, physicians collected biological samples from consenting suspected cases in the entire population, defined as having a cough lasting eight days or more. The pertussis vaccine studies were in accordance with the Helsinki Declaration (Préziosi et al 1997). The children who did not receive vaccination in the trials were under active surveillance as well. Samples included nasopharyngeal aspirates for isolating the bacteria and to detect DNA using PCR. Acute and convalescent blood samples were drawn to measure IgG titers to pertussis toxin (PT) or filamentous hemagglutinin (FHA) by ELISA. Surveillance for pertussis focused on children under age 15 years. All suspected cases and their co-residents were followed actively by a physician. The usual demographic data, including age, gender, hut, compound, hamlet, and village were known for each child in the area. Pertussis vaccination status and dates of vaccination were also known. The primary analysis of the efficacy trials was based on unconditional vaccine efficacy estimators (Simondon et al 1997).

For each suspected case, the date of symptom onset, duration of cough, type of cough, a wide range of symptoms, results of each biological diagnostic test done, and physician diagnosis were recorded. Focusing on the year 1993, an epidemic year that produced a large number of cases and extensive exposure to pertussis, Prézios and Halloran (2003b) and Halloran, et al (2003b) analyzed the data to estimate not only VE_S but also VE_I and VE_T for pertussis. Prézios and Halloran (2003b) considered a number of different case definitions and the relation to estimated VE_S, VE_I, and VE_T. Halloran et al (2003b) considered different statistical methods for the secondary attack rate analysis (see Chapter 12.3) using just one case definition. In the latter paper, a case of pertussis was defined as requiring clinically, at least 21 days of cough with paroxysms and biologicially, either *B. pertussis* isolated from a nasopharyngeal aspirate or significant increase or decrease in PT or FHA antibodies as measured by ELISA or presence of a bacteriologically confirmed case in the same compound within 28 days. The latter criterion is called an epilink.

Préziosi and Halloran (2003b) chose the compound as the transmission unit within which it was assumed that susceptibles were exposed to infection by the first case in the unit. The compound is the "home", ie, the residential unit where individuals make privileged contacts and where random mixing is a reasonable assumption. The compound is the transmission unit of choice in some African rural settings (Garenne et al 1993; Aaby et al 1996).

A potentially infectious contact, or exposure, was defined as a susceptible living in the same compound during the infectious period of the index case. Exposed susceptibles were children with no history of pertussis living in a compound with an index case. Onset of pertussis symptoms was assumed to be the onset of infectiousness, thus the latent period equals the incubation period. Co-primaries were those cases whose onset of cough was <7 days after that of the index case, assumed to be too soon after the index case to have been infected by the index case. To allow for uncertainty in duration of infectiousness, a secondary case was defined as a case whose date of onset was ≥ 7 days after that of the index case and less than a variable cutoff, specifically no cutoff, 56, 42, or 28 days.

Generally, when estimating protective efficacy, VE_S, from SARs, co-primaries are simply ignored in the analysis, entering as neither susceptibles nor infectives (Orenstein, et al 1988; Fine et al 1988). However, the particular interest here was in the effect of vaccine status on infectiousness of the index case. Because primaries and co-primaries often had different vaccine status, compounds with co-primaries were excluded from the analysis. Chu et al (2004) developed MCMC methods to estimate heterogeneous transmission with multiple infectives.

A total of 518 of the 1800 compounds (29%) were detected as having potential cases of pertussis in 1993. In 189 (36%) of those compounds, pertussis was confirmed. They represented 232 primary and co-primary cases and 1217 susceptibles. Among those were excluded compounds with co-primary cases ($n = 33$ [17%]), compounds with no susceptibles ($n = 5$ [3%]), and compounds with a partially vaccinated primary case ($n = 42$ [22%]). Thus a total of 109/189 (58%) of the qualifying compounds were eligible for analysis. The 109 compounds represented 109 primary cases and 790 susceptibles, of whom 152 (19%) were partially vaccinated and 638 (81%) were either unvaccinated or completely vaccinated. Table 10.1 gives the data and SARs using different cutoffs. The result of at least one biological confirmation criterion was available in over 97% of the suspected cases meeting the clinical def-

Table 10.1 Number of exposed susceptibles, secondary pertussis cases, and secondary attack rates (SAR) by pertussis vaccination status of the index case and the exposed susceptible children and cutoff for counting secondary cases (Halloran et al 2003b)

	Exposed Susceptibles and Secondary Cases					
	Vaccinated		Unvaccinated		Combined	
Index Case	Cases/Exposed	SAR	Cases/Exposed	SAR	Cases/Exposed	SAR
Vaccinated						
Cutoff: none	11/127	0.09	9/67	0.13	20/194	0.10
56 days	10/127	0.08	6/67	0.09	16/194	0.08
42 days	10/127	0.08	5/67	0.07	15/194	0.08
28 days	3/127	0.02	3/67	0.04	6/194	0.03
Unvaccinated						
Cutoff: none	61/246	0.25	73/198	0.37	134/444	0.30
56 days	55/246	0.22	67/198	0.34	122/444	0.27
42 days	52/246	0.21	66/198	0.33	118/444	0.27
28 days	41/246	0.17	52/198	0.26	93/444	0.21
Combined						
Cutoff: none	72/373	0.19	82/265	0.31	154/638	0.24
56 days	65/373	0.17	73/265	0.28	138/638	0.22
42 days	62/373	0.17	71/265	0.27	133/638	0.21
28 days	44/373	0.11	55/265	0.21	99/638	0.16

inition. From the same study, Préziosi and Halloran (2003a) estimated the effect of pertussis vaccination on clinical severity, VE_P (Chapter 9).

10.2.4 England

During World War II, several investigations were undertaken by the Whooping-cough Immunization Committee of the Medical Research Council to assess the prophylactic value of pertussis vaccination, with disappointing results. Between 1946 and 1950, the committee conducted an essentially randomized, controlled trial in children between 6 and 18 months old when recruited. They tested five batches of vaccine from three manufacturers, two from the Michigan Department of Health, two from Glaxo Laboratories, and one from Parke Davis and Co. in 10 separate field trials (Medical Research Council 1951). Each child in the study was visited monthly by a nurse-investigator. Information was obtained on exposure to pertussis, incidence of upper-respiratory track disease, other immunizations, and other childhood diseases. If it was found by the visit or routine report by the parent that a child had been exposed to pertussis or had developed suspicious symptoms, repeated visits were made, and the mother was asked to take notes as well.

A total of 6710 children completed the trial, with 3358 in the vaccinated and 3352 in the unvaccinated group. In the vaccine group, there were 149 cases in 102,961 child-months at risk, and in the unvaccinated group, there were 687 cases

Table 10.2 Total number of cases of pertussis and secondary attack rates by type of exposure according to vaccine group from the study by the Medical Research Council in England 1946–1950

	Home Exposure			Other Exposure			No
Vaccination Status	No. of Exposures	No. of Cases	Rate (%)	No. of Exposures	No. of Cases	Rate (%)	Exposure History
Vaccinated	203	37	18.2	566	47	8.3	65
Unvaccinated	173	151	87.3	561	213	38.0	323

in 102,180 child-months at risk, a risk ratio of 1 to 4.6. The results give a $VE_{S,IR} = 1 - 1.45/6.72 = 0.78$ (95% CI, 0.74–0.82). Analysis of information on the exposures of children to pertussis was divided into two categories. First, home exposures were children exposed in their own home to one or more siblings, and second, other exposures were children exposed in "day nurseries, in nursery schools, at parties, in cinemas, in buses, and while playing outside the home with other children." In this study, the number of exposures was recorded, not the number of children exposed, as some children were exposed more than once. Table 10.2 gives the summary data, not broken down by the 10 areas and five vaccine batches. When analyzed by vaccine batch, the two vaccines from the Michigan Department of Health gave a considerably greater degree of protection than the other three.

After this study, England continued to monitor efficacy of pertussis vaccine. As the controversy over the vaccine continued, a fresh assessment was made. During an outbreak that began in 1977, from January 1978 through June 1980, England undertook a national assessment of the efficacy of pertussis vaccination in 21 area health authorities (PHLS Epidemiologic Research Laboratory 1982). The 21 areas comprised about one-quarter of the total health authorities in England at that time. Case notification rates for children with three doses of DTP or three doses of DT were studied in that period. The vaccination status both of the population under six years of age and of the notified cases was provided from computer records by each area health authority (AHA). Home visits by nurses and health visitors from the AHA were made to notified cases to assess the severity of the case, the family circumstances, and to take perinasal swabs. Information was collected on age, sex, history of pertussis in the distant past, and history of recent illness that could have been pertussis. Particular attention was given to children under six years of age. A subsequent home visit about six weeks later was also made to record symptoms in contacts under six years. Nurses were asked to report all cases of cough whether or not associated with typical paroxysms. A household contact who developed spasmodic cough was considered a case. The original analysis included only two-child households. About 90% of the notified cases were visited.

In the DTP group, a total of 2261 cases were notified in about 250,163 child-years at risk (0.9%). In the DT group, a total of 9515 cases were notified in 187,595 child-years at risk (5.1%) over the course of the study. Efficacy, $VE_{S,IR}$, based on the total number of cases for each year of birth was greater than 0.80. However,

Table 10.3 Secondary attack rates in home contacts according to age and vaccine group, England (from PHLS Epidemiological Research Laboratory 1982)

Age of Contact (Years)	3 DTP Contacts	3 DTP No of Cases	3 DTP Rate (%)	3 DT Contacts	3 DT No of Cases	3 DT Rate (%)	Relative Rate DTP:DT
0– < 1	28	12	43	56	34	61	1:1.4
1– < 2	108	35	32	399	316	79	1:2.5
2– < 3	97	36	37	384	299	78	1:2.1
3– < 4	108	34	31	284	170	60	1:1.9
4– < 6	476	92	19	428	165	39	1:2.0

the analysis based on the secondary attack rates in households was lower in the study. Table 10.3 shows the relative secondary attack rates in two-child families in which symptoms in the contact began at least one week after those of the index case. Efficacy was consistently around 0.50, except in the children less than one year, where the number of cases is small. In this study, the co-primaries were those within 7 days of the index case and secondary cases were those that occurred within about 42 days of the index case and at least 7 days after the index case. The efficacy was higher with a more severe case definition, reaching 71% in children with 10 paroxysms or more.

Fine et al (1988) reanalyzed this study and considered why estimates of pertussis vaccine efficacy might be lower in household contact studies than when assessed in cohort analyses in general populations. They restricted their analyses to households with at least one child under six years of age. The primary case was defined as the first recent case in the household, which in many households was not the index case. Co-primaries were defined as cases within one week of the primary case. Incidence cases were those that occurred more than one week after the primary cases. These included more than potentially secondary cases. Incidence cases were further divided into retrospective, prospective, and current incidence cases depending on whether they occurred before, after, or around the time of the initial visit to the household. The analysis included 9242 households with 10,406 contacts, of whom 6436 (61.8%) developed pertussis at the same time or after symptom onset in the primary case. The 1520 co-primary cases were excluded from further analysis. A surprising 94% of all incidence cases were retrospectively ascertained.

There were two key findings. First, vaccine efficacy was lower, although not significantly, in retrospectively than in prospectively ascertained cases. The overall, age standardized efficacy was 0.35 (95% CI 0.25–0.44) in retrospectively ascertained cases, and 0.59 (95% CI 0.42–0.70) in prospectively ascertained cases. Secondly, the efficacy was lower, although not significantly, in contacts exposed to vaccinated primary cases than in contacts exposed to unvaccinated primary cases. Thus, the two stratified VE_I estimates in equation (10.2) differed. This latter finding is not consistent with the biological argument that the bacterial exposure from a vaccinated case would be lower than from an unvaccinated case (Préziosi and Halloran 2003b). They speculate that it could be due to household clustering of vaccine failures or false-positive diagnoses.

10.2.5 Sweden

After pertussis vaccination was discontinued in 1979 in Sweden, pertussis became endemic again (Romanus et al 1987). Thus it was possible to conduct randomized, placebo-controlled trials of pertussis vaccination in Sweden. A trial of two acellular pertussis vaccines compared with placebo was conducted in Sweden 1986–1987. The efficacies were lower than expected, which could have been due to more sensitive case ascertainment, so further efficacy trials were planned directly comparing the acellular with whole cell vaccines. Several pertussis vaccine trials were conducted in Sweden in the 1990s.

In a double-blind, placebo-controlled trial in the Göteborg area of western Sweden, 3450 infants were randomized to vaccination with DT or the same DT with pertussis toxoid at 3, 5, and 12 months of age. The study children were born between June 1991 and May 1992 (Trollfors et al 1995). Trollfors et al (1998) were interested in estimating the indirect protection of close contacts of the children in the vaccine trial. A household study was nested within the primary efficacy study described in Section 6.4.2. Parents and siblings in households were followed for a median of two years starting 30 days after the third vaccination up to January 31, 1995. The numbers of older siblings of the DTP and DT were 938 and 965, of younger siblings 514 and 523, and of parents 3237 and 3229, respectively. The vaccination status of parents and siblings of the study children was not recorded. This is an example of the mini-community design (Section 10.7.5).

Later acellular pertussis vaccine candidates contained further antigens. Storsaeter et al (1998) did a study to evaluate immunological surrogates of protection after household exposure to pertussis. The idea was to use household exposure as a natural challenge experiment in studying surrogates of protection. The study was nested in a primary efficacy study (Gustafsson et al 1996). The household study is reported in Section 15.3.2. Further examples of studies of the efficacy of acellular pertussis vaccination after household exposure are Trollfors et al (1997) in Sweden and Schmitt et al (1996) in Germany.

10.3 Influenza

Prospective, longitudinal household studies have a long history in the study of transmission of influenza and other acute respiratory diseases. Household studies of influenza have generally not been used for estimating vaccine efficacy, although they have been used for evaluating the effects of post-exposure prophylaxis of influenza antiviral agents. Household studies of influenza are particularly useful for studying transmissibility and the serial interval. We present a number of household-based studies of influenza transmission for their historical significance and to promote future prospective household-based studies of influenza and other respiratory diseases. This sort of study of had essentially been discontinued. The novel influenza virus (H1N1) pandemic that started in 2009 has raised the consciousness about the important role of prospective household studies in estimating the transmissibility and the serial interval of influenza. We present the household-based studies of influenza antivirals to illustrate further methodological issues.

10.3.1 Seattle USA

Intensive surveillance of families with school-age children for influenza virus infections was conducted from 1975 to 1979 in Seattle, Washington, USA (Fox et al 1982b). The study followed the Virus Watch method that basically involves continuing virological surveillance of families. The Virus Watch in Seattle began by recruiting families with newborn infants in 1965 to 1969 with a focus on respiratory and enteric viruses detectable by cell culture methods and that were not well understood at that time. The Virus Watch method was specifically adapted for the study of influenza viruses to yield a better description of their behavior. Families with at least one child were recruited in fall 1975 (Group I) or fall 1976 (Group II) and followed for three years. In Group I, 112 families were recruited, and in Group II, 116 familes were recruited. By the 1978–1979 season, the families had dwindled to 44 and 73, yielding a total of 639 family-seasons of observation over four influenza virus epidemic seasons.

The protocol required collection of blood samples by venipuncture at four-month intervals, information concerning onset and manifestation of symptoms, and duration of illness in any family member, using illness records kept by the mother. Nose–throat swab specimens for virus isolations were to be collected from all family members on a regular basis, biweekly or, during influenza outbreaks, weekly, particularly when onset of a new case occurred. The plan was quite ambitious and could not be fully implemented. Many illnesses were missed, although there is no way to estimate how many. Between 9% (Group I) and 13% (Group II) of reported illnesses had no specimens collected, and between 26% (Group I) and 32% (Group II) of illnesses were recognized only because specimens were collected. Fox et al (1982a) analyzed the pattern of infection in invaded households and the relation of age and prior antibody to occurrence of infection and related illness. Susceptibility to each type or subtype was rigorously defined so that the resulting secondary attack rates would reflect virus infectivity. Susceptibles were defined on the basis of a pre-episode hemagglutination-inhibiting antibody titer of 1:$\leq$20 for A/H3N2 virus and 1:$\leq$10 for A/H1N1 and type B viruses. Of 102 contacts susceptible to A/H3N2, 53% became infected when exposed in the household. Of 147 contacts susceptible to A/H1N1, 44% were infected when exposed. Of 55 contacts susceptible to type B, 47% became infected.

Table 10.4 Observed distribution of influenza A(H3N2) infections in 1977–1978 and 1980–1981 combined epidemics in Tecumseh, Michigan, USA (Addy et al 1991)

No.	No. of Susceptibles per Household				
Infected	1	2	3	4	5
0	110	149	72	60	13
1	23	27	23	20	9
2		13	6	16	5
3			7	8	2
4				2	1
5					1
Total	133	189	108	106	31

10.3.2 Tecumseh, USA

Active community surveillance of acute respiratory illness took place in Tecumseh, Michigan, USA, during the five-year period 1976–1981 (Monto et al 1985). Beginning in October 1976, recruitment over a three-month period resulted in 1000 individuals, approximately 10% of the community, being under surveillance by the end of December. The households were recruited in a stratified manner until the required number was reached. Initially there were no restrictions on eligibility. Because of attrition, further recruitment was necessary. In 1978 the requirement that a family have at least one child of school age or younger was added. Then in 1979, families were recruited at the birth of the child until the end of the study in 1981. Throughout the five years of the study, families on surveillance were called weekly to identify the onset of acute illness. Specimens for virus isolation were collected when an illness was reported within two days of symptom onset. Blood specimens were collected from all on surveillance at six-month intervals. In addition, specimens for virus isolation were collected by Tecumseh physicians from patients with febrile respiratory illness. Table 10.4 contains a summary of the distribution of influenza A(H3N2) infections in 1977–1978 and 1980–1981 combined epidemics in Tecumseh, Michigan given in Addy et al (1991). Addy et al (1991) give the household frequency data in Table 10.4 stratified by age group 0–17 years and 18+ years as well. Table 10.5 contains a summary of the data stratified by age group and preseason antibody titer (Longini et al 1988). The criterion for classifying individuals as susceptible is a preseason hemagglutination inhibition test detecting no antibody in a dilution of 1 in 128 or less. People with higher titers were considered immune and were not included in the tables. Households with more than five susceptibles were deleted from all analyses. Longini et al (1988) give the household level frequency data stratified by pre-season antibody level and age group.

Table 10.5 Infection attack rates by pre-season antibody titer level stratified by age group: influenza A(H3N2) epidemic seasons 1977–1978 and 1980–1981 combined in Tecumseh, Michigan, USA (Longini et al 1988)

Pre-Season Antibody Titer	Infection Status			
$(1:x)$	No. Infected	No. Not Infected	Total	Attack Rate
Children (0–17 years)				
Low level ($x < 8$)	100	200	300	0.333
High level ($8 \leq x \leq 64$)	20	180	200	0.100
Total	120	380	500	0.240
Adults (18+ years)				
Low level ($x < 8$)	96	440	536	0.179
High level ($8 \leq x \leq 64$)	42	402	444	0.095
Total	138	842	980	0.141

10.3.3 Cleveland, USA

A large longitudinal 10-year study of illness of families in Cleveland, Ohio, USA was conducted from January 1, 1948 through May 31, 1957 (Dingle et al 1964). The study had two primary objectives. The first was to answer questions such as how much illness actually occurs, what is the etiology of the illnesses, how important is the family unit in spreading the illness, do families have a characteristic pattern of illness, and do individuals and families vary in susceptibility to illness. The second objective was to study specific diseases, using clinical, epidemiological, and laboratory results. The study had four parts. First, illnesses or events occurring in each individual and family were observed and recorded. Second, known entities such as streptococcal infections, influenza, or noninfectious diseases were differentiated and their behavior studied. Third, possible entities of unknown etiology were investigated. Fourth, problems such as the spread of infectious agents in the population, evaluation of therapeutic or prophylactic agents, and the occurrence of noninfectious processes were studied. Stable, middle-class families with at least one child were recruited. Extensive medical examinations were done on each family when it entered the study and at regular intervals, either six-month or one-year in children, and annually in adults. Records were kept by each mother, who notified the investigators at the time of each illness, however minor. Each family was visited weekly by a field worker, who obtained a throat culture from each member of the household. The family physician was called when necessary. During the study, an epidemic of poliomyelitis occurred in 1952, and stool specimens were collected. Some diseases, such as chickenpox, were recognized more reliably than others.

A total of 96 families and 443 individuals were in the study at one time or another. In May 1957, the first reports of the new antigenic variant of influenza virus A occurred in Asia. In anticipation of the influenza pandemic, the Cleveland study was reactivated in September 1957. Sixty of the families agreed to participate again for collection of detailed clinical and epidemiological data (Jordan et al 1958). Table

Table 10.6 Influenza attack rates by age during the Asian influenza pandemic of 1957 in Cleveland, Ohio, USA, as measured by virus isolation (Jordan et al 1958)

Age Groups		Respiratory Illness	Test for Virus		Virus Isolated	
(Years)	No.	No.	No.	Percent	No.	Percent
0–4	28	44	35	79.6	12	42.9
5–9	76	113	80	70.8	44	57.9
10–14	68	108	83	76.6	40	58.8
15+	17	27	19	70.4	8	47.1
Adults	119	100	71	71.0	22	18.5
Totals	308	392	288	73.5	126	40.9

10.6 contains the influenza illness attack rates by age as measured by virus isolation during the Asian influenza pandemic in the 60 families.

10.3.4 Influenza Epigrippe, France

The Epigrippe study was conducted during the 1999–2000 influenza season in France (Carrat et al 2002). Households were recruited for follow-up by 161 general practitioners. In total 946 households were recruited. For a household to be included, a member of the household had to visit a general practitioner with a history of fever (≥38°C) in the last 48 hours and respiratory signs. The household had to have at least one other member, everyone had to give consent to participate in the study, and the patient seeking care had to be the first case in the household and not be hospitalized as a result of the illness. In all index cases, nasal swabs were obtained at the first visit. Biological confirmation of influenza virus was by immunofluorescence test and/or culture and/or PCR. Households followed up with diaries of symptoms for 15 days after recruitment of the index case. Influenza was defined clinically in contacts. Of the 946 index cases, 510 tested positive for influenza virus. Follow-up information was obtained on 334 (65%) of the households with positive index cases. Cauchemez et al (2004) analyzed the data that included the 334 confirmed index cases and households and 350 clinical influenza cases in 790 contacts. Influenza in symptomatic contacts was not confirmed biologically, nor was there any biological confirmation of possible asymptomatic infections. A case of influenza in the contacts was defined as having clinical influenza for at least one day.

Table 10.7 Some characteristics of the four studies as reported in the four papers (Halloran et al 2007a)

	Zanamivir		Oseltamivir	
	Zan I Hayden et al 2000	Zan II Monto et al 2002	Osel I Hayden et al 2004	Osel II Welliver et al 2001
Centers	15	59	multi	76
Where	US, Canada, UK, Finland	S. Africa, Europe New Zealand, NA, Australia	North America, Europe	North America, Europe
Study period	Oct 98–Apr. 99	June 2000–Apr. 2001	2000–01	1998–99
Predominant types	B (~30%) A(H3N2)	B (~33%) A(H1N1) (north) A(H3N2) (south)	B (~33%) A(H1N1)	B (~47%) A(H3N2)
Randomized:				
No. families (IC)	337 (321)	487	277	374
No. contacts	837	1291	812	962
Inf. index cases*:				
Control arm				
Households (IC)†	87 (81)	153	84	79
No. contacts	215	398	228	206
Treatment arm				
Households (IC)	78 (76)	129	89	84
No. contacts	195	368	248	209

* Includes only households with laboratory-confirmed index cases.
† IC = index case.

10.3.5 Influenza antivirals

Four randomized household-based studies of the efficacy of post-exposure prophylaxis in preventing clinical influenza in household contacts were conducted, two of zanamivir (Hayden et al. 2000; Monto et al. 2002), called Zan I and Zan II, and two of oseltamivir (Hayden et al 2004; Welliver et al 2001), called Osel I and Osel II (Halloran et al 2007a). Table 10.7 contains a summary of some characteristics of the four studies. All four studies were household-based, multicenter, randomized, controlled trials, where treatment was randomized by household (cluster-randomized design). Households with a suspected case of influenza illness were enrolled as a whole in each study. Assignment of the index case to treatment or control varied across the studies, resulting in differences in the effect measures estimated in each study. Ages for eligibility of index cases and contacts also varied across studies.

- Zan I (Hayden et al 2000): Randomized, double-blind, placebo-controlled trial. Households were randomized to study drug (zanamivir) or placebo. Index cases and eligible contacts within a household all received either drug or placebo. Children under age 5 years did not receive study drug.

- Zan II (Monto et al 2002): Randomized, double-blind, placebo-controlled trial. Households were randomized for eligible contacts to receive the study drug (zanamivir) or placebo. Index cases did not receive antiviral therapy. Children under age five years did not receive study drug.
- Osel I (Hayden et al 2004): Randomized, open-label, trial. Households were randomized for eligible contacts to receive either antiviral post-exposure prophylaxis or antiviral treatment when illness developed (expectant treatment). All index cases received study drug (oseltamivir) treatment for five days. Children under one year were excluded from participating.
- Osel II (Welliver et al 2001): Randomized, double-blind, placebo-controlled trial. Households were randomized for eligible contacts to receive study drug (oseltamivir) or placebo. Index cases did not receive antiviral therapy. Children under 12 years were excluded from participating as contacts, but could be (untreated) index cases.

In all four studies, the primary endpoint in the household contacts was laboratory-confirmed clinical influenza illness. A secondary endpoint was laboratory-confirmed influenza infection, whether symptomatic or asymptomatic. All four studies did extensive laboratory testing of the enrolled index cases and their contacts. Because contacts were tested for influenza infection regardless of whether they had symptoms, it is possible to estimate pathogenicity from the data (Chapter 9). Contacts were supposed to complete diary cards once or twice daily for 14 days or more, depending on the study, with details of symptoms and temperature. The definitions of clinical symptomatic influenza cases essentially included fever and symptoms, although they varied across the four studies. The period for inclusion of secondary cases in the original analyses varied across the studies.

Analogous to the vaccine efficacies in equations (10.2), from the appropriate SAR_{jk}s, in principle, we can estimate the stratified antiviral efficacies, AVE_S, AVE_I, and AVE_T. Three main design issues are illustrated by these studies that are applicable for vaccine studies as well. First, household randomization restricts the efficacy parameters that can be estimated (Section 10.6.5). Second, asymptomatic infections in contacts were ascertained, so that pathogenicity and the effect of prophylaxis on pathogenicity, AVE_P, could be estimated. Third, each of the efficacies AVE_S, AVE_I, and AVE_T could be based on laboratory-confirmed influenza illness, $\mathrm{AVE}_{\cdot d}$, or simply laboratory-confirmed infection, $\mathrm{AVE}_{\cdot i}$, in the eligible contacts.

10.4 Measles Vaccination

Measles vaccines are generally much greater than 90% efficacious against clinical disease. One of the considerations is at what age infants or children should be vaccinated. Maternal antibodies transferred before birth protect very young infants and interfere with the live vaccine virus being able to induce an immune response in the infant. If vaccinated too young when maternal antibodies are still present, vaccination will not be effective. On the other hand, if vaccinated too late, maternal antibody protection will have waned, and the child could easily contract measles before being vaccinated. In the United States, vaccination against measles occurs between 12 and 15 months. However, in developing countries, this is often too late because exposure is more widespread. Considerable research has been directed at understanding the optimal age to vaccinate infants in developing countries. In the 1990s, new vaccines with high titers of vaccine virus were tried that were thought could induce antibodies at a younger age.

10.4.1 Niakhar, Senegal

The clinical efficacy of three measles vaccines was studied in a randomized trial in Niakhar, Senegal, in the same population described in Section 10.2.3. Garenne et al (1993) evaluated the efficacy of measles vaccines after controlling for the level of exposure to infection within the compounds. They conducted two analyses of efficacy, one based on the unconditional cases per person-time at risk, the other based on the secondary attack rate within the compound. The first analysis was based on a randomized vaccine trial conducted from August 1987 to July 1990 to compare two high-titer vaccines, the Edmonston–Zagreb and the Schwarz, and the standard Schwarz (Garenne et al 1991). The randomized trial covered the cohorts of children born between February 1987 and January 1989. The children were randomized into the three vaccine groups, with the two high-titer vaccines being administered at 5 months and the standard Schwarz at 10 months. The unvaccinated group were those children who were not available to be vaccinated on their scheduled day. An unvaccinated control arm was unethical. A total of 1566 children were vaccinated, with vaccine coverage of 81.6% of the resident target population. The analysis controlling for the level of exposure within the compound was nested in the randomized study.

Three measles outbreaks occurred during the study. In the first, 27 cases occurred between May and September 1988, then 161 cases between October 1988 and July 1989, and then 413 cases between August 1989 and July 1990. When a family suspected a case of measles or a case was seen in the clinic, a specifically trained physician went to the compound. The physician visited the compound twice a week until the last case was cured. For serological confirmation, an initial blood sample was obtained by fingerprick in susceptible children in the family during the first visit, with a second sample obtained from clinical cases at least four weeks after the onset of rash.

Exposure was defined as being susceptible (those who had never had measles) and being present in a compound where there was a clinical case of measles. Secondary cases were defined as those occurring in the same compound 7 to 18 days after the index case. The mean time lag between index and secondary cases was 12.2 days, similar to that found in previous analyses (Hope-Simpson 1952; Bailey 1957). Different levels of exposure within compounds were defined using a linear score: 1 = living in a different compound; 2 = living in same compound but eating from a

Table 10.8 Incidence and secondary attack rates of measles in a randomized trial of three measles vaccines in 30 villages 1987–1989, Niakhar, Senegal. HT = high titer. (Garenne et al 1993)

Group	Prospective study			Compound Exposure Study		
	Resident January 1, 1990	Cases Reported/ Confirmed	Incidence Rate per 1,000 p-yrs	Contacts	Cases Reported/ Confirmed	SAR (%)
Schwarz	740	1/0	0.80	54	1/0	1.85
HT EZ	552	5/3	4.12	53	3/2	5.66
HT Schwarz	274	5/2	6.67	24	2/1	8.33
Unvaccinated	348	54/21	40.63	46	30/13	65.22

different kitchen; 3 = eating from the same kitchen but sleeping in a different hut; 4 = sleeping in the same hut. Reported clinical cases could be either directly or indirectly confirmed. Direct confirmation required fulfilling the clinical case definition and having at least a fourfold rise in HIA to measles virus during the acute phase. Indirect confirmation was by epilink, that is, when it occurred in a compound where another case was directly confirmed.

10.5 Pneumococcal Carriage Studies

Pneumococcal diseases are a major health problem all over the world. The etiologic agent is *Streptococcus pneumoniae* (Pnc), a bacterium surrounded by a polysaccharide (sugar) capsule. There are about 90 different serotypes of Pnc differentiated by the composition of the capsule. Pneumococcal bacteria are prevalent in populations. Generally the pneumococcal bacteria colonize the nasopharyngeal area without causing symptoms. Symptomatic disease can be either invasive or noninvasive. Invasive disease includes pneumonia, meningitis, and bacteremia with fever. Noninvasive disease includes otitis media and bronchitis. Generally, the cases of disease, especially invasive disease, are not considered infectious for others, at least not important for transmission. In contrast, the asymptomatic carriers are considered to be the main sources of infection. People have the ability to acquire colonization in the nasopharynx and to clear it repeatedly without developing complete immunity. Given the numerous serotypes, a person may acquire one type of infection, clear it, then acquire either the same type or another.

The original pneumococcal vaccines were based on the polysaccharide capsule and contained up to 23 of the serotypes. The first to be licensed in the United States was in 1977, with an improved version in 1983 (Plotkin and Plotkin 2008). Immunogenicity was not great, so a new generation of conjugate vaccines was developed based on purified polysaccharide joined to a harmless variety of diphtheria toxin. The conjugate pneumococcal vaccine was licensed in the United States in 2000. These vaccines contain 7 to 11 serotypes and induce a T-cell-dependent immune response. They have been shown to be effective in children and a strong population effect is being observed. In preparation for introducing the new vaccines, a series of household-based carriage studies was conducted in a number of different countries. The studies were to study the acquisition and clearance of the different serotypes, their relative prevalence, and possible difference in their acquisition and clearance rates. One question of scientific interest was whether vaccination against the vaccine serotypes would increase not only the relative but also absolute prevalence of nonvaccine serotypes.

In pneumococcal carriage studies, the time of onset and the time of clearance of carriage are not observed, so households are not generally ascertained on an index case. Households may be ascertained on some aspect of the index person, such as having a young infant in the household. Household members are examined at regular intervals to determine whether they are carrying the bacteria. Follow-up is active. The data are longitudinal, also called panel data, with repeated sampling of the same individuals at fixed, or nearly fixed, time intervals.

10.5.1 Finland

Auranen et al (2000) analyzed data from the FinOM cohort study concerning the epidemiology of acute otitis media with a special emphasis on *Streptococcus pneumoniae* (Pnc) bacteria (Syrjänen et al 2001). Healthy unselected babies born to Finnish-speaking mothers and not previously immunized with a pneumococcal vaccine were consecutively enrolled at their first routine visit to a local well-baby clinic in Tampere, Finland between April 1994 and August 1995. Nearly all babies in Finland attend such clinics. During the enrollment period, 53% of the families with a newborn chose to participate in the study. The infants were followed for nasopharyngeal carriage of Pnc over a period of two years. Auranen et al (2000) analyzed a subset of 97 infants and their families for which carriage information was collected from all family members. The 97 infants were enrolled consecutively between December 1994 and May 1995.

During the follow-up, 14 younger siblings of the index children were born. All family members ($N = 370 + 14$) were examined for Pnc carriage when the index child was 2, 3, 4, 5, 6, 9, 12, 15, 18, and 24 months old, for a total of 10 time points over the two-year follow-up period. Time is defined for each family from birth of the index child. At each observation, the absence or presence of Pnc was identified for the seven Pnc serotypes that were to be included in the new vaccine. The proportion of recorded observations was 86% of the potential number, which is high for such extensive follow-up. In 40 of the 97 families, there was no observed carriage in anyone in the family during the follow-up period.

From September 2001 to May 2002, a further carriage study was conducted in Finland. It was the first longitudinal study of pneumococcal carriage to record serotype specific exposure to pneumococcal bacteria simultaneously with families and day care centers, the two most important mixing groups (Leino et al 2008). The acquisition of pneumococcal carriage by day care attendees was strongly associated with previous exposure to a homologous serotypes in the day care center. In the 36 acquisitions with known exposure within the day care center or the family, the child had been exposed in the day care center in 35 cases and in the family in in 9 cases. The three day care centers were much larger than families, leading to the suggestion that the larger size and younger age of the children in the day care centers were about to main micro-epidemics better than the small families. The authors suggest that the day care centers serve as core populations to enhance pneumococcal transmission within the population as a whole. A child-to-child basic reproductive number was estimated as 1.4 (Hoti et al 2009) .

10.5.2 France

A five-month longitudinal study of three- to six-year old children in 81 schools was conducted in France from January to May 2000 (Guillemot et al 2005). Children were examined for Pnc carriage using oropharyngeal swabs approximately once a month over a five-month period (Figure 10.1). The mean time between consecutive swabs was 37 days (sd 15 days). During the observation period 9857 swabs were collected for serotyping. The 4488 three- to six-year old childen attending the schools represented 88% of the children in the area under study. Of these, 2445 (55%) gave at least one swab. The mean number of swabs was four (range: one to five) among children providing at least one swab. All children attending the schools were included in the analysis as a density factor, even if they had not provided a single observation of follow-up (Cauchemez et al 2006d). The analysis was restricted to the 16 serotypes isolated in at least 30 swabs in the selected schools. The analysis divided the serotypes into two groups, those contained in the seven-valent vaccine and those not. The study preceded the introduction of the vaccine into France, so all participating children were unvaccinated. Cauchemez et al (2006d) analyzed this study using methods similar to Auranen et al (2000).

10.5.3 United Kingdom

A study of 121 preschool children <3 years old and all household members was conducted in the United Kingdom during the follow-up period from October 2001 to July 2002 (Hussain et al 2005). Enrollment was through primary health care registers in Hertfordshire. Families were visited once a month over a 10-month period. All family members were examined for carriage using nasopharyngeal swabs. At least one swab was obtained from 489 individuals in 121 families for a total of 3753 swabs, of which 932 (25%) were positive for Pnc. Melegaro et al (2004) modeled the household transmission similarly to Auranen et al (1996). However, they used

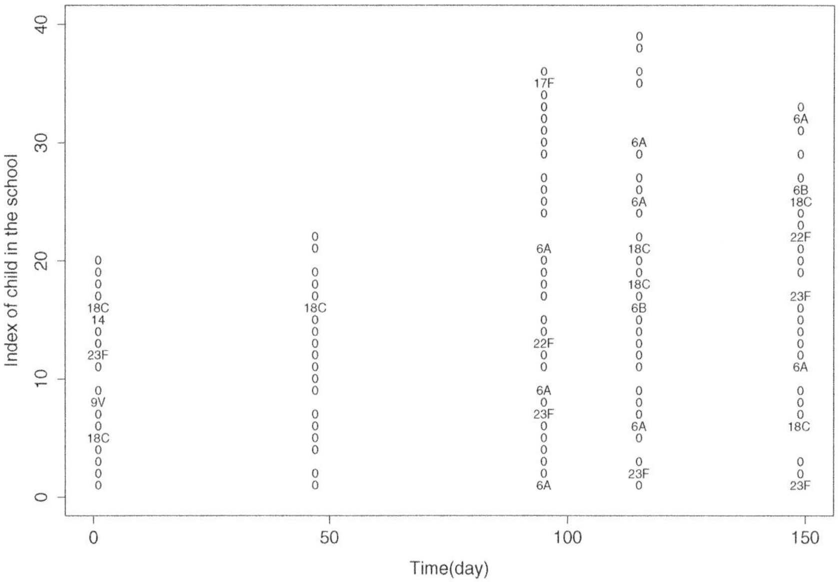

Fig. 10.1 Longitudinal data in a school participating in a pneumococcal carriage study. A "0" represents a sample in which no pneumococcal serotypes was detected. The other symbols represent the pneumococcal serotype abbreviation of the detected bacteria. Similar to Cauchemez et al (2006d).

maximum likelihood estimation to estimate the transition rates between carriage and noncarriage (Section 11.4.1).

10.5.4 Bangladesh

A study in a community-based project in a transitional area in Savar, Bangladesh enrolled 99 children born between May 2000 and April 2001 and their families (98 because 2 newborns were twins) (Granat et al 2007). The families were visited every two weeks until the index child was four months old, then monthly up to one year of age, for a total of 16 visits. The goal of the study was to describe the development of pneumococcal carriage in a developing country setting. Swabs were taken from the infant and from other children and family members present and consenting during the visit. A total of 1459 samples (92% of those planned) were collected from the 99 index children and 2865 from the other family members. Approximately 50% of the infants had acquired pneumococcal carriage by eight weeks of age. The point prevalence of pneumococcal carriage in the first five years was about 50% and declined after that to between 7 and 8% in adults.

10.6 Design Considerations

10.6.1 Transmission units and contacts

The scientific question of interest will influence the design of the study in households or other transmission units. A transmission unit is a place or social relationship within which individuals are assumed to make contact sufficient for transmission. The concept of a contact sufficient for transmission is very broad and must be defined in each particular study. The transmission mode of an infectious agent determines what types of contact are potentially infectious. Contacts can be defined between two individuals, or an individual and a vector. Contacts can be defined within small transmission units, such as households. Within small transmission units, mixing is often assumed to be random. A small transmission unit can be defined as two individuals in a social relationship, such as a steady sexual partnership, or a household with just two susceptible people. The definition of a contact within a study can depend on the definition of the transmission units. The individuals in a small transmission unit exposed to an infectious case can be thought of as a *mini-cohort* (Orenstein et al 1988) that has its own reference date for exposure to infection. An advantage is that vaccination status is less likely to change over the time of follow-up. Individuals living in the same household are likely to be more homogeneously exposed to infection. Comparing vaccinated and unvaccinated persons matched on household could be less prone to bias from differences in exposure to infection (Struchiner et al 1994). A small transmission unit can also be thought of as a *mini-community* if the indirect effects of vaccination of a fraction of the people in the transmission unit are of interest.

Different definitions of a potentially infective contact and transmission unit, for the same infectious agent, even within the same study, are possible. In a study of chickenpox transmission, a potentially infective contact could be defined as being in the same school on one day with someone with chickenpox. Alternatively, it could be defined as living in the same house during the presumed infectious period of the person with chickenpox. In the first case, the transmission unit is the school, and in the latter, it is the household. In the first case, the contact is defined over one day, and in the latter, it is defined over the entire infectious period. In tuberculosis, a contact could be defined as riding on the same bus with someone with open tuberculosis, or as living in the same household with someone with tuberculosis. In the former case, the transmission unit is the bus, and in the latter, it is the household.

There could be different definitions of a contact for one definition of transmission unit. In an HIV study, a potentially infective contact could be defined as each sex act between two sexual partners in a steady relationship, one of whom is infected with HIV. Alternatively, the partnership over its entire duration or over the duration of the study could be defined as one potentially infective contact.

Different levels of potentially infective contacts can be defined. In the measles vaccine study in Niakhar, Senegal, four levels of exposure within a compound were defined and given a linear score. In another study of measles transmission in Niakhar, Senegal, the SARs estimated in schools, in homes, and in huts differed (Cisse et al 1999). Kendrick and Eldering (1939) differentiated definite and indefinite exposures.

When collecting data on households, the identities and number of the people living in the household should be collected. Also, if there is interest in estimating transmission parameters or the secondary attack rate, it important to ascertain for each member of the household whether they were actually present in the household during the period of interest.

10.6.2 Ascertainment

The method of ascertaining households for inclusion in a study is central. Households can be ascertained when a case develops within the household, the case-ascertained design (Yang et al 2006), or a group of households can be ascertained before a case develops and followed prospectively over time. The index case of a household can be ascertained in a number of ways. A case may appear in a clinic for treatment, then the family is enrolled in the study. A case may be notified to the local authorities, and the family visited for inclusion in the study.

Prospective enrollment of households can occur in several ways. Population-based active surveillance in households at regular intervals is one method. An example is the population-based surveillance in Niakhar, Senegal. Enrollment of families prospectively, such as in the influenza studies in Tecumseh, Michigan, USA, and Seattle, Washington, USA, is another approach. In the Finnish pneumococcal carriage study, families were enrolled when the infant attended the well-baby clinics.

Ideally one would have a random sample of households in the study, whether ascertained on an index case or enrolled prospectively. Ascertainment of a household by the index case is prone to ascertainment bias. A household with a higher number of potential cases has more chance of being ascertained than a household with a smaller number. If the size of the household has an influence on the results of the analysis, then the result will be subject to ascertainment bias. It could be that households with two or more cases would more likely be ascertained than households with single cases, so the secondary attack rate would be estimated to be higher than if a random sample had been observed. However, following a large number of households prospectively could be very expensive compared to a study based on ascertaining index cases. The potential biases need to be weighed against the efficiency of the study.

In an individually randomized vaccine trial, the households of the individuals in the vaccine study can be included in a further study, an example of the augmented study design (Section 10.7.4). If the household is included whether or not the trial participant or anyone in the household is infected, then the household is also randomized. If the household is included in a nested household study only if a case develops in the household, whether or not the first case is the vaccine trial participant or a sibling, the nested study is subject to potential selection bias (Halloran and Struchiner 1995; Becker et al 2006).

A second issue is how cases within the household are ascertained. If the index case is the first case in the household, then it is also the primary case. Then all further cases in contacts will be ascertained prospectively. If there are cases in a household that preceded the index case, then these cases will be ascertained retrospectively. In the PHLS pertussis vaccination study (Section 10.2.4), index cases were those cases notified to the area health authority. The household was visited, and cases within the household were ascertained both retrospectively and prospectively. Fine et al (1988) found that vaccine efficacy based on the retrospective incidence cases was lower, though not significantly, than that based on prospective incidence cases. They proposed three possible reasons for the observation. First, a higher number of cases in a household could result in a higher probability of ascertainment (ascertainment bias). Second, there may have been more diagnostic errors in the retrospective incidence cases (misclassification bias). False-positives would reduce the efficacy estimates. The third explanation draws on the idea of the all-or-none protective effects, or at least heterogeneous protection. If the vaccine failed in some of the people, the cases in the vaccinated unprotected people would occur early after the primary case. So the retrospective incidence cases would be enriched in vaccine failures. The vaccinated children observed prospectively would be enriched in highly protected children. Fine et al (1988) question whether retrospective incidence cases and prospective incidence cases should be lumped together in the same analysis due to potentially different sources of bias. The pertussis analysis is somewhat extreme in that a substantial portion of the retrospective incidence cases occurred more than 10 weeks before the initial visit to the household.

Onset of symptomatic disease is easier to ascertain than onset of infection. In active surveillance of symptomatic disease, surveillance could be at regular intervals and time of onset of disease retrospectively ascertained. Potential cases can be ascertained prospectively by asking family members to keep symptom diaries. When symptoms appear, they may be instructed to contact the study coordinator, or the families may be contacted regularly to check about onset of symptoms. In the carriage studies where symptoms do not occur, participants are tested at regular intervals for carriage. With infection or carriage data, the infection times between observations cannot be ascertained, but may be imputed using statistical methods (Chapter 11).

If ascertainment of households is on an index case, then the duration of follow-up for each household needs to be determined, depending on the natural history of the infectious agent. Household exposure studies can be used as natural challenge studies when trying to identify immunological surrogates of protection (Storsaeter et al 1998). In this situation, a decision needs to be made about the choice of timing of the immunological measurement.

10.6.3 Case definition

The problem of case definition is similar to other types of study design. When households are ascertained on an index case, a different case definition is sometimes used for the secondary cases than for the index case. Retrospectively ascertained cases can often not be confirmed biologically.

10.6.4 Data structure

There are three basic data structures for outcomes of interest for household studies. The three are time-of-onset data, final value data, and longitudinal data. In time-of-onset data, one observes the time of onset of symptoms or infection of each of the cases in the household. In final value data, only whether an infection or illness occurred between the beginning and end of the study period is observed for each person in the household. In longitudinal data, the members of households are followed over time and observed (sampled) repeatedly at intervals. Combinations of the types of data are possible. For example, active surveillance of households could occur at intervals. However, if a case occurs, and shows up in a clinic, then an observation occurs outside of the usual longitudinal follow-up. Time-of-onset data can be reduced to final value data for the analysis. Also, one can decide to ignore the household structure in the analysis and just analyze the data using unconditional approaches based on survival analysis or final value data.

Another important aspect of the data structure depends on the method of ascertainment. If ascertainment of a household is on an index case or index infection, then there is at least one case (infection) in each household.. If ascertainment is prospective in that households are included before developing the first case, then some of the households may have zero cases. The statistical analysis may need to account for the difference in the two data structures resulting from the ascertainment method.

10.6.5 Assignment mechanism

In evaluating the effect of interventions, the assignment mechanism is key. We consider first that we are interested in estimating VE_S, VE_I, and VE_T from a household-based study. As is evident from equations (10.1) and (10.2), which of these efficacy parameters will be estimable depends on which secondary attack rates or transmission probabilities can be estimated. This in turn depends on who in the households are vaccinated and who are not. For example, to estimate the secondary attack rate from an infected vaccinated person to a susceptible unvaccinated person, SAR_{10}, some of the households must have vaccinated primary cases and unvaccinated contacts. To estimate SAR_{11}, some of the households must have vaccinated primary cases and vaccinated contacts.

Table 10.9 Estimable antiviral efficacies from each of four household-based, household-randomized, influenza antiviral efficacy studies. AVE_I is not estimable from any of the studies alone (Halloran et al 2007a)

	Zanamivir		Oseltamivir	
	Zan I Hayden et al 2002	Zan II Monto et al 2002	Osel I Hayden et al 2004	Osel II Welliver et al 2001
$AVE_{S01/00} = 1 - \frac{SAR_{01}}{SAR_{00}}$	–	$AVE_{S01/00}$	–	$AVE_{S01/00}$
$AVE_{S11/10} = 1 - \frac{SAR_{11}}{SAR_{10}}$	–	–	$AVE_{S11/10}$	–
$AVE_{I11/01} = 1 - \frac{SAR_{11}}{SAR_{01}}$	–	–	–	–
$AVE_{I10/00} = 1 - \frac{SAR_{10}}{SAR_{00}}$	–	–	–	–
$AVE_T = 1 - \frac{SAR_{11}}{SAR_{00}}$	AVE_T	–	–	–

Most household-based studies of vaccine efficacy conducted up to now have been either observational studies or studies nested within individually randomized studies. In these studies, the allocation of vaccination within households generally is not under the control of the investigator. Theoretical and simulation studies have shown that to estimate VE_S, VE_I, and VE_T in the same study, discordant or individual randomization within households is better than randomization by household (Datta et al 1999; Yang et al 2006). If everyone in a household is randomized either to vaccine or control, only VE_T will be estimable.

Consider the four household-based influenza antiviral trials described in Section 10.3.5. The Zan II and Osel II studies both did not treat the index case, then randomized all contacts in the household to either drug or control. Thus, in both of these studies the stratified $AVE_{S01/00} = 1 - SAR_{01}/SAR_{00}$ is estimable (AVE for antiviral efficacy). In the Osel I study, the index cases were all treated, and then all household contacts randomized to either drug or control. In Osel I, the other stratified $AVE_{S10/11} = 1 - SAR_{11}/SAR_{10}$ is estimable. In contrast, the Zan I study randomized everyone in a household, index cases and contacts, to either drug or control. In Zan I, $AVE_T = 1 - SAR_{11}/SAR_{00}$ is estimated. Without careful examination, one might believe that all three studies were estimating the same parameter, but there are not so subtle differences that could be important for interpreting the studies. Table 10.9 provides an overview of the efficacy estimates that can be obtained from each study. None of the four studies alone provides information to estimate AVE_I, the effect of the drug in reducing the infectivity of the infected index case. By combining the two oseltamivir studies or the two zanamivir studies, one can obtain estimates of AVE_I, although combining separate studies with other subtle design differences is not ideal.

In the pertussis vaccine study in Niakhar, there were sufficient numbers of discordant vaccinated and unvaccinated children to estimate all of the vaccine efficacies (Section 12.3). If it is possible to control allocation of vaccination or other intervention within households at the design phase, careful consideration should be given to exactly what one would like to estimate. A study needs to be larger to get a good estimate of VE_I than to estimate VE_S. VE_I is estimated based on exposure to vaccinated compared with exposure to unvaccinated cases. If a vaccine has a strong protective effect, it may not be possible to get a good estimate of VE_I. However, if VE_S is high, VE_I has less public health importance and less influence on the results of simulation models.

10.7 Related Designs

10.7.1 Case-contact design

An alternative to ascertaining clearly defined transmission units is the *case-contact* design. In the case-contact approach, an index case is identified, then the people who have made contact with the index case are identified. For example, in tuberculosis, SARS, HIV, or the novel influenza (H1N1) pandemic, through contact tracing, the people who have made contact with the infective person might be identified and their infection status ascertained. One difficulty in estimating the transmission probability from such a study is in determining the temporal order of infection in the contacts. Case-contact studies are studies in which individuals exposed to a case are followed to find if they are infected or diseased. In this type of study, there is no explicit transmission unit such as a household or a school.

10.7.2 Cluster designs

In dengue studies, ascertainment of clusters by index cases has been used for focal mosquito control. Traditionally, a radius of 100 meters around the household of the index cases was targeted for intensive mosquito intervention. The rationale was that the usual mosquito vector of dengue virus *Aedes aegypti* has a short flight range. More recently, index cases have been used to locate clusters of people with the purpose to identify early infections in people to study the immunopathogenesis of dengue infection (Beckett et al 2005). People within a short radius of the index case are bled and followed for 14 days. The idea is that the people around an index case would be enriched for infected people compared to the general population, so that the cluster approach is more efficient than a cohort study to identify newly infected people.

Secondary attack rates in neighborhood clusters can also be used to evaluate vaccine efficacy in urban or semi-urban settings (Orenstein et al 1985). The study can be conducted by identifying neighborhood clusters, each with at least one known case. The study participants are those of the age of interest who live close to the known case. The proximity could be defined as living no more than one house away from the front doorway of the house with a case. The cluster starts at the known case in the neighborhood. The adjacent households are visited. If a case occurred in a house in the period of interest, then the houses next to it are visited until no further cases are found. Thus, all participants live within about an equal proximity to a case. The exposure is less well defined than in a household study, but perhaps better than in a population-based study. A second visit to the neighborhood will be necessary to confirm suspected cases and to detect further secondary cases.

10.7.3 Susceptibles exposed to infective contacts

In contrast to studies within transmission units, another study design approach to estimate the transmission probability or VE_S conditioning on potential exposure to infection is to assemble a cohort of susceptibles. The study then follows the susceptibles and collects information on their contacts with infectives or potential infectives. One can use either information about the infection status of the actual contacts or information about prevalence of infection and contact structure in the population from which the contacts are drawn. This type of study could be particularly useful for studies of sexually transmitted diseases or diseases transmitted by injecting drug users where contacts can be fairly easily defined. Also, the transmission probability per contact might be low. Study subjects might give information on the average number of contacts rather than the exact number of contacts they each make per unit time. From this, the expected number of contacts during the study period can be estimated. The data required are infection outcome, number of potentially infective contacts, and covariate status, for example, vaccination status, for each person in the study. Yang et al (2009a) developed a model to estimate the VE_S of an HIV vaccine that used reported number of contacts and information on the prevalence of infection in the population. One of the study populations was an cohort of injecting drug users in Thailand. The contacts were drug injections with needles. Injections with shared needles were potentially infectious. The second study population was primarily men who have sex with men. The model allowed for errors in the reported number of contacts in each time interval.

10.7.4 Augmented vaccine studies

It is possible to design studies prospectively that intentionally make use of multilevel information in estimating vaccine efficacy. One such design is the *augmented* trial design (Longini et al 1996; Datta et al 1998). In the augmented study design, individuals are recruited and possibly randomized to intervention. Then the trial can be augmented by including information on contacts and transmission units such as households or partnerships of the primary trial participants. This is one method to preserve the individual level analysis and randomization. The primary analysis can still focus on estimating VE_S, although estimation of VE_I is also possible. The individual recruitment and randomization are similar to standard randomized studies that aim to estimate relative risks based on one of the unconditional measures, such as incidence rate. However, then individuals with whom the primary study participants make contact, such as in a household or partnership, are also recruited. That is, the transmission unit of the participant is recruited into the study, and augments the original primary study. The augmented participants may or may not be also randomized to intervention. Studies of vaccine efficacy based on household exposure that are nested in individually randomized clinical trials of vaccines are examples of augmented designs in which households of trial participants are recruited once a case develops in the household. The augmented study design can be thought as an extension of the idea of small transmission units within a community, as in Chapter 11, or the augmenting transmission units can be thought of as independent units, as in Chapter 12.

10.7.5 Mini-community designs

In a study design we call the *mini-community design*, households of individual study participants are recruited into the study, regardless of whether a case has developed in the household. The scientific goal of this type of study is to estimate the indirect effect of vaccination of the study participants on protecting the other household members. The goal is to estimate unconditional estimates of the type VE_{IIa} for indirect effects. In these studies, follow-up is over some defined period of calendar time. The goal is therefore different than in studies based on the secondary attack rates or transmission probabilities. Similar to the community-randomized trial design, one hopes and assumes that the households are independent of one another.

If just one child in a family is in a trial, then the proportion of the family vaccinated may be too low to observe an indirect effect. That is, other siblings or household members might provide enough source of infection to mask any reduction in transmission due to the vaccinated child. If the interest is in estimating indirect effects of vaccination in families, one could consider vaccinating a larger fraction of the household. For example, in a study in South Africa, interest is on studying whether vaccinating children in the family with pneumococcal conjugate vaccine could protect HIV-infected household members against pneumococcal disease. In this study, all children in some households and none in others could be vaccinated to have the maximal contrast in indirect effects.

The mini-community design is an example of a community-randomized design (Chapter 13), just that the communities are very small. The mini-community design seems particularly useful for infectious agents with a high ratio of asymptomatic infection or carriage to symptomatic disease, such as with pneumococcal bacteria. Further methodological development of the mini-community design is an open topic for future research.

Problems

10.1. (a) Describe the main differences in the design of prospective versus case-ascertained household studies.
(b) What are the advantages and disadvantages of the two approaches?
(c) What are the differences in the potential sources of bias?

10.2. (a) Consider the data in Table 10.4. Ignoring the household structure, compute the attack rate for each different household size and the study population as a whole.
(b) Is there any trend in the attack rates by size of household? Would you expect one? Why or why not?

10.3. (a) Consider the data in Table 10.8. Define the rate of exposure to measles as the number of children exposed divided by the number at risk on January 1, 1990. Compute the rate of exposure for the three vaccine groups and the unvaccinated group. Are there any differencs in the exposure rates among the groups?

10.4. Consider designing a household-based study of a new vaccine targeted to children under 6 years old. The study will include only households with at least two children under 6 years old. Using a placebo as control is ethical for this vaccine. What vaccine efficacy measures will be estimable if you randomize by household? by individual?

Chapter 11
Analysis of Households in Communities

11.1 Overview

In this chapter, we consider analyses that assume the households or other transmission units are nested in a community. Community-acquired infection serves as a source of initial infection within households as well as possible further cases in the household. Infected household members can infect others in the household. To start, we discuss general aspects of these models. All models in this chapter are variants of the basic models presented in this section. They use different data structures, assumptions, and methods of estimation, but the underlying parameters are similar. The data can be final-value data, time-to-event data, or longitudinal (panel) data.

Each model has two general types of parameters, one for infection from the community, and the other for transmission from an infective to a susceptible within the household. The first is an unconditional parameter, that is, it does not condition on exposure to infection. The second is a conditional parameter. The models can be formulated in discrete time or continuous time. For some data structures, such as data on sexual contacts, contacts can be substituted for time. Models formulated in discrete time have a parameter for the probability of infection from the community per unit time and a parameter for the probability of transmission from an infective to a susceptible within the household per unit time. Continuous-time models have analogous rate parameters. One parameter describes the rate of community-acquired infection, the other the rate of transmission from an infective to a susceptible within a household. Both continuous- and discrete-time parameters can be transformed into the probability of acquiring infection from the community over the period of time of interest, called the community probability of infection, CPI, and the secondary attack rate within the household, SAR.

The approaches in this chapter are not used as often as the conventional secondary attack rate (Chapter 12) for vaccine evaluation, but they could be. Standard software is not available for most of the models in this chapter. Estimation generally requires statistical knowledge and computer programming skills.

M.E. Halloran et al., *Design and Analysis of Vaccine Studies*, Statistics for Biology and Health, DOI 10.1007/978-0-387-68636-3_11,

11.1.0.1 Discrete-time model

Consider a study from time period 0 to time period T. Let a be the probability a susceptible household member becomes infected from the community in one time unit. Let $b = 1 - a$ be the corresponding escape probability. Then the probability of escaping infection from the community over the T time periods is $B = b^T = (1-a)^T$, and the community probability of infection is

$$\mathrm{CPI} = 1 - B = 1 - b^T = 1 - (1-a)^T. \tag{11.1}$$

Let $q = 1 - p$ be the probability of escaping infectious contact in a household within one time unit. Then if a person is infectious for T_I time units, the probability of escaping infection from an infective within a household is $Q = q^{T_I} = (1-p)^{T_I}$, and the secondary attack rate is

$$\mathrm{SAR} = 1 - Q = 1 - (1-p)^{T_I}. \tag{11.2}$$

11.1.0.2 Continuous-time model

In the continuous-time model, a parameter α denotes the instantaneous risk of infection from the community and a parameter β denotes the instantaneous risk of infection from an infective in the household. In the simplest form, if the study duration is from time 0 to time T and the duration of infectiousness is T_I, then

$$\begin{aligned} \mathrm{CPI} &= 1 - \exp(-\alpha T), \\ \mathrm{SAR} &= 1 - \exp(-\beta T_I). \end{aligned} \tag{11.3}$$

11.1.0.3 Vaccine effects and other covariates

Vaccination status and other covariates can be easily entered into the models. Either separate values of each parameter can be estimated for each category or parameters representing the effects of covariates can be included in the model. Typically the parameter θ denotes the relative per-contact susceptibility of a vaccinated compared to an unvaccinated person, so that $\mathrm{VE}_{S,p} = 1 - \theta$. Similarly, the parameter ϕ denotes the relative infectiousness per contact of a vaccinated compared with an unvaccinated person, so that $\mathrm{VE}_I = 1 - \phi$. If p is the per-time unit (or per-contact) transmission probability between two unvaccinated people in a household, then θp is the per-time unit (or per-contact) transmission probability to a vaccinated susceptible from an unvaccinated infective. Let unvaccinated and vaccinated status be denoted 0,1. The secondary attack rate from an unvaccinated infective individual to a vaccinate susceptible is $\mathrm{SAR}_{01} = 1 - (1 - \theta p)^{T_I}$.

If only the infective person is vaccinated, then $\text{SAR}_{10} = 1-(1-\phi p)^{T_I}$. If both people are vaccinated, then $\text{SAR}_{11} = 1-(1-\theta\phi p)^{T_I}$. This latter model assumes that the vaccine effects on infectiousness and susceptibility in reducing the transmission probability are independent and multiplicative. Alternatively, one could use another parameter φ to denote the vaccine effect on the transmission probability if both the infective and the susceptible in the contact are vaccinated, so that $\text{SAR}_{11} = 1-(1-\varphi p)^{T_I}$. The vaccine parameters enter similarly into the continuous-time models. For example, assuming multiplicative and independent effects, $\text{SAR}_{11} = 1-\exp(-\theta\phi\beta T_I)$.

The CPI involves only the susceptibles directly. One could introduce another parameter θ_c denoting a different effect of vaccination on reducing susceptibility to infection from the community. However, introducing more parameters into a model sometimes cannot be supported by the amount of data available. Often the assumption is made that the effect of vaccination on protecting against infection from the community and from an infective in a household are the same, so that just one parameter θ is estimated. This is a strong biological assumption, because exposure within a household could be more intense (Fine et al 1988).

Other covariates such as age can be entered similarly into the model. Often, such as in influenza or pneumococcal studies, child- and adult-specific transmission probabilities or rates are estimated. Covariates such as vaccination or treatment status can change over time in models that incorporate time. The parameters a and p, or α and β, can also be time-dependent. Information about the prevalence of infection can be used to estimate the community probability or rate of infection as varying over time, so that a or α can be functions of time. Infectiousness of an infective within a household can vary with time after being infected, so p or β can be functions of time after being infected. If an estimate of prevalence of infection in the population is available, then, in models based on contacts, the transmission probability in the community at large can also be estimated (Hudgens et al 2001).

Note that if we define $\text{VE}_{S,p} = 1-\theta$, this will not necessarily equal

$$VE_{S,SAR} = 1 - \frac{SAR_{01}}{SAR_{00}} = 1 - \frac{1-(1-\theta p)^{T_I}}{1-(1-p)^{T_I}}. \tag{11.4}$$

See Problem 11.1.

11.1.0.4 Estimation

Estimation is most often in a likelihood or Bayesian framework. The likelihood component of the Bayesian model is sometimes exactly the same as that in the likelihood framework. In general, however, a Bayesian framework that uses Markov chain Monte Carlo (MCMC) methods for estimation allows for relaxation of some of the assumptions of a straight likelihood approach. The relaxation of the assumptions often comes at the expense of making other assumptions, particularly in the form of informative priors on some of the parameters.

In the next two sections, we consider models for final-value data and time-of-onset data for diseases in which individuals acquire infection or disease just once over the course of the study. These correspond to either the SEIR or SIR models. In Section 11.4 we present models for longitudinal data for infections with repeated acquisition and clearance of infection, such as in pneumococcal carriage studies. These correspond to SIS models.

11.2 Final-Value Data

The data required are the number of susceptibles in each household at the beginning of the observation period and the number of infections that occurred in each household by the time the observation period is over. Household final-value data for influenza infection are in Tables 10.4 and 11.1. Data further categorized by covariates, such as vaccination, antibody titers (Table 10.5), or age, allow the estimation of the effects of covariates.

Assume that observations are made on infections in a community, starting in time period $t = 0$ and ending in time period $t = T$. This period could correspond to an epidemic season or some other period of epidemiological interest. The main criterion is that all, or nearly all, of the outbreaks in the sample of households should essentially have run their course within $[0,T]$. The final-value data on n households are observed, where a_{jk} = observed number of households with k original susceptibles of which j become infected, $k = 1,2,\dots,K$ and $j = 0,1,\dots,k$, where $\sum_k \sum_j a_{jk} = n$. For example, $a_{13} = 4$ means that there are four households with three household members in which one person became infected. This analysis requires biological confirmation of susceptibility before and infection status after the period of observation. Categorical covariates such as vaccination status or age could also be observed. For example, people could be either unvaccinated or vaccinated, denoted 1 and 2. Then $a_{(j_1,j_2)(k_1,k_2)}$ = observed number of households in which (j_1, j_2) of (k_1,k_2) susceptibles in each household become infected.

11.2.1 Discrete-time model

Longini and Koopman (1982) present a model for the distribution of the total number of cases in households from a homogeneous community and use a maximum likelihood approach for estimation. To derive the final-size distribution of household infections, three key assumptions are made: (1) sources of infection from the community are distributed homogeneously; (2) household members mix at random within the household; and (3) each household member can be infected either from within the household or from the community.

Infection from the community is modeled by defining a_t as the probability a susceptible household member becomes infected from the community in time period

t, and $b_t = 1 - a_t$ is the corresponding escape probability. Define B as the probability that a susceptible individual is not infected from the community during the period of observation. A general expression for B is

$$B = \prod_{t=0}^{T} f(b_t), \tag{11.5}$$

where $f(\cdot)$ is a bounded function describing infection rates in the community. A simple form for $f(\cdot)$ is $f(b_t) = b_t$.

Now consider the effect of secondary spread within a household following introductions from the community. An individual is infected in time period t_0 and will pass through a series of stages in time periods $t_1, t_2, \ldots,$ until becoming immune. Define p_t as the probability that an infective who was infected at time $t = t_0$ will make infectious contact in the household with another individual in time period t. Then $\{p_t\}$ describes the pattern of infectiousness over time. The structure of $\{p_t\}$ is

$$\begin{array}{lll} p_t = 0 & \text{when } t_0 \le t \le t_l, & \text{the latent period,} \\ p_t > 0 & \text{when } t_{l+1} \le t \le t_m, & \text{the infectious period,} \\ p_t = 0 & \text{when } t_{m+1} \le t < t_\infty, & \text{the immune period.} \end{array}$$

Let $q_t = 1 - p_t$ be the daily probability of escaping infectious contact. Then if there is an infected individual in the household who became infected at time $t = t_0$, let Q_{t_r} be the probability that a susceptible individual has escaped infection within the household at time t_r, $t_0 \le t_r < t_{m+1}$. The probability Q that the susceptible individual escapes infectious contact from the infective during his entire period of infectiousness is

$$Q = \prod_{t=t_0}^{t_m} q_t = Q_{t_m}.$$

As described in Section 11.1, the secondary attack rate SAR $= 1 - Q$, and the community probability of infection CPI $= 1 - B$.

11.2.1.1 Final-size distribution

Assume all households under consideration are free of infected members at the beginning and end of the period of observation. Let $\Pr(j|k)$ be the probability that j of k initial susceptibles within a household are infected during the course of the epidemic. Write $m_{jk} = \Pr(j|k)$ to simplify notation.

When $k = 1$, it follows from the above assumptions that $m_{01} = B$ and $m_{11} = 1 - B$. When $k = 2$, $m_{02} = B^2$. For m_{12}, there are two possible ways it can occur. Either the first susceptible individual becomes infected with probability B, and the second susceptible escapes infection from both the community and the infective in the household, or the first susceptible escapes infection from both sources and the second becomes infected in the community. Thus

$$m_{12} = 2(1-B)BQ = 2m_{11}BQ.$$

For m_{22}, similarly

$$m_{22} = 2(1-B)(1-Q)B + (1-B)^2 = 1 - m_{02} - m_{12},$$

because the probabilities must sum to one. In general, there are $\binom{k}{j}$ ways to get j infected individuals from k originally susceptible ones. The general expression for m_{jk} is

$$m_{jk} = \binom{k}{j} m_{jj} B^{k-j} Q^{j(k-j)}, \quad j < k, \text{ and } m_{kk} = 1 - \sum_{j=0}^{k-1} m_{jk}. \tag{11.6}$$

The density function (11.6) provides the final-size distribution for the modified Reed–Frost model of Sugiyama(1960).

If it is assumed that there is spread only within the household, then $B = 1$. If there are initially i infectives within the household, then equation (11.6) becomes

$$m_{jk} = \binom{k}{j} m_{jj} Q^{i+j(k-j)}, \quad j < k,$$

and $i + j$ is the final number of infectives in the household, equivalent to equation (4.7).

When $Q = 1$, there is no spread in households, and the disease in question is presumably not infectious. Then (11.6) reduces to the binomial distribution:

$$m_{jk} = \binom{k}{j} (1-B)^j B^{k-j}, \quad j \leq k. \tag{11.7}$$

This is the distribution of infection in households we would expect if the disease were not contagious, and we would analyze final attack rate data in a community of households. If household structure is ignored or there is no household spread, then CPI $= 1 - B$ is the incidence proportion, or attack rate.

In some cases, the zero class a_{0k} is not present. This occurs when households are surveyed only after an initial infective has appeared, the case-ascertained design. Then the zero-truncated distribution is used. The general expression for m_{jk} is then

$$m_{jk} = \binom{k}{j} m_{jj} B^{k-j} Q^{j(k-j)} / (1 - B^k), \quad j < k. \tag{11.8}$$

11.2.1.2 Likelihood Estimation

The parameters Q and B can be estimated by maximum likelihood (ML). The likelihood function is

$$L(Q,B) = \prod_k \prod_j m_{jk}^{a_{jk}}.$$

The explicit form of the log-likelihood function from (11.6) is

$$\ln L = c + \sum_k \sum_j a_{jk}\{\ln m_{jj} + (k-j)\ln B + j(k - j\ln Q\}). \tag{11.9}$$

The ML estimates $\widehat{Q}$ and $\widehat{B}$ are solutions of the score functions that can be solved iteratively by the method of scoring. The information matrix provides variances and covariances. Estimates from the data provide starting values. In the truncated case, the ML procedure can proceed, using a different approach to get initial guesses. Becker (1989, pp. 182–193) discusses a similar model with an approximate approach for estimation. Becker (1989) and Haber et al (1988) use a generalized linear model approach.

11.2.1.3 Analysis of data from an Asian influenza epidemic

Table 11.1 presents data from an Asian influenza epidemic from households with three initially susceptible people. The data are the number of households that had either 0, 1, 2, or all 3 people infected by the end of the epidemic.

Using model (11.6), $\widehat{B} = 0.856$, $\text{var}(\widehat{B} = 0.0009)$ and $\widehat{Q} = 0.834$, $\text{var}(\widehat{Q} = 0.0063)$. Thus, the estimated probability of a susceptible individual being infected by an infective in his household during the course of his infectious period is $\widehat{SAR} = 1 - \widehat{Q} = 0.166$. Assuming the latent period is $l = 2$ days and infectious period $T_I = 4$ days, and $p_t = p$ for $t = 3,4,5,6$, then the estimated daily probability of escaping infection in the household is $\hat{q} = \widehat{Q}^{1/T_I} = 0.834^{0.25} = 0.956$. The estimated daily probability of infection in a household $\hat{p} = 1 - \hat{q} = 0.044$.

The estimated $\widehat{\text{CPI}} = 1 - \widehat{B} = 0.144$. The approximate percentage of cases from the community can be calculated by setting $Q = 1$. Then from (11.7), if there no spread within the household, the expected number of cases would be

$$nk(1 - \widehat{B}) = 14.4,$$

but the total number of observed cases allowing spread within the household ($\widehat{Q} = 0.834$) is 19. Hence, approximately 75% of total cases were due to infection from the community.

To further illustrate the role of the mixing assumptions in this model, we can estimate the usual attack rate from these data by simply ignoring the household structure. Suppose we do not have information on households. There are 42 households with three people each, so the total population is 126 people. From Table 11.1, 19 people became infected. The attack rate is AR$= 19/126 = 0.151$. The attack rate is interpreted as the probability of becoming infected without any further assumptions about the dynamics of interaction in the community or households. The estimated AR is higher than the estimated community probability of infection, CPI. The sim-

Table 11.1 Observed and expected distributions of Asian influenza data (Sugiyama 1960) in households of size three as analyzed by Longini and Koopman (1982)

Number of Cases	Observed Number of Households	Expected Number of Households
0	29	29.17
1	9	7.87
2	2	3.62
3	2	1.34
Total	42	42.00

Table 11.2 Comparison of CPI and SAR from the influenza A(H3N2) epidemic seasons 1977–1978 and 1980–1981 combined, in Tecumseh, Michigan, stratified by age group and pre-season antibody titer (Longini et al 1988)

Age		Pre-Season Antibody Titer (1 : x)	
		Low Level ($x < 8$)	High Level ($8 \leq x \leq 64$)
Children (0–17 years)	$\widehat{\text{CPI}}$	0.231 ± 0.032	0.094 ± 0.028
	$\widehat{\text{SAR}}$	36.6 ± 6.2	3.4 ± 4.7
Adults (18+ years)	$\widehat{\text{CPI}}$	0.131 ± 0.018	0.089 ± 0.015
	$\widehat{\text{SAR}}$	18.2 ± 4.4	1.6 ± 3.7

ple AR is higher than the CPI because the AR includes the portion of the infected individuals who, under the model that included the SAR, were estimated to have been infected within households. This example illustrates the importance of considering the mixing assumptions within a population when developing models for estimating meaningful population parameters in infectious disease epidemiology.

11.2.1.4 Extension to covariates

Longini et al (1988) extended the model to include categorical covariates such as age group, antibody level, or vaccine status. Assuming that people are equally infectious regardless of stratum, they computed the SAR and CPI for children and adults stratified further by the level of pre-season antibody. The summary data are in Table 10.5 and the estimates are in Table 11.2. An antibody efficacy similar to vaccine efficacy can be computed as

$$\text{Antibody efficacy} = 1 - \frac{\text{Risk(high antibody titer)}}{\text{Risk(low antibody titer)}}, \tag{11.10}$$

using the estimates of SAR and CPI in Table 11.2 and AR in Table 10.5 as the measures of risk (See Problem 11.2).

11.2.1.5 Using Markov chain Monte Carlo methods

O'Neill et al (2000) used Bayesian inference to estimate the probability of escape from infection in the community and from an infective in a household. The likelihood part of their Bayesian model was the same as in Longini and Koopman (1982), with a different recursive approach to obtain the final-size distribution. Using uniform prior distributions for the parameters B and Q, the posterior density should be equivalent to the likelihood. A Metropolis–Hastings algorithm was used for Bayesian inference. Figure 11.1 shows the joint posterior distribution of the two parameters of interest for the Tecumseh data in Table 10.4, where in the figure $q_c = B = 1 - \text{CPI}$, $q_h = Q = 1 - \text{SAR}$. Applying a simple numerical maximization technique to the MCMC output yielded estimates for the Tecumseh data that were virtually identical to those in Addy et al (1991) (Section 11.2.2, Table 11.3). Both O'Neill et al (2000) and Addy et al (1991) obtained $q_c = Q = 0.8677$. O'Neill et al (2000) obtained $q_h = B = 0.8408$ and Addy et al (1991) give $q_h = B = 0.8406$.

11.2.2 Generalized stochastic model

A stochastic infectious disease model was developed by Ball (1986) in which the distribution of the length of the infectious period is allowed to have any distribution that can be described by a Laplace transformation. Addy, et al (1991) extended this model to allow for infection from an unspecified source in the community or transmission within a household. The model allows for discrete covariates, such as age group or vaccine status, for heterogeneous susceptibility and infectivity. The model for the probability of escaping infection in the community, $\text{B} = 1 - \text{CPI}$, is formulated in discrete time. However, the transmission parameter to be estimated is β_{ik}, the rate at which a susceptible of type i has contact with an infective of type k. The final size distribution is found recursively. In the special case of a constant infectious period, the final size distribution is the same as equation (11.6).

If T_I is a constant duration of infectivity and β does not vary, then $\exp(-\beta T_I)$ is the probability of escaping infection by an infective. Then $\text{SAR} = 1 - \exp(-\beta T_I)$. When T_I is variable, the SAR is calculated by taking the expectation, and then $\text{SAR} = 1 - E\{\exp(-\beta T_I)\} = 1 - \phi(\beta)$, where $\phi(\cdot)$ is the Laplace transform of the length of the infectious period. The standard error of the SAR is calculated using the delta method on the Laplace transform, if T_I is variable. Estimates were obtained using maximum likelihood. The results of the analysis of the Tecumseh influenza data in Table 10.4 are in Table 11.3 for constant T_I assuming homogeneity and, in the second analysis, allowing for age-group-specific transmission rates.

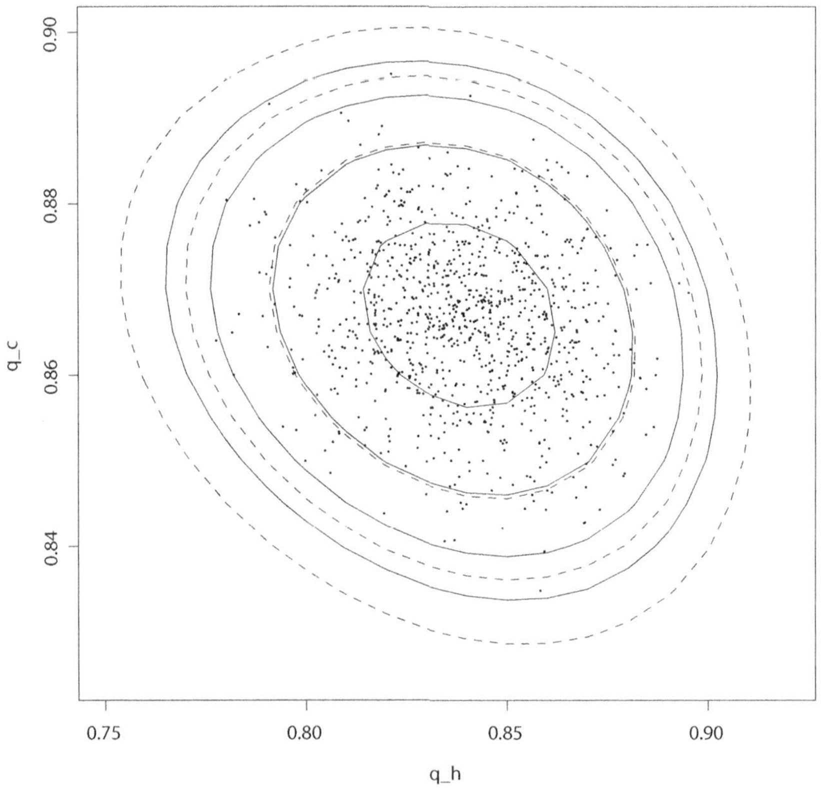

Fig. 11.1 Joint posterior distribution, $q_c = B = 1 - CPI$, $q_h = Q = 1 - SAR$, analyzing Tecumseh influenza data from Addy et al (1991). MCMC sample values (1000 values, at sampling interval 10): ——, contour lines surrounding highest posterior density credible intervals at 50%, 90%, 99%, and 99.9% levels; - - - -, posterior probability density function values of 10%, 1%, and 0.1% of its maximum (courtesy of P. O'Neill, from O'Neill et al 2000, Appl Stat, 49:517–542. Reprinted with permission).

11.2.3 Other final-value analyses

Becker and Angulo (1981) use household data that includes smallpox vaccination status from an epidemic of variola minor, a mild form of smallpox (Angulo 1976) to estimate the protective effects of smallpox vaccination. Becker et al (2003) reanalyze those data and use Bayesian inference to estimate the probability that smallpox vaccination is completely protective and the relative susceptibility and infectiousness in those only partially protected. Magder and Brookmeyer (1993) use a generalized linear model and EM algorithm to estimate the community probability of transmission and transmission parameters for HIV in intravenous drug users. In a

Table 11.3 Maximum likelihood estimates and standard errors for parameters of model of influenza A(H3N2) infections in 1977–1978 and 1980–1981 combined epidemics in Tecumseh, Michigan assuming contant period of infectiousness $T_I = 4.1$ days. For transmission parameters, the first subscript refers to the susceptible, the second to the infective. SAR given in %. (Addy et al 1991)

	Estimate	Transformation
Homogeneity:		
	$\beta = 0.0423 \pm 0.0061$	SAR$= 15.9 \pm 2.1$
	$B = 0.8677 \pm 0.0097$	CPI$= 0.1323 \pm 0.0097$
Log-likelihood	$= -532.974$	
Child= 1, Adult= 2		
	$\beta_{11} = 0.0805 \pm 0.0208$	$\text{SAR}_{11} = 28.1 \pm 6.1$
	$\beta_{12} = 0.0354 \pm 0.0291$	$\text{SAR}_{12} = 13.5 \pm 10.3$
	$\beta_{21} = 0.0268 \pm 0.0135$	$\text{SAR}_{21} = 10.4 \pm 5.0$
	$\beta_{22} = 0.0401 \pm 0.0127$	$\text{SAR}_{22} = 15.2 \pm 4.4$
	$B_1 = 0.8184 \pm 0.0254$	$\text{CPI}_1 = 0.1816 \pm 0.0254$
	$B_2 = 0.8897 \pm 0.0128$	$\text{CPI}_2 = 0.1103 \pm 0.0128$
Log-likelihood	$= -522.333$	

study during a dengue epidemic in Mexico, Dantes et al (1988) used model (11.6) to estimate the SAR and CPI in three Mexican cities.

11.3 Time-of-Onset Data

The data required are the number of susceptibles in each household at the beginning of the observation period and the time of onset of each case or infection that occurred in each household by the time the observation period is over. For covariates that change during the observation period, such as vaccination or treatment status, the time of beginning and possibly end, in the case of treatment, are needed.

11.3.1 Likelihood approach

Yang et al (2006) developed likelihood methods to estimate the prophylactic effects of interventions in households using time-of-onset data. The methods were an extension of the discrete-time data approach (Rampey et al 1992). The methods were motivated by the influenza antiviral household studies in Table 10.7 and used to analyze the two oseltamivir trials. They are also applicable to vaccines and other prophylactic agents. The model assumes the distributions of the latent period and the infectious period are known. The latent period is assumed to be of the same duration as the incubation period, so that a person is assumed infectious once symptoms develop. The model does not take asymptomatic infection into account.

Let the trial start on day 1 and end on day T. The simplest data for each participant are the first date with symptoms of the disease of interest, the assigned treatment, and the treatment period. Let p be the transmission probability per daily contact within the household between a susceptible person and an infective person if both have not received the treatment. Let b be the daily probability that a susceptible untreated person is infected by a source of infection from the community.

Analogous to vaccine efficacies, the antiviral efficacies can be estimated. Let $\text{AVE}_S = 1 - \theta$, where θp is the reduced transmission probability resulting in illness if the susceptible person is taking an antiviral agent and exposed to an untreated infected person in the household. The model assumes that efficacy is the same for contacts outside the household, ie, the reduced transmission probability resulting in illness for a person taking an antiviral agent is θb. $\text{AVE}_I = 1 - \phi$, where ϕp is the reduced transmission probability if the infective person is treated. AVE_T is the total effect on transmission when both people in a transmission pair are treated. The analysis considered the two different assumptions of independence and multiplicativity of θ and ϕ as well as that a separate parameter φ be estimated if both the infective and the susceptible in a contact received treatment. Here we present just the former.

11.3.1.1 Notation and escape probabilities

Let $\tilde{t}_i$ denote the day of illness onset for an infected person i. Let $r_i(t) = (0 \text{ untreated}, 1 \text{ treated})$ indicate the treatment status of person i on day t. Let the function $f(t|\tilde{t}_j)$ denote the probability that person j is infectious on day t given the day of illness onset $\tilde{t}_j$. Assuming independence between θ and ϕ, the probability that a susceptible person i escapes infection by an infective family member j on day t is given by

$$q_{ij}(t) = 1 - \theta^{r_i(t)} \phi^{r_j(t)} p f(t|\tilde{t}_j).$$

Let D_i denote the set of people in the same household with person i. Then

$$e_i(t) = (1 - \theta^{r_i(t)} b) \prod_{j \in D_i} q_{ij}(t) \quad \text{and} \quad Q_i(t) = \prod_{\tau=1}^{t} e_i(\tau)$$

are the escape probabilities for person i on day t and up to day t, respectively. The probability that person i is infected on day t is given by

$$Z_i(t) = Q_i(t-1)(1 - e_i(t)). \tag{11.11}$$

Allowance must be made that we do not observe the exact infection times, but just the onset of illness. Assuming the duration of the latent (and incubation) period is known, then it is possible to compute the maximum and minimum duration of the latent period. Let $\underline{t}_i$ and $\bar{t}_i$ be the earliest and latest potential infection day for person i. Let $g(\tilde{t}_i|t)$ be the probability of illness on day $\tilde{t}$, given infection on day t. Then the contribution to the likelihood of person i is

Table 11.4 Maximum likelihood estimates by age (1–17 vs 18+) for pooled oseltamivir trials conducted in 1998–1999 and 2000–2001, North America and Europe (Yang et al 2006)

Assumption $\varphi = \theta\phi$	Parameter	MLE	95% C.I.	SAR	Estimate	95% C.I.
Yes	b_c †	0.0023	(0.0015, 0.0035)			
	b_a	0.00055	(0.0003, 0.001)			
	p_{cc}	0.038	(0.023, 0.063)	SAR_{cc} ‡	0.15	(0.074, 0.21)
	p_{ca}	0.012	(0.007, 0.021)	SAR_{ca}	0.049	(0.021, 0.075)
	p_{ac}	0.018	(0.008, 0.040)	SAR_{ac}	0.071	(0.014, 0.13)
	p_{aa}	0.022	(0.014, 0.034)	SAR_{aa}	0.086	(0.047, 0.12)
	AVE_S	0.85	(0.52, 0.95)			
	AVE_I	0.66	(-0.10, 0.89)			
	AVE_T	0.95	(0.77, 0.99)			

†, ‡ Subscript c denotes child (1–17), a denotes adult (18+), and ca denotes child-to-adult transmission.

‡ SAR_{vu} is based on the average 4.1 days of infectious period, ie, $\text{SAR}_{vu} = 1 - (1 - p_{vu})^{4.1}$.

$$L_i(b, p, \theta, \phi, \varphi | \tilde{t}_j, j \in D_i) = \begin{cases} Q_i(T) & \text{if } i \text{ is not infected} \\ \sum_{t=\underline{t}_i}^{\bar{t}_i} g(\tilde{t}_i | t) Z_i(t) & \text{otherwise.} \end{cases} \tag{11.12}$$

MLEs can be obtained using usual methods. Results are in Table 11.4. Yang et al (2006) compared randomization schemes and prospective versus retrospective ascertainment designs.

11.3.2 Bayesian latent variable approach

Cauchemez et al (2004) adapted the Bayesian hierarchical model of Auranen et al (2000) developed to analyze pneumococcal carriage studies (Section 11.4.1) to influenza household studies. The essential difference is that unlike in the pneumococcal carriage studies, individuals can have only one episode of influenza. That is, the model for influenza assumed an SIR model, rather than an SIS as in Section 11.4.1. A main difference in this influenza model compared to that in Section 11.3.1 is that the distribution of the duration of the infectious period for influenza is estimated whereas in the previous model it was assumed known. An additional difference is that it is assumed that individuals became infectious as soon as infected, that is, there is no latent period. Similar to the likelihood model in 11.3.1, this model does not take asymptomatic infections into account

The influenza Epigrippe study in France motivating the analysis is described in Section 10.3.4. The data were times of ascertainment of culture-confirmed index cases in physicians' practices and the time of onset of clinical influenza (not biologically confirmed) in individuals within ascertained households. Similar to Auranen et al (2000), the unobserved start and end of the infectious period for each case of influenza were imputed using a data augmentation algorithm. Let $I(t)$ be the collection of infectives in a household. Let α_i be the rate of transmission from the community for individual i. Let ε_i measure the susceptibility to infection of individual i, and β_j measure the ability of j to infect others. Let $\varepsilon_i\beta_j/n$ be the rate of transmission from an infective j to a susceptible i in a household of size n. For an individual i susceptible just before t, the rate of transmission to i is

$$\lambda_i(t) = \alpha_i + \varepsilon_i \sum_{j \in I(t)} \beta_j/n, \tag{11.13}$$

similar to model (11.16). The duration of the infectious period for infective j was assumed to follow a gamma distribution, with mean μ_j, standard deviation σ_j, and density d_{μ_j,δ_j}. The distribution of the infectious period was estimated from augmented data for the unobserved dates of the start and end of the infectious period. An MCMC approach was used for estimation. The prior distribution for both μ and σ was a gamma distribution with mean 3 and standard deviation 2. The vague prior distribution for both α and β was the exponential distribution Exp(0.001).

The community probability of infection (CPI)f is defined as the probability that participant i would be infected from the community during the 15-day follow-up period of the household,

$$\mathrm{CPI}_i = 1 - \exp(-15\alpha_i).$$

The secondary attack rate, SAR, defined as the probability that an infective j infects susceptible i in a household of size n is

$$\mathrm{SAR}_{ij}(n) = 1 - \int_0^{+\infty} \exp\left(-\varepsilon_i \frac{\beta_j}{n}\right) \mathrm{d}_{\mu_j,\delta_j}(t)\mathrm{d}t. \tag{11.14}$$

The interest was in exploring the role of children in the infection process, so parameters were stratified by children under 15 years and adults.

The mean duration of the influenza infectious period was estimated at 3.8 days (95% CI 3.1–4.6) with standard deviation of 2.0 days (95% CI 1.1–2.8) for a 95% credible interval for the infectious period of (0.8,8.6) days for influenza. The overall household SAR attack for clinical influenza (not biologically confirmed) decreased from 0.43 (95% CI 0.39–0.48) in households of size 2 to 0.21 (95% CI 0.18–024) in households of size 5. This result could be partly model-dependent. The overall CPI over the 15 days of follow-up was 0.08 (95% CI 0.04–0.12). They found similar age-specific trends in transmission parameters as other researchers.

11.3.3 Other time-of-onset analyses

A data-augmentation method was developed to analyze the two zanamivir trials in Table 10.7 (Yang et al 2007b). Similar models were used as the basis for a resampling-based test to detect person-to-person transmission of an infectious disease (Yang et al 2007c) and to detect human-to-human transmission of Avian A (H5N1) influenza (Yang et al 2007a). The software TranStat is publicly available for this purpose. Yang et al (2009b) developed a Bayesian approach to analyze the influenza household studies with time of onset data that takes data on asymptomatic infection into account.

11.4 Longitudinal Data

Many bacterial infections are characterized by repeated acquisition and clearance of infection. Asymptomatic carriage of pneumococcal bacteria, meningococcal bacteria, and *H. influenza b* (Hib) bacteria are three examples. To estimate the acquisition and clearance rates, one needs longitudinal data where a collection of individuals in households is sampled over time at a number of time points. Several field studies that gathered longitudinal data from repeated sampling within families or schools are described in Section 10.5. The problem with longitudinal data of asymptomatic carriage is that neither the acquisition nor clearance times are observed. Different approaches to statistical models can deal with this problem making a variety of assumptions.

Motivated by two studies of Hib carriage in Finland, Auranen et al (1996) proposed the use of a susceptible–infected–susceptible (SIS) model for estimating the acquisition and clearance parameters. At any given time, individuals can be in either the noncarrier, susceptible state S, or the asymptomatic, infectious carrier state C. People can make the transition between states, $S \to C$ and $C \to S$. The mini-epidemic in the family is represented by an individual-based stationary Markov model that describes the dynamics of infection in the family. The approach is also appropriate for use with pneumococcal carriage studies. Other problems with pneumococcal studies include combining multiple serotype data, missing data, competition, and errors in diagnosis.

The key parameters in the model are the hazard rates of transitions $S \to C$ and $C \to S$. Let $C(t)$ be the number of carriers in the family at time t. The basic model before allowing for covariates, for the transition $S \to C$ is a combination of the effective contact rate within the family β and the rate of infection from the community α. The rate of transition $S \to C$ for susceptible i, the acquisition rate, is

$$\lambda^{(i)}(t) = \alpha^{(i)} + \beta^{(i)}C^{(i)}(t). \tag{11.15}$$

One can also make the transition rates age-group dependent, such as children and adults. The constant rate of transition $C \to S$, the clearance rate, is denoted by $\mu^{(i)}$. The spread of carriage within a family is modeled by a Markov process. The state at time t is the combined state of the individuals in the family. The possible transitions within a family in any time interval can be described by a matrix of transition probabilities. However, the matrix is of large dimension leading to possible computational difficulties. This approach is discussed in more detail in Section 11.4.2.

A second approach was suggested by Auranen et al (2000) that makes use of Bayesian data augmentation. For each individual, the unobserved times of acquiring and clearing carriage are included in the model as latent unobservable variables. If the acquisition and clearance times of each individual were known, the conditional likelihood of the data would be simple. Markov chain Monte Carlo methods are used to augment the data with the acquisition and clearance times. The approach considers histories of infection events separately for each individual.

Pneumococcal carriage studies and the models in this section fit well within the context of a general framework of estimating vaccine effects. Vaccine parameters for susceptibility and infectiousness, also vaccine-dependent clearance rates, could be added to the models. The question of how to use these approaches in pivotal trials of vaccines for licensure is open (Käyhty et al 2006).

11.4.1 Bayesian latent variable approach

Auranen et al (2000) modeled the sequences of binary observations on pneumococcal (Pnc) carriage by constructing latent point processes of acquiring and clearing carriage. The longitudinal pneumococcal carriage study motivating this analysis is described in Section 10.5.1. The model allows for carriage of different serotypes s. The study identified seven Pnc serotypes that were going to be included in the planned vaccine. The analysis was confined to the three most prevalent types, 6B, 19F, and 23F. The data for children under 5 years old are summarized in Table 11.5. The observed numbers of changes in the carriage status over the observation intervals are presented. The data are stratified according to age class, 0 to 2 years and 2 to 5 years. They are also stratified by the background carriage in the family at the start of the observation period. The table summarizes the data over the three serotypes. Pnc carriage was almost always clustered by serotype within a family.

The hierarchical model has three stages: the observation model, the transmission model, and the prior model. In the observation model, the augmented data need to be consistent with the observed data. Any observation of carriage of that serotype needs to take place during one of the augmented periods of carriage that results from the imputed acquisition and clearance times. Figure 11.2 illustrates the data augmentation approach. The model assumes conditional independence between consecutive observations of the same individual as well as between observations of different family members. The transmission model allows dependence of the process within the family.

The transmission model is of the form in model (11.15). Let α be the rate to acquire carriage of serotype s from the community, β be the rate of transmission from an infective in a family to a susceptible, μ be the clearance rate (no serotype specific rates), and n be the size of the family. $C_i^{(s)}(t)$ is a 0,1 indicator if individual i is a carrier of serotype s at time t, and $C_i(t)$ indicates any of the serotypes. Let T_i

Table 11.5 The number of observed changes in the individual pneumococcal carriage status over the observation intervals (Auranen et al 2000)

Carriage among other family members at start of observation interval		Age Class 0–2 years Carriage at Next Observation			Age Class 2–5 years Carriage at Next Observation		
	Carriage	No	Yes	Total	No	Yes	Total
No carriage in in family	No	562	33	595	107	10	117
	Yes	16	12	28	8	4	12
Total		578	45	623	115	14	129
At least one carrier in family	No	24	1	25	12	6	20
	Yes	6	10	16	6	7	13
Total		30	11	41	20	13	33

denote the time of birth of individual i , so that $t - T_i$ is the age of subject i. The intensities of the point processes of acquiring and clearing carriage are

$$\tilde{\lambda}_i^{(s)} = \left[\alpha(t-T_i) + \beta(t-T_i)\sum_{k=1}^{n} C_k^{(s)}(t)\right] \times \{1 - C_i(t)\}$$

$$\tilde{\mu}_i(t) = \mu C_i(t). \tag{11.16}$$

Model (11.16) makes several assumptions. The acquisition rates α and β are assumed to depend on the age of the noncarrying susceptible. The acquisition rates are assumed to be the same for all three serotypes. The model allows carriage of only one serotype at a time. The duration of carriage is assumed to be an exponential random variable that is the same for all three serotypes. The model also requires an initial carriage state for each individual that is related to the proportion π of Pnc carriers, assumed to be a single parameter across all age groups and for all serotypes. The proportion π needed to be estimated because the initial observation was missing on some of the participants. The rate μ of clearing carriage was assumed to be μ_1 for children under 2 years old and μ_2 for family members 2 years and older.

The full Bayesian model, notation, and methods for computation were presented in Auranen et al (2000). The parameters to be estimated were α, β, μ, and π from the imputed acquisition and clearance times, the serotype data, and the initial carriage status data. The priors on the parameters were assumed to be independent. Vague priors were used on all of the parameters, with means informed in part by the data. The acquisition rates α_f and β_f were assumed to be same for all family members older than 5 years, with rate ratio $\varphi_f = \beta_f/\alpha_f$. An age-dependent $\alpha(a)$ was assumed for children less than 5 years old. The function was formulated as piecewise constant over the interval 2 and 60 months of age. The rate ratio $\varphi = \beta(a)/\alpha(a)$ was assumed to be constant.

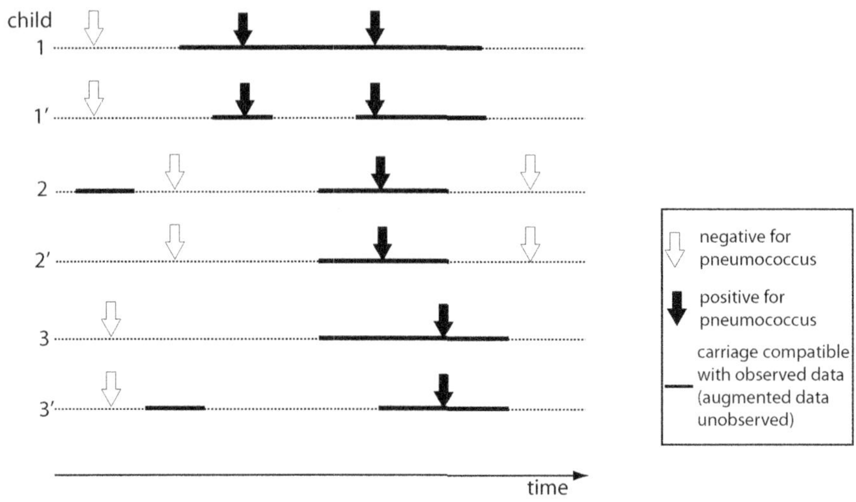

Fig. 11.2 Data augmentation strategy to estimate transmission parameters of *Streptococcus pneumoniae* in a longitudinal study of pneumococcal carriage. The observed data are presence or absence of pneumococcal bacteria in the nasopharynx. The data are augmented with the times of acquisition and clearance of carriage which give the period of carriage. The figure shows two different possible augmentations compatible with the observed data.

The age-dependent community acquisition rate $\alpha(a)$ in children under 5 years old increases up to approximately 0.3 new infections per year at age 18 months, which corresponds to the increased prevalence of carriage. Further estimates are in Table 11.6. The posterior mean of the ratio φ of the within-family (with at least one carrier in the family) and the community rate of acquisition was 25 in children under 5 years. In family members older than 5 years, the posterior mean rate of community acquisition was 0.037 per year and the rate ratio φ_f was 15. The posterior mean duration $(1/\mu_1)$ of carriage was longer in children less than 2 years old than in older family members $(1/\mu_2)$. The model was assessed using a number of approaches. A clear pattern in the data was the temporal clustering of pneumococcal carriage within families.

Cauchemez et al (2006d) used a similar approach to Auranen et al (2000) to analyze a longitudinal study in France in schools described in Section 10.5.2. The primary scientific question of the analysis was whether the seven Pnc vaccine serotypes have a competitive advantage over the nonvaccine serotypes. The analysis proposed to study this question by comparing the mean duration of carriage $(1/\mu)$ and within school child-to-child transmission rate (β) of the seven vaccine serotypes with those of the nonvaccine serotypes, denoted by V and U, respectively. No children had yet been vaccinated. The vaccine serotypes are 6B, 9V, 14, 18C, 19F, and 23F. Vaccine serotype 4 was not included in the analysis because it was isolated in only 10 samples. The nonvaccine serotypes included in the analysis are 6A, 3, 19A, 11A, 15A, 23A, 17F, 10A, and 9L.

Table 11.6 Summary of the marginal posterior distribution of the parameters estimated for the Finnish pneumococcal carriage study in households. Parameter definitions are in the text (Auranen et al 2000)

Parameter	Mean	Median	90% Equal-Tail Credible Interval
α_f (per year)	0.037	0.037	0.016–0.061
φ	25	23	14–44
φ_f	15	10	3-42
μ_1 (per month)	0.45	0.44	0.30–0.66
μ_2 (per month)	0.71	0.69	0.49–1.01
$1/\mu_1$ (months)	2.3	2.3	1.5–3.3
$1/\mu_2$ (months)	1.5	1.4	1.0–2.0
π	0.023	0.022	0.011–0.037

The model is similar to that in (11.16), except the term for transmission within school included the term $1/n$, where n is the number of children in the school regardless of whether they took part in the study. The term $1/n$ serves as a density factor and reduces transmission the larger the school is. Thus the individual rate to acquire serotype s at time t was $\beta C_s(t)/n$, rather than just $\beta C_s(t)$, where $C_s(t)$ is the number of children carrying serotype s at time t.

An expression for the secondary attack rate, SAR, the probability that a child carrying the bacteria transmits to a noncarrying child during the carriage period, is presented. Comparing the SAR for the vaccine types to that of the nonvaccine types allows comparison of the overall fitness for transmission because it is a function of the mean duration of carriage and the child-to-child transmission rate. Let L be the duration of carriage with density $f(L) = \mu \exp(-L\mu)$ and $1 - \exp(-\beta L/n)$ be the probability that a carrying child during time period L transmits to a noncarrying child in the school. Then

$$SAR = \int_0^{\infty} (1 - \exp(-\beta L/n) f(L) dL,$$

which reduces to $SAR = (1 + n\mu\beta^{-1})^{-1}$. The results are summarized in Table 11.7. There was no evidence that the vaccine serotypes had different transmission characteristics than the nonvaccine serotypes. Cauchemez et al (2006c) further investigated heterogeneity among the 15 serotypes using a clustering step to select a parsimonious description of the transmission characteristics.

11.4.2 Markov transition model

Another approach to estimating the acquisition parameters α and β in equation (11.15) and the clearance rate μ is by explicit formulation of the transition matrix for the Markov process in the households (Auranen et al 1996). The spread of carriage

Table 11.7 Summary of the marginal posterior distribution of the parameters estimated for the study of pneumococcal carriage in schools in France. Parameter definitions are in the text (Cauchemez et al 2006d)

	Vaccine Serotype		Nonvaccine Serotype		Ratio	
	Mean	95% Credible Interval	Mean	95% Credible Interval	Mean	95% Credible Interval
$1/\mu$ (days)	23	21–25	22	20–24	1.06	0.94–1.28
β (% day^{-1})	4.6	4.2–5.0	5.1	4.5–5.6	0.91	0.80–1.05
SAR (%)						
$n = 30$	3.4	3.2–3.7	3.6	3.3–3.8	0.97	0.88–1.06
$n = 50$	2.1	1.9–2.2	2.2	2.0–2.3	0.97	0.88–1.06
$n = 100$	1.1	1.0-1.2	1.1	1.0–1.2	0.97	0.88–1.06

within the family is modeled by the transition between states in a Markov process. The state of the family at time t is the combined state of the individuals in the family. The number of possible states depends on the number of individuals in the family. In a family with three members, there are eight possible states. Letting 1 indicate a carrier and 0 a noncarrier, the possible states are 000, 001, 010, 011, 100, 101, 110, and 111. A family in which at one observation time, the second person is a carrier, the other two noncarriers, and at the next observation time, both the second and third are carriers, makes the transition from state 010 to state 011. The corresponding intensity matrix Q with elements q_{ij} is

$$\begin{array}{ccccccccc}
 & 000 & 001 & 010 & 011 & 100 & 101 & 110 & 111 \\
000 & q_{11} & \alpha^{(3)} & \alpha^{(2)} & 0 & \alpha^{(1)} & 0 & 0 & 0 \\
001 & \mu^{(3)} & q_{22} & 0 & \alpha^{(2)}+\beta^{(2)} & 0 & \alpha^{(1)}+\beta^{(1)} & 0 & 0 \\
010 & \mu^{(2)} & 0 & q_{33} & \alpha^{(3)}+\beta^{(3)} & 0 & 0 & \alpha^{(1)}+\beta^{(1)} & 0 \\
011 & 0 & \mu^{(2)} & \mu^{(3)} & q_{44} & 0 & 0 & 0 & \alpha^{(1)}+2\beta^{(1)} \\
100 & \mu^{(1)} & 0 & 0 & 0 & q_{55} & \alpha^{(3)}+2\beta^{(3)} & \alpha^{(2)}+\beta^{(2)} & 0 \\
101 & 0 & \mu^{(1)} & 0 & 0 & \mu^{(3)} & q_{66} & 0 & \alpha^{(2)}+2\beta^{(2)} \\
110 & 0 & 0 & \mu^{(1)} & 0 & \mu^{(2)} & 0 & q_{77} & \alpha^{(3)}+2\beta^{(3)} \\
111 & 0 & 0 & 0 & \mu^{(1)} & 0 & \mu^{(2)} & \mu^{(3)} & q_{88}
\end{array}$$

The elements on the diagonals represent the intensity of staying in the same state. The $q_{ii} = 1 - \sum_{j \neq i} q_{ij}$ (Karlin and Taylor 1975). The element (4,8) represents the transition from state 011 to state 111. Individual number 1 has the transition rate $\alpha^{(1)} + 2\beta^{(1)}$, representing the rate of acquisition from the community and the exposure by the two carriers in the household. To simplify estimation, the model only allows one family member to make a transition during the time period of the time step. The 0s in the matrix represent transitions that are not allowed, and thus have 0 intensity. The matrix can represent households of any size and include age- or covariate- (vaccination status) dependent rates. For the Hib analysis, Auranen et al (1996) had two levels of the three rate parameters, one for children under seven years old and one for everyone older than seven. They used a Bayesian approach to estimate the model parameters.

Melegaro et al (2004) used a similar model to estimate the acquisition and clearance rates for a household study of pneumococcal carriage in the United Kingdom (Hussain et al 2005) presented in Section 10.5.3. A density correction factor $(n-1)^w$ was added, where $(n-1)$ is the number of other family members in a household size n, and w corresponds to the level of density dependence. When $w=0$, the model represents density-independent transmission.

The population was divided into two age groups, children under 5 years and everyone else greater than 5 years, denoted by $i=1,2$. $C_1(t)$ and $C_2(t)$ are the number of carrier children (<5 yrs) and adults in the household. Then the probability of a transition in a short time interval δt for an individual in age class i is

$$\Pr_i(S \to C)_{\delta t} = \left(\alpha_i + \frac{\beta_{1i}C_1(t) + \beta_{2i}C_2(t)}{(n-1)^w}\right) \cdot \delta t,$$

$$\Pr_i(C \to S)_{\delta t} = \mu_i \cdot \delta t.$$

Melegaro et al (2004) use a Markov model with 1-day intervals to analyze 28-day interval data assuming only one person can change in the household per day. The parameters were estimated using a likelihood approach. The estimate of the density parameter w was significantly greater than 0 ($w = 1.2$, 95% CI 0.2–2.2) suggesting that transmission within households depends on density.

In a further analysis, Melegaro et al (2007) extended the model to estimate serotype-specific transmission parameters. Five distinct data sets were constructed, one for each of the target serotypes. The carriage status of each study participant was recorded at each monthly visit as 0 (noncarrier), 1 (carrier of the target serotype), 2 (carrier of any other serotype), or 9 when the swab was not taken or the laboratory result was not reported. Estimation used a likelihood approach.

Problems

11.1. $VE_{S,p}$ and $VE_{S,SAR}$

(a) Consider a vaccine that reduces the per-day transmission probability to a susceptible from 0.1 in an unvaccinated person to 0.03 in a vaccinated person. What is $VE_{S,p}$ based on the transmission probability?

(b) Now consider that index case exposes the susceptibles on average four days. Use equation (11.4) to compute the expected $VE_{S,SAR}$. Compare $VE_{S,p}$ and $VE_{S,SAR}$ and consider the consequences for interpreting such estimates.

11.2. Comparing antibody efficacies

(a) Compute the antibody efficacies based on the SAR, CPI, and AR for children and adults using equation (11.10) and the results in Tables 10.5 and 11.2.

(b) Compare the estimates and explain why the antibody efficacy based on the SAR is higher than those based on the CPI and AR.

11.3. Likelihood for B and Q for final value data
Write out the log-likelihood function (11.9) explicitly in terms of B and Q for a data set with households of size $k = 1,2,3$, with number of infectives $j = 0,\ldots,k$.

11.4. Final size distribution if not contagious
(a) Assuming there is no spread within households and that CPI = 0.3, based on equation (11.7), compute the final size distribution of infection in a community of 1000 households of size 3.
(b) Repeat for CPI = 0.4.
(c) What statistical method could be used to test whether there is within-household spread?

11.5. Asymptomatic infections
In the analyses of time-of-onset of influenza data in Section 11.3, the asymptomatic influenza infections are not taken into account. How might symptomatic infections be ascertained in these studies? Presumably the time of onset of asymptomatic infections would not be observed. How could this be dealt with in the analysis?

11.6. Estimating transmission parameters for longitudinal data
What are the essential similarities and differences in the assumptions of the Bayesian latent variable approach and the Markov transition approach to modeling and estimating the transmission parameters for the longitudinal pneumococcal carriage studies?

Chapter 12
Analysis of Independent Households

12.1 Introduction

In this chapter, we consider methods of analysis that assume that the households are independent of one another. The most commonly used approach is to estimate vaccine efficacy based on the conventional secondary attack rate. We also consider the estimation of indirect effects of vaccination using household studies. The Reed–Frost model in Chapter 4 is another example of a model that assumes households or transmission units are independent.

12.2 Conventional SAR Analysis

The data structures for the conventional secondary attack rate analysis are similar to those for the analysis using time of onset data assuming that households are within communities in Section 11.3. Data on the time of onset of disease for each case in the household as well as knowledge of who is susceptible are required. To estimate the conventional household SAR, the main task is to set up the analysis. Decisions need to be made on

1. who in the household is eligible to be a secondary case, and
2. who of the eligible household members are the secondary cases.

The first contributes to the denominator of the secondary attack rate, the second contributes to the numerator.

One decides who is the index, or primary case in the household, and which of the other cases in the household could reasonably have been infected by the primary case. Occasionally one differentiates the index case, the case that results in ascertainment of the household, from the primary case, the earliest temporal case in the household. To decide which of the subsequent cases in the household could have been infected by the primary case, one needs estimates or assumptions about the minimum and maximum incubation periods, the latent period and its relation

M.E. Halloran et al., *Design and Analysis of Vaccine Studies*, Statistics for Biology and Health, DOI 10.1007/978-0-387-68636-3_12,

to the incubation period, and the maximum time that a person remains infectious. These values will vary according to the disease of interest. Using this information, one then needs to define the time interval after the primary case that would include the secondary cases. Based on the time of onset data within each household, each case is defined as being either a secondary case or not. Co-primary cases are people who developed disease too soon after the primary case to have been infected by the primary case. They are not counted as secondary cases, and are generally simply excluded from the analysis. They are not included in the denominator of the SAR. Primary cases are also not included in the analysis. The estimated household secondary attack rate is the total number of secondary cases in all households divided by the total number of at-risk susceptibles in all households. In some cases, tertiary or higher generation cases may be included in the analysis by calling the secondary cases the primary case for further chains of transmission. Tertiary cases or higher cases are included in the denominator of exposed individuals for the secondary attack rate, but not in the number of cases in the numerator. Chapter 10 contains several examples of studies with intervals for determining the eligible susceptible household members and the secondary cases.

Pertussis vaccination. Préziosi and Halloran (2003b) defined exposed susceptibles as children with no history of pertussis living in a compound with an index case (Section 10.2.3). Onset of pertussis symptoms was assumed to be the onset of infectiousness, thus the latent period was assumed to equal the incubation period. Co-primaries were those cases whose onset of cough was <7 days after that of the index case. To allow for uncertainty in duration of infectiousness, a secondary case was defined as a case whose date of onset was ≥ 7 days after that of the index case and less than a variable cutoff, specifically no cutoff, 56, 42, or 28 days. Similar assumptions were made by Kendrick and Eldering (1939) (Section 10.2.2). In the PHLS Epidemiologic Research Laboratory (1982), the co-primaries were those within 7 days of the index case and secondary cases were those that occurred within about 42 days of the index case and at least 7 days after the index case (Section 10.2.4). In a reanalysis of this study, co-primaries were defined as cases within one week of the primary case (Fine et al 1988). Incidence cases were those that occurred more than one week after the primary cases. These included more than potentially secondary cases.

Measles. For measles, Orenstein et al (1985) recommend 18 days of follow-up in a household after the onset of rash in the primary case. Garenne et al (1993) defined secondary cases as those occurring in the same compound 7 to 18 days after the index case (Section 10.4.1). Exposed susceptibles were children who had never had measles living in a compound where there was a clinical case.

Mumps. In a secondary attack rate analysis of mumps vaccine efficacy in an outbreak investigation, Kim-Farley et al (1985) defined co-primaries as cases in family members occurring within 10 days of the onset of disease in the index case. Cases with onset of disease more than 30 days after the index case were considered tertiary cases. Children with previous history of mumps disease, unknown vaccine histories, or unknown dates of vaccination were excluded from the analysis.

In the conventional secondary attack rate analysis, the assumption is that the households or other small transmission units are independent of one another. There is an asymmetric assumption that the index case and co-primaries get infected from outside the unit, and the other susceptibles are exposed only within the unit. This assumption is very different than the assumption in Chapter 11 in which individuals can acquire infection from the community even if there is an infective in the household. If the transmission probability or secondary attack rate is estimated without taking into account the opportunity to become infected outside of the transmission unit, it will overestimate the actual probability of becoming infected per contact. In general, ratio measures, such as the vaccine efficacy based on the ratio of secondary attack rates, are less biased by this problem. Kemper (1980) discusses biases in conventional SAR estimation. The drawback in using models such as those in Chapter 11 is that they contain strong modeling assumptions about the mixing in the community. An advantage of the conventional SAR studies or case-contact study designs is that they do not make assumptions about the community at large. The analysis is also relatively simple once the biological assumptions about the time intervals containing the secondary cases have been made.

12.2.1 Vaccine efficacy from conventional SAR

As described in Chapter 2, the secondary attack rates can be differentiated by the vaccine status of the primary case and/or the vaccine status of the secondary cases. In general, there are at least seven measures potentially of interest. Considering the estimates of VE based on the relative secondary attack rates, there are three main unstratified vaccine effects:

$$VE_{S.1/.0} = 1 - \frac{SAR_{.1}}{SAR_{.0}}, \quad VE_{I1./0.} = 1 - \frac{SAR_{1.}}{SAR_{0.}},$$
$$VE_T = 1 - \frac{SAR_{11}}{SAR_{00}}. \tag{12.1}$$

The traditional measure of $\text{VE}_{S,SAR}$ to estimate the protective effect of vaccination in household studies corresponds to $\text{VE}_{S.1/.0}$. When not ambiguous, we use the notation $\text{VE}_{S,SAR}$ for traditional estimates. If one stratifies on the vaccine status of the infective person or the susceptible person, then there are four further stratified measures of VE_S and VE_I:

$$VE_{S01/00} = 1 - \frac{SAR_{01}}{SAR_{00}}, \quad VE_{S11/10} = 1 - \frac{SAR_{11}}{SAR_{10}},$$
$$VE_{I10/00} = 1 - \frac{SAR_{10}}{SAR_{00}}, \quad VE_{I11/01} = 1 - \frac{SAR_{11}}{SAR_{01}}. \tag{12.2}$$

The confidence interval for any of the VE_{SAR} measures is generally based on the log relative risk. If a_0, a_1 are the number of cases and n_0, n_1 are the number exposed in the relevant comparison groups, then the relative risk is $RR = a_1 n_0 / a_0 n_1$. The standard deviation of the log relative risk is

$$\sigma = \left(\frac{1}{a_1} - \frac{1}{n_1} + \frac{1}{a_0} - \frac{1}{n_0} \right)^{1/2}.$$

The vaccine efficacy estimate and 95% confidence interval are

$$VE_{SAR} = 1 - \frac{a_1/n_1}{a_0/n_0}, \tag{12.3}$$
$$95\%\ \text{CI} \quad [1 - \exp(\log(RR) + 1.96 * \sigma), 1 - \exp(\log(RR) - 1.96 * \sigma)].$$

For example, in the Medical Research Council study of pertussis vaccination (Table 10.2), there were $a_1 = 37$ pertussis cases among $n_1 = 203$ home exposures in the vaccinated children, and $a_0 = 151$ cases among $n_0 = 173$ home exposures in the unvaccinated children. In the report, the vaccination status of the exposing children is not included, so only the traditional unstratified $\text{VE}_{S,SAR}$ can be computed. The $\text{VE}_{S,SAR}$ estimate and 95% confidence interval are 0.79 [95% CI 0.72, 0.84].

This simple approach does not take into account that several children may be exposed to the same infective, so that there may be correlation within households. Becker et al (2006) consider estimation of vaccine effects, in particular, VE_I and VE_S from pairs of individuals within households. Quite often, one infectious person exposes several people, possibly within a transmission unit, such as a household. Correlation within transmission units or unmeasured heterogeneity across transmission units could result, for example, from differences in infectivity, difference in mixing within the unit, or genetic variation. This conventional method to estimate the confidence intervals for vaccine efficacy fails to take the structure of the clustered binary data into account.

12.3 SAR Analysis Taking Correlation into Account

Préziosi and Halloran (2003b) and Halloran et al (2003b) were particularly interested in estimating the effect of pertussis vaccination on reducing infectiousness of vaccinated cases, VE_I. They analyzed the pertussis vaccination study in Niakhar, Senegal, described in Section 10.2.3. The data are summarized in Table 10.1. Many of the compounds had several children, so correlation within compound might be important. They developed methods for estimating the VE measures based on the SAR that take correlation within transmission units into account. We present these methods using the pertussis vaccination study in Niakhar, Senegal, as an example.

12.3.1 Notation

Let n be the number of compounds with a unique index case and m_i be the number of susceptibles in the ith compound. Let y_{ij} be the binary (0,1) pertussis outcome of the jth susceptible exposed to the index case in the ith compound for any given case definition. Let $x_{ij} = (x_{ij1}, \ldots, x_{ijp})'$ denote a $p \times 1$ vector of explanatory variables associated with y_{ij}. In particular, let $x_{i\cdot 1}$ denote the vaccine status of the index case in compound i, and x_{ij2} the vaccine status of the jth exposed susceptible individual in compound i. Complete pertussis vaccination requires at least three doses of vaccine. This analysis considers only unvaccinated and fully vaccinated children, with $x_{i\cdot 1} = 0$ and $x_{i\cdot 1} = 1$ for an unvaccinated and fully vaccinated index case. Similarly, x_{ij2} is 0 or 1 for the unvaccinated and fully vaccinated susceptibles.

Let N_{vs} be the total number of susceptibles in the n compounds with vaccine status s exposed to index cases with vaccine status v, and a_{vs} be the total number of cases in the N_{vs} susceptibles. In this analysis, $V, S \in \{0, 3\}$. The subscript 0 denotes unvaccinated, 3 indicates three doses of vaccine. Additional levels of vaccination are possible, such as $V, S \in \{1, 2\}$ for partially vaccinated people, but are not considered here. The $\cdot$ subscript represents collapsing over strata. The number of cases and susceptibles in each grouping of interest is

$$
\begin{aligned}
a_{vs} &= \sum_{i=1}^{n} \sum_{j=1}^{m_i} I_{V=v} I_{S=s} y_{ij}, & N_{vs} &= \sum_{i=1}^{n} \sum_{j=1}^{m_i} I_{V=v} I_{S=s}\,, \\
a_{..} &= \sum_{i=1}^{n} \sum_{j=1}^{m_i} y_{ij}, & N_{..} &= \sum_{i=1}^{n} m_i\,, \\
a_{.s} &= \sum_{i=1}^{n} \sum_{j=1}^{m_i} I_{S=s} y_{ij}, & N_{.s} &= \sum_{i=1}^{n} \sum_{j=1}^{m_i} I_{S=s}\,, \\
a_{v.} &= \sum_{i=1}^{n} \sum_{j=1}^{m_i} I_{V=v} y_{ij}, & N_{v.} &= \sum_{i=1}^{n} \sum_{j=1}^{m_i} I_{V=v}\,.
\end{aligned}
$$

Let SAR_{vs} denote the secondary attack rate from an index case with vaccine status v to a susceptible with vaccine status s. Pooling across compounds, the standard two SARs not stratified by vaccine status of the index case used in estimating protective $\text{VE}_{S,SAR}$ are $\text{SAR}_{\cdot s} = a_{\cdot s}/N_{\cdot s}$, $s = 0, 3$. If not stratified by vaccine status of the susceptible, $\text{SAR}_{v\cdot} = a_{v\cdot}/N_{v\cdot}$, $v = 0, 3$. The nonparametric estimates of the four SARs stratified by vaccine status of index cases and susceptibles are $\text{SAR}_{vs} = a_{vs}/N_{vs}$, $v, s = 0, 3$.

The three main unstratified nonparametric VEs in equation (12.1) and stratified nonparametric VEs in equation (12.2) can be estimated using these SARs with the standard confidence intervals as in equation (12.3).

12.3.2 Vaccine efficacy based on the logistic model

To take correlation within compounds into account, a marginal model or a random-effects model could be used. The parametric form in both cases is the logistic model, with the SAR as the usual probability p of an event. The model-based approach allows inclusion of covariates, such as age, either of the index case as compound-level environmental variables or of the susceptibles as individual variables. In marginal models, inference about population averages is the focus (Diggle et al 1994, pp. 131–135). If there is heterogeneity across compounds in the baseline transmission, then the estimated baseline coefficients represent an average over the heterogeneities. The correlation structure is some function of the marginal mean and possibly additional parameters.

In the random-effects model, a slightly different baseline transmission is estimated for each compound, with the degree of heterogeneity estimated in the variance of the random effect. The vaccine effects in each compound are interpreted in relation to that compound's baseline transmission. In considering vaccine efficacy, the primary scientific question is about the population average, or marginal, VE measures. Thus, the marginal model is the model of choice. The coefficients for the marginal and random-effects models are indicated by β and β^*.

12.3.2.1 The marginal model

The marginal model for the logit of the SAR_{ij} of the jth person in the ith household is

$$\mathrm{logit}(SAR_{ij}) = \beta_0 + \beta_1 x_{i\cdot 1} + \beta_2 x_{ij2} \,, \tag{12.4}$$

where $x_{i\cdot 1}$ denotes the vaccine status of the index case in compound i and x_{ij2} denotes the vaccine status of the jth exposed susceptible in compound i. The vaccine status of the index case, $x_{i\cdot 1}$, enters the analysis as a compound-level, environmental variable. To obtain VE estimates on the SAR scale, we transform the parameters from the logistic model to the probability scale. The stratified SARs from model (12.4) are

$$\begin{aligned} SAR_{00} &= \frac{\exp\beta_0}{1+\exp\beta_0}, & SAR_{03} &= \frac{\exp(\beta_0+\beta_2)}{1+\exp(\beta_0+\beta_2)}, \\ SAR_{30} &= \frac{\exp(\beta_0+\beta_1)}{1+\exp(\beta_0+\beta_1)}, & SAR_{33} &= \frac{\exp(\beta_0+\beta_1+\beta_2)}{1+\exp(\beta_0+\beta_1+\beta_2)}. \end{aligned} \tag{12.5}$$

Parameter estimates from the above model provide estimates for the stratified $\mathrm{VE}_{S00/03}$ and $\mathrm{VE}_{S30/33}$, the stratified $\mathrm{VE}_{I00/30}$ and $\mathrm{VE}_{I03/33}$, as well as VE_T. Plugging the expressions for the SARs into equations (12.2), and for VE_T in equation (12.1), the expressions for the VE measures are

$$VE_{S03/00} = \frac{1-\exp(\beta_2)}{1+\exp(\beta_0+\beta_2)}, \qquad VE_{S33/30} = \frac{1-\exp(\beta_2)}{1+\exp(\beta_0+\beta_1+\beta_2)},$$
$$VE_{I30/00} = \frac{1-\exp(\beta_1)}{1+\exp(\beta_0+\beta_1)}, \qquad VE_{I33/03} = \frac{1-\exp(\beta_1)}{1+\exp(\beta_0+\beta_1+\beta_2)},$$
$$VE_T = \frac{1-\exp(\beta_1+\beta_2)}{1+\exp(\beta_0+\beta_1+\beta_2)}. \tag{12.6}$$

To obtain estimates of the unstratified $\mathrm{VE}_{I3./0.}$ and $\mathrm{VE}_{S.3/.0}$, additional submodels are fit, such as $\mathrm{logit}(SAR_{ij}) = \beta_0' + \beta_1' x_{i\cdot 1}$ and $\mathrm{logit}(SAR_{ij}) = \beta_0'' + \beta_2'' x_{ij2}$ and transformed back to obtain

$$VE_{I3./0.} = \frac{1-\exp(\beta_1')}{1+\exp(\beta_0'+\beta_1')}, \qquad VE_{S.3/.0} = \frac{1-\exp(\beta_2'')}{1+\exp(\beta_0''+\beta_2'')}. \tag{12.7}$$

Alternatively, one could use the parameter estimates from the full model (12.4) and substitute the respective means of $x_{i\cdot 1}$ and x_{ij2}. The marginal model taking correlation of transmission within compound into account can be estimated using generalized estimating equations (GEE) (Liang and Zeger 1986).

Appropriate confidence intervals on the transformed scale are obtained using the bootstrap (Efron and Tibshirani 1993). Bootstrap samples were selected using the compound as the sampling unit. Three different bootstrap confidence intervals were computed, namely the percentile, the bias-corrected (BC), and the bias-corrected and accelerated (BC_a) intervals. Figure 12.1 shows the point estimates and histograms of 2000 bootstrap estimates of the VE_I, VE_S, and VE_T parameters based on the GEE model. Bootstrap confidence intervals sampling on compounds were also computed for the VE estimators based on the nonparametric SARs described in the previous section. Analytic confidence intervals for the GEE estimates of VE on the transformed scale were obtained using the multivariate delta method (Agresti 1990).

12.3.2.2 The random-effects model

The random-effects model for the logit of the SAR_{ij} of the jth person in the ith household is

$$\mathrm{logit}(SAR_{ij}|U_i) = (\beta_0^* + U_i) + \beta_1^* x_{i\cdot 1} + \beta_2^* x_{ij2}\,. \tag{12.8}$$

The simplest model assumes the random effect $U_i \sim N(0,\sigma^2)$. On the logistic scale, the parameter β_0^* would be interpreted as the log odds of transmission from an unvaccinated index case to an unvaccinated susceptible for a typical compound with random effect $U_i = 0$. The parameter β_1^* would be the log odds ratio of transmission occurring when the index case is vaccinated compared to when it is unvaccinated within any given compound. The parameter β_2^* would be the log odds ratio of transmission occurring when a susceptible in the compound is vaccinated compared to a susceptible in that same compound who is unvaccinated.

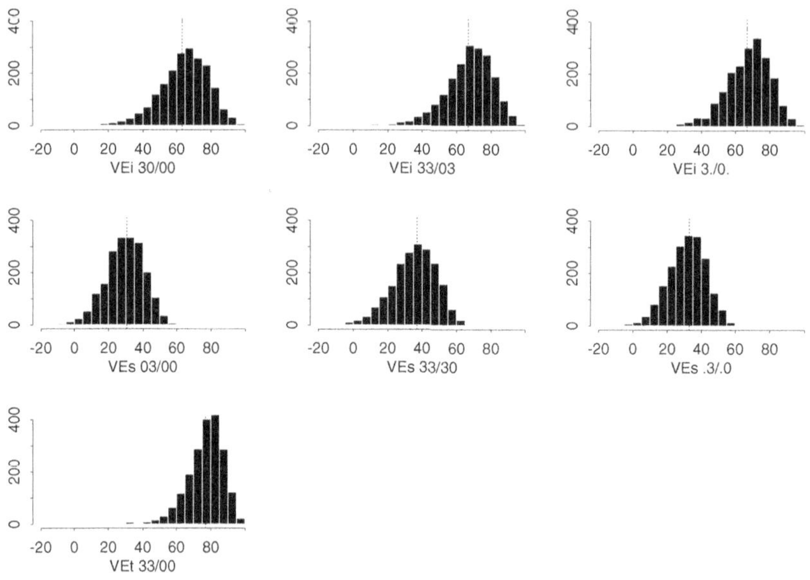

Fig. 12.1 Histograms of 2000 bootstrap estimates of (top row) VE for infectiousness, VE_I stratified and unstratified; (middle row) VE for susceptibility, VE_S, stratified and unstratified; and (bottom) total VE, VE_T, based on the GEE logistic regression parameters. The dotted line in each histogram indicates the estimate for the actual data set. (Halloran et al 2003b, Journal of the American Statistical Association, 98:38–46. Reprinted with permission.)

The compound-specific SAR_{ij}s are obtained by incorporating the random effect into the expression. For example, the compound-specific SAR_{00i} from an unvaccinated index case to an unvaccinated susceptible is

$$SAR_{00i}|U_i = \exp(\beta_0^* + U_i)/[1 + \exp(\beta_0^* + U_i)].$$

The marginal SAR_{00} is the estimated expectation of the SAR_{00} obtained by numerical integration over the estimated distribution of the random effects. The VE_i estimates for each compound i are obtained from expressions analogous to (12.6). The marginal VE estimates are the estimated expectations obtained by numerical integration over the estimated distribution of the random effects. To obtain estimates of the unstratified $VE_{I3./0.}$ and $VE_{S.3/.0}$, random effects submodels similar to those described above can be fit.

Two methods were used to estimate the random effects model. The first is a Bayesian hierarchical model (Carlin and Louis 2008), and the second is a nonlinear mixed model (Davidian and Giltinan 1995). The population mean VE measures were computed by averaging over the compounds at each iteration. The 95% poste-

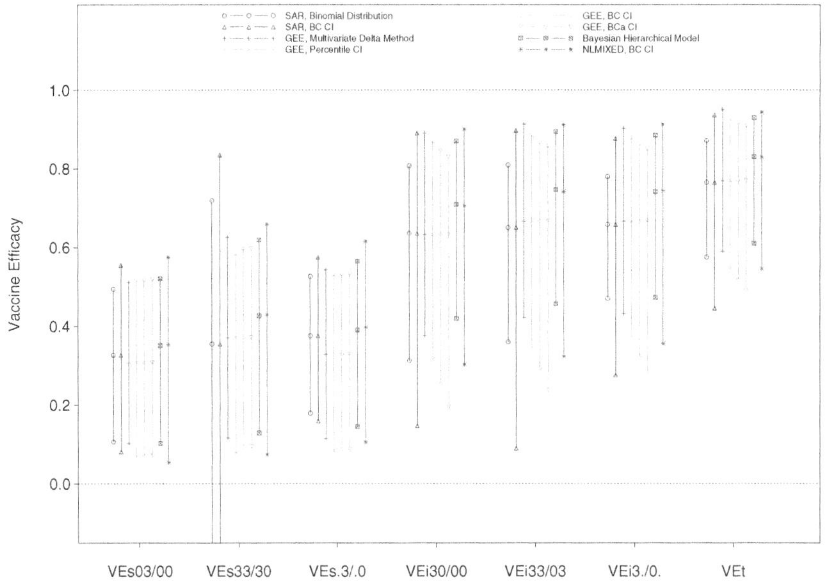

Fig. 12.2 Comparison of approaches to estimating SARs and confidence intervals. (Halloran et al 2003b, Journal of the American Statistical Association, 98:38–46. Reprinted with permission.)

rior credible intervals for the VE measures are available directly on the transformed scale from the approximation to the posterior distribution from the MCMC chains.

12.3.3 Pertussis vacccine efficacy

Figure 12.2 shows the different point estimates and confidence intervals for VE_S, VE_I, and VE_T. Table 12.1 contains selected results. The point estimates for VE_I and VE_T obtained from the nonparametric SAR and from the GEE are nearly identical. The bootstrap CIs for the nonparametric VE estimates are wider than the simple CIs based on the log relative risk. In particular, the bootstrap CIs for VE_I, and to a lesser extent, VE_T are wider. For example, the BC bootstrap 95% CI of $VE_{I3./0.}$ is 1.94 wider than the simple 95% CI. The difference is less pronounced with CIs of VE_S, with the ratio of the lengths being between 1.2 and 1.3. Thus, the conventionally used CI substantially underrepresents the variability in the data. The greater sensitivity of the variability of the VE_I and VE_T estimators to compound-level effects might result from the vaccine status of the index case being a compound-level environmental variable. The nonparametric estimate of $VE_{S33/30}$ is unstable because the

Table 12.1 Pertussis vaccine efficacy estimates from the Niakhar region, Senegal, 1993 (Halloran et al 2003b)

	Vaccine Efficacy (VE) × 100% (95% Confidence Interval)						
	VE for Susceptibility			VE for Infectiousness			Total VE
Estimator	$VE_{S03/00}$	$VE_{S33/30}$	$VE_{S.3/.0}$	$VE_{I30/00}$	$VE_{I33/03}$	$VE_{I3./0.}$	VE_T
SAR (BC*)	33 (8,55)	36 (−62,88)	38 (16,57)	64 (15,89)	65 (9,90)	66 (28,88)	77 (45,94)
SAR (simple)	33 (11,49)	36 (−48,72)	38 (18,53)	64 (31,81)	65 (36,81)	66 (47,78)	77 (58,87)
GEE (BC)	31 (7,52)	37 (9,60)	33 (9,53)	63 (25,85)	67 (29,87)	67 (32,86)	77 (52,92)
NLMIXED (BC)	35 (5,57)	43 (7,66)	40 (11,61)	71 (32,90)	74 (32,91)	74 (36,91)	83 (54,94)
Bayes median	35 (10,52)	43 (13,62)	39 (15,56)	71 (42,87)	75 (46,89)	74 (47,88)	83 (61,93)

* BC = bias-corrected bootstrap confidence interval.

total number of secondary cases was only 20, compared with 134 cases for $VE_{S03/00}$, so both the simple and the BC bootstrap CIs are quite wide.

The bootstrap CIs of the GEE estimates of VE_I are also wider than those based on the simple CI for the nonparametric VE estimates, however, not as wide as the bootstrap CIs of the nonparametric VE estimates. For example, the GEE percentile, BC, and BC_a bootstrap 95% CIs for $VE_{I3./0.}$ compared to the simple SAR 95% CI are 1.63, 1.74, and 1.83 wider, respectively. Thus, the parametric model in the GEE helps stabilize the estimation compared to the nonparametric approach.

The multivariate delta method CIs on the GEE estimates are symmetric and similar in length to the percentile bootstrap CIs. However, the normality assumption of the VE_I and VE_T estimators is clearly violated, so we do not recommend using the multivariate delta method. Also, CIs based on the multivariate delta method could theoretically exceed one, which could cause difficulty because vaccine efficacy is bounded at 1.

12.3.4 Varying case definition and cutoff

Préziosi and Halloran (2003b) considered the effect of varying the case definition and the cutoff date on the seven VE estimates. The data are summarized in Table 10.1. The primary focus of the analysis was on estimating VE_I. The primary method of analysis was the GEE approach using the bias-corrected and accelerated (BCa) bootstrap confidence intervals described in the previous section. Based on the main case definition and no cutoff of secondary cases, vaccine efficacy for infectiousness VE_I was estimated to be 0.85 (95% CI 0.46–95) for children vaccinated with three doses of a whole cell (94%) or an acellular (6%) pertussis vaccine. See Problem 12.3.

Table 12.2 Antiviral efficacies for oseltamivir (Halloran et al 2007a). Osel I is presented in Hayden et al (2004), Osel II in Welliver et al (2001)

	Based on Laboratory-Confirmed Infection with Symptoms			
Effect	$AVE_{.d}$	95% C.I.	Drug Cases/Exposed	Control Cases/Exposed
$AVE_S = 1 - SAR_{11}/SAR_{10}$ (Osel I alone)				
1 – 7 Days	81	35, 94	3/237	16/241
2 – 7 Days	81	35, 94	3/237	16/241
$AVE_S = 1 - SAR_{01}/SAR_{00}$ (Osel II alone)				
1 – 7 Days	91	64, 98	2/205	22/195
2 – 7 Days	91	62, 98	2/205	21/194
$AVE_I = 1 - SAR_{10}/SAR_{00}$ (Osel I/Osel II)				
1 – 7 Days	81	45, 93	4/180	22/190
2 – 7 Days	80	43, 93	4/180	21/189
$AVE_T = 1 - SAR_{11}/SAR_{00}$ (Osel I/Osel II)				
1 – 7 Days	91	63, 98	2/195	22/190
2 – 7 Days	91	61, 98	2/195	21/189

12.4 Estimating Influenza Antiviral Efficacies

Halloran et al (2007a) used the conventional secondary attack rate to estimate the influenza antiviral efficacies from the four randomized household studies of influenza antiviral presented in Chapter 10 and analyzed by Yang et al (2006, 2007b, 2009b), as described in Chapter 11. Each of the efficacies can be based on (1) laboratory-confirmed influenza illness, $AVE_{.d}$, or (2) laboratory-confirmed infection, $AVE_{.i}$, in the eligible household contacts. Here we present only the estimates based on laboratory-confirmed influenza illness, $AVE_{.d}$, for the two oseltamivir studies (Table 12.2). Influenza has a very short incubation period. The interval for co-primaries was assumed to be either one day or two days after ascertainment of the index case. As discussed in Chapter 10, the randomization schemes in the studies restrict which SAR_{ij}s, and thus which antiviral efficacies could be estimated from the individual studies. The estimate of $AVE_{S,d}$ in the Hayden et al (2004) study is based on different SAR_{ij}s from that in the Welliver et al (2001) study. The AVE_I and AVE_T estimates are obtained by combining the two studies.

12.5 Mini-Community Design for Indirect Effects

In the mini-community design, the household or other small transmission unit serves as the unit in which to estimate indirect effects of vaccination, similar to studies in larger communities to estimate indirect, total, and overall effects (Chapter 13). The gradient from small transmission units, such as households, to compounds as in Niakhar, to day care centers, to schools, to towns or whole countries is fairly continuous. Thus, this section could also have been put into Chapter 13, but here we focus on households. Similar to many household-based vaccine efficacy studies, these mini-community studies can be nested in either randomized clinical trials or observational studies where the primary analysis is based on unconditional measures. Unlike the other efficacy measures in this chapter, the estimates of the indirect effects of vaccination do not condition on the index case being a case of infection or disease. In the indirect effect measures, the analysis conditions only on the vaccination status of the index child or children in the household. The outcomes of interest are the disease or infection status of the other members of the household. Then the estimates of the indirect effects in the other members of the household are based on one of the unconditional risk measures, such as attack rate or cases per person-time in the other members of the household. If based on incidence rates per person-time, then

$$\mathrm{VE}_{IIa} = 1 - \frac{\frac{\text{no. of cases in household members of vaccinated children}}{\text{person-time of household members of vaccinated children}}}{\frac{\text{no. of cases in household members of unvaccinated children}}{\text{person-time of household members of unvaccinated children}}}. \tag{12.9}$$

12.5.1 Pertussis

Trollfors et al (1998) nested a study of the indirect effects of pertussis vaccination in households in the Swedish study described in Section 10.2.5. They estimated the indirect effects based on equation (12.9) using the ratio of the incidence rates (pertussis cases divided by total time at risk) in parents and younger siblings of recipients of DTaP or DT. They used four different case definitions, the first being similar to the WHO definition, and the second based on criteria developed by themselves. They further divided the cases by $\geq$21 days of paroxysmal cough and cough $\geq$7 days. Other criteria were similar to those discussed in Section 12.3.4. The results are in Table 12.3. Unfortunately, the original paper does not include the amount of person-time computed for each group.

Problems

12.1. Computing mumps $\mathrm{VE}_{S,SAR}$

(a) Table 12.4 shows the data from a family-based mumps vaccine efficacy study after an outbreak in Ashtabula County, Ohio, in 1982. In study 1, vaccine status was verified by the parents. In study 2, it was verified by the provider. Compute the

Table 12.3 Number of pertussis cases in parents and younger siblings of study children and indirect protection achieved by vaccination of the study child with pertussis toxoid (from Trollfors et al 1998)

	Pertussis Cases		Indirect Protection	
	DTaP	DT	(%)	95% CI
Parents				
WHO definition				
≥21 days of paroxysmal cough	11	26	60	16, 82
≥7 days of cough	23	35	38	−9, 65
Göteborg definition				
≥21 days of paroxysmal cough	14	32	58	20, 80
≥7 days of cough	26	44	44	7, 67
Younger siblings				
WHO definition				
≥21 days of paroxysmal cough	10	18	43	−31, 76
≥7 days of cough	11	10	37	−40, 73
Göteborg definition				
≥21 days of paroxysmal cough	10	26	61	15, 83
≥7 days of cough	11	26	56	9, 81

secondary attack rates and $VE_{S,SAR}$ with confidence intervals for both studies.
(b) Compare the estimates.

Table 12.4 Data from family-based mumps vaccine efficacy study in families of students with mumps illness in the sixth, seventh, and eighth grades in School A, Ashtabula County, Ohio, February 5 through April 23, 1982 (Kim-Farley et al 1985)

	Study 1	Study 2
Case definition	Parotitis ≥2 days	Parotitis ≥2 days
Case finding	Parents	Parents
Vaccine status	Parents	Provider verified
Cases/exposed (vaccinated)	4/36	2/30
Cases/exposed (unvaccinated)	32/74	30/69

12.2. Computing measles VE_{SAR}
(a) Table 12.5 contains data from a measles epidemic in Senegal 1994–1995 (Cisse et al 1999). Compute the estimates based on the SARs of the main VE_S, VE_I, and VE_T, the two stratified VE_Ss and the two stratified VE_Is. Compute their confidence intervals using the standard approach.
(b) Compare the main and the stratified estimates.

12.3. Pertussis vaccine efficacy with different cutoffs
(a) Table 10.1 contains the number of secondary pertussis cases using four different

Table 12.5 Number of exposed susceptibles, secondary cases, and secondary attack rates (SAR) by vaccination status of the index case and the exposed susceptible children (Cisse et al 1999)

	Exposed Susceptibles and Secondary Cases					
	Vaccinated		Unvaccinated		Combined	
Index Case	Cases/Exposed	SAR	Cases/Exposed	SAR	Cases/Exposed	SAR
Vaccinated	6/83	0.07	3/17	0.18	9/100	0.09
Unvaccinated	41/374	0.11	47/124	0.38	88/498	0.18
Total	47 /457	0.10	50/141	0.35	97/598	0.16

follow-up cutoffs. Compute different VE_{SARs} using different cutoffs.
(b) Discuss how and why the SARs and the VE_{SAR} estimates change as the cutoff period increases.

12.4. Different analyses
(a) Create a hypothetical community composed of small transmission units. Assign to each individual a covariate status (0,1) and also an infection time and infection status at the end of an epidemic. Consider the various approaches for estimating the effect measures, such as the conventional secondary attack rate, the secondary attack rate, and the community probability of infection simultaneously, and the simple cumulative incidence (attack rate).
(b) How do the data being used for each approach differ? What parameters can be estimated? What is the interpretation of the measures under each approach?

Chapter 13
Assessing Indirect, Total, and Overall Effects

13.1 Study Designs for Dependent Happenings

Due to the dependent happenings in infectious diseases (Ross 1916), widespread vaccination in a population can reduce transmission and produce indirect protective effects, even in unvaccinated individuals. The public health importance of a vaccine is related to the direct protection of the vaccinated individuals as well as the indirect protection conferred by increased herd immunity at the population level. In recent years, interest in estimating the indirect, total, and overall effects of vaccination programs has increased. Most often, the effects have been evaluated using surveillance data by comparing the incidence before and after implementation of a vaccination strategy in a population. In some cases, dramatic effects have been observed such as with pneumococcal vaccines (Musher 2006). Up until now, planned, prospective community-randomized studies to evaluate indirect, total, and overall effects of vaccination strategies are rare. However, interest in implementing such studies, either pre- or post-licensure is increasing. Although mathematical models offer useful guidance on examining potential population effects of vaccination strategies (Chapters 4 and 5), they cannot replace data from an actual study when such a study is feasible.

Struchiner et al (1990) and Halloran and Struchiner (1991) developed a conceptual framework for four classes of study designs to evaluate the direct, indirect, total, and overall effects of interventions called the study designs for dependent happenings. In Chapter 2 we introduced the general concepts of direct, indirect, total, and overall effects of vaccination and the four basic study designs to evaluate them (Figure 2.3). In this chapter, we present the concepts of direct, indirect, total, and overall effects using an informal potential outcomes approach to causal inference. Throughout this chapter we distinguish two levels of intervention, vaccination strategies, allocations or programs at the population level, and vaccination of individuals within populations. We present some of the observational approaches to assessing indirect, total, and overall effects, and their advantages and disadvantages. We then present community-randomized studies as an approach to estimation

M.E. Halloran et al., *Design and Analysis of Vaccine Studies*, Statistics for Biology and Health, DOI 10.1007/978-0-387-68636-3_13,

and inference of indirect, total, and overall effects. We consider basic designs, approaches to randomization, sample size determination, and general considerations of analysis. Finally we formally define causal estimands of direct, indirect, total, and overall effects and their estimators for group randomized studies.

13.1.1 Definitions and study designs

Following Halloran and Struchiner (1991), the *direct effect* of vaccination in an individual is the difference between the outcome in the individual receiving the vaccine and what the outcome would have been if the individual had not been vaccinated, all other things being equal. This definition of a direct effect corresponds to the notion of potential outcomes in causal inference in that it is defined for the unobservable difference between the response in the observed person and what it would have been in the same person without the intervention. An example of a direct effect is the reduction in the probability of becoming infected that results from being vaccinated, given exposure to infection.

The *indirect effect* of a vaccination program or strategy on an individual is the difference between what the outcome is in the individual not being vaccinated in a community with the vaccination program and what the outcome would have been in the individual, again not being vaccinated, but in a comparable community with no vaccination program. It is, then, the effect of the vaccination program on an individual who was not vaccinated. The combined *total effect* in an individual of being vaccinated and the vaccination program in the community is the difference between the outcome in the individual being vaccinated in a community with the vaccination program and what the outcome would be if the individual were not vaccinated and the community did not have the vaccination program. The total effect, then, is the effect of the vaccination program combined with the effect of the person having been vaccinated. The *overall effect* of a vaccination program is the difference in the outcome in an average individual in a community with the vaccination program compared to an average individual in a comparable population with no vaccination program.

A simple indirect effect is the reduction in the probability per unit time of becoming infected that results from reduced exposure to infection consequent to a mass immunization program. Thus, an unvaccinated person in a population experiences a changed hazard or incidence compared with what it would have been if the commmunity had had no immunization program. The analogous total effect would be the effect experienced by a vaccinated person who has both the benefits of being vaccinated and the indirect effect of the reduced transmission. The overall effect would be the weighted average of the reduction in incidence in the vaccinated and unvaccinated individuals compared to if there were no immunization program.

These effects can be defined more generally, by allowing that vaccination occurs in the comparison population as well, however, with a different level of coverage or different allocation strategy. The definitions also apply to subpopulations of interest within comparison populations, for example, school children only. The indirect, total, and overall effects are defined within the context of a particular intervention program or allocation strategy. For example, one would expect that the indirect effects of vaccinating 30% of the population would differ from the indirect effects of vaccinating 60% of the population compared to no vaccination. Common to these effects is the need to imagine a community in which vaccination had not taken place or a community with an alternative vaccination strategy.

The four different kinds of effects of vaccination motivated the definition of broad categories of study designs (Struchiner et al 1990) based on different pairs of comparison populations and subpopulations, according to whether the studies measure direct, indirect, total, or overall effects as shown in Figure 2.3. The community with the vaccination strategy is population A, and the community with no vaccination, or the alternative, possibly baseline vaccination strategy is population B. In the simple case of having only two comparison populations, the study designs for dependent happenings are analogous to studies that compare outcomes before (population B) and after (population A) implementation of a vaccination strategy in the population. However, because the community level effect is of interest, for statistical inference, one generally will prefer to have several communities in which the intervention takes place and several comparison communities. Then there would be several A communities and several B communities. If the allocation of the vaccination program to the communities is randomized, then the study becomes a group- or cluster-randomized design as discussed in Section 13.3.

When several communities are included in the study, the indirect effects of a particular allocation of vaccination is then the comparison of the incidence or other outcome of interest in the unvaccinated people in the A communities compared to the comparable unvaccinated people in the control B communities. These comparisons are called type IIa designs. The indirect vaccine effectiveness measures are designated VE_{IIa}. The total vaccine effects of the combination of being vaccinated and the allocation is the outcome in the vaccinated people in the A communities compared to that of the comparable unvaccinated people in the unvaccinated B communities. These comparisons are called type IIb designs, and the total vaccine effectiveness measures are designated VE_{IIb}. The overall effectiveness of the vaccine and allocation compare the average outcomes in the vaccinated communities with those of the control communities. These comparisons are called type III designs, and the overall effectiveness measures are designated VE_{III}.

These study designs for dependent happenings are quite general. They do not specify the outcome measure, the parameter of effect, temporal aspects, sampling methods, or methods of analysis. In addition, each of these designs makes a comparison between comparable populations, in that, in the absence of an effect, the outcomes of the compared populations could be expected to be similar. In particular, in infectious diseases, one needs to emphasize the need for comparability of exposure to infection. That is, if there were no intervention program, the individuals in the comparison communities would be exposed comparably to infection. This is often not the case, especially when several communities are included in the study,

Table 13.1 Comparisons pre- and post-introduction of a vaccination strategy to estimate indirect, total, or overall effects

Comparison
Change in incidence or attack rates in target population (overall effects), possibly stratified by vaccination status (indirect and total effects)
Reduction in incidence in age groups that did not receive vaccination strategy (indirect)
Reduction in incidence greater than vaccine coverage (overall)
Change in age distribution of disease
Increased prevalence of colonization and disease by nonvaccine strains

in which case the design can incorporate matching or stratification as described in Section 13.3.4.

Table 2.2 contains examples of the VE_{IIa}, VE_{IIb}, and VE_{III} based on the usual unconditional measures incidence rate, hazard rate, and cumulative incidence. Many other measures could be used, including average age of infection or the basic reproductive number, R_0. The change in the average age of infection could be in the unvaccinated people (indirect effect), the vaccinated people (total effect), or the average of the whole population (overall effect.)

13.2 Observational Studies

13.2.1 Pre- and post-vaccination comparisons

A common approach to estimating indirect, total, and overall effects of introducing a new vaccination program to a population is to compare the pre-vaccination with the post-vaccination incidence. These comparisons depend on good data on cases of the illness of interest and some method to determine the denominators. To determine indirect or total effects, one also needs to know the vaccination status of the reported cases. One might also want to know the level of vaccine coverage and the age-appropriate and age-specific vaccine uptake.

Comparisons of pre- and post-vaccination outcomes include comparison of incidence or attack rates before and after introduction of vaccination (overall effects), possibly also stratified by vaccine status (indirect and total effects), reduction in incidence greater than vaccine coverage, reduction in incidence in age groups that did not receive vaccination, change in the age distribution of disease, and increased prevalence of colonization and disease by nonvaccine strains (Table 13.1).

If the reduction in overall incidence, including both the vaccinated and unvaccinated individuals combined, is higher than the level of coverage, there is a strong indication of indirect effects of vaccination. Thus, even with a 100% efficacious vaccine, if coverage were 60%, one would not expect a greater than 60% reduction in incidence if there were no indirect effects. Thus, an observed 80% reduction in incidence would be evidence for indirect benefits of vaccination. Another indication that herd immunity is playing a role is a reduction in incidence in age groups that are too young or too old to be in the age group targeted by the strategy. Reduction of incidence in these groups is evidence of a purely indirect effect of the vaccination program. The mean and median age of first infection will generally increase as transmission is reduced, because it will take on average longer for a person (child) to be exposed. As transmission is reduced, incidence in all age groups may decrease, but the relative proportion of cases in the older age groups could increase. The change in age of first infection is also an indication that the reproductive number R is changing. In cases of infectious agents with many circulating strains, only some of which are contained in the vaccine, such as *Streptococcus pneumoniae*, there is interest in whether the prevalence of colonization and incidence of disease due to the nonvaccine strains will increase as the prevalence of vaccine strains is reduced.

If an observed change in outcome, such as a change in incidence rate, is to be attributed to the vaccination strategy when comparing only the pre- and post-vaccination situation, one needs to make an assumption of minimal secular trends. When the pre- and post-vaccination differences are small, and one is comparing only one pre- to one post-vaccination population, one cannot be sure that some other cause than vaccination is not responsible for any observed changes. For example, change in sanitation or simple cyclical variation of the infection rates might decrease incidence. Also, if the duration of observation is short, for instance, a comparison of influenza one year and then the following year in which a vaccination campaign was done, one cannot be sure that a lower influenza incidence in the second year was not simply due to a milder influenza season.

Another approach to estimating effects of widespread vaccination is to compare data from different regions with different levels of coverage. Ali et al (2005) reanalyzed an individually randomized trial of cholera vaccine by comparing incidence in areas with different vaccine coverage levels (Section 13.2.5). However, the level of vaccine uptake may be related to other factors correlated with the level of incidence. Thus the estimates of indirect effects could be confounded, unless the coverage levels were randomized.

13.2.2 Pertussis

13.2.2.1 Pertussis in Niakhar, Senegal

Préziosi et al (2002) studied pertussis in a prospective cohort of children in rural Niakhar, Senegal over a 13-year period before and after introduction of a pertussis vaccination program. Children under age 15 years who were residents of the Niakhar study area were followed prospectively between January 1984 and December 1996 for the occurrence of pertussis. (See Section 10.2.3 for further details.) From 1980 to 1985, sporadic immunizations were performed, reaching fewer than 5% of the

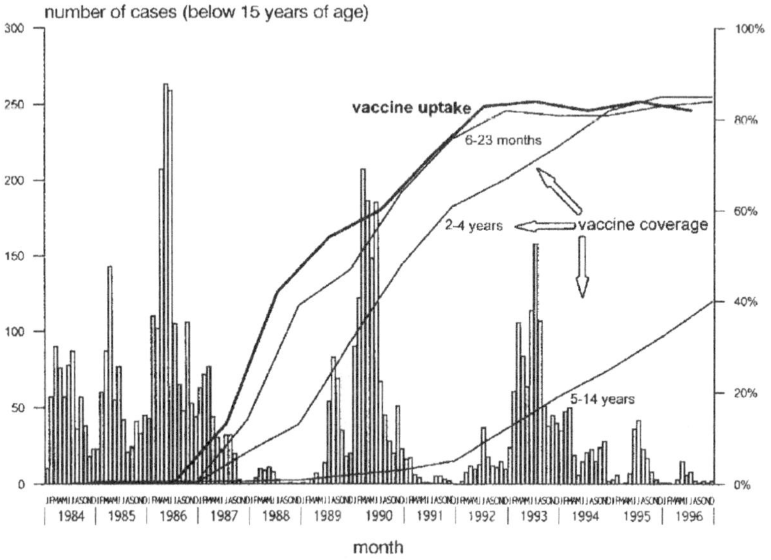

Fig. 13.1 Pertussis cases per month, vaccine uptake, and age-specific vaccine coverage per year, Niakhar, Senegal, 1984–1991 (Préziosi et al 2002, Am J Epidemiol 155:891–896. Reprinted with permission.)

children. From November 1986 to January 1987, Senegalese authorities conducted Expanded Program of Immunization (EPI) mass immunization campaigns targeting children under age five years. After August 1987, infants were immunized by monthly visits of the EPI mobile teams, with rigorous record keeping. From 1987 to 1989, children received whole cell pertussis vaccine as part of DTP-IPV at approximately 3, 5, and 10 months of age. From 1990 to 1996, clinical trials of the relative efficacy of whole cell pertussis and acellular pertussis vaccines were conducted with vaccination at 2, 4, and 6 months of age. A child who had received three doses of pertussis vaccine regardless of vaccine type was considered to be fully immunized.

Vaccine uptake was measured by the number of children who received three doses of pertussis vaccine before the end of the calendar year of their first birthday, divided by the number of live births. Vaccine coverage was evaluated by the number of fully immunized children resident on December 31st of the year, divided by the corresponding number of residents per age group. Pertussis incidence rates were calculated using a person-time incidence density approach. One unit was added to each monthly total to avoid null values and a moving average over five months was used to smooth variations.

EPI vaccine uptake rose from 13% in 1986 to 72% in 1990, and finally reached a level of 82 to 84% (Figure 13.1). High vaccine coverage (>80%) was achieved in the youngest age group (6 months to 1 year) by 1991, but remained relatively low at 40% in the 5 to 14 age group even up to 1996. Pertussis was endemic, with annual peaks and epidemics every three to four years, centered on 1986, 1990, and 1993.

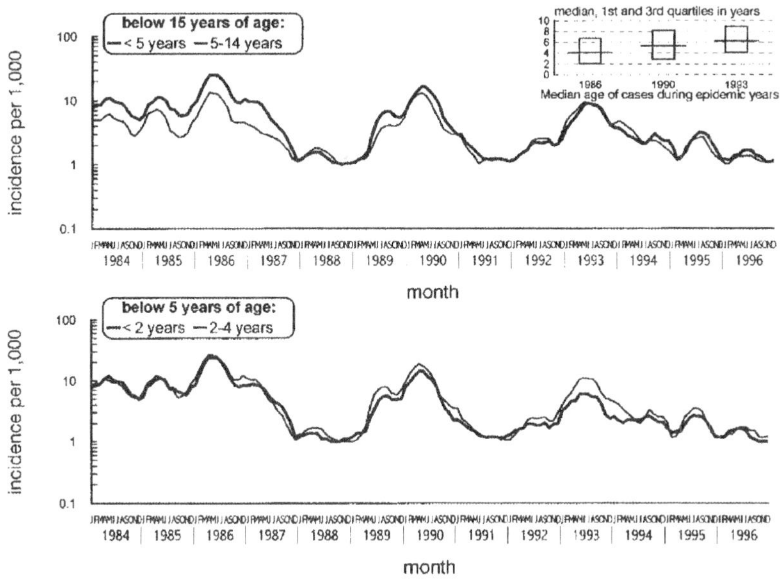

Fig. 13.2 Age-specific incidence rates of pertussis per period, Niakhar, Senegal, 1984–1996 (Préziosi et al 2002, Am J Epidemiol 155:891–896. Reprinted with permission.)

Both the number of cases between epidemics and the magnitude of the epidemic peaks decreased. From late 1987 onward, the number of cases reported dropped between epidemic years (Figure 13.2).

The decrease in incidence was observed in every age group, but especially in children under age 5 years. The greatest decline was in children under age 2 years. The declining trend was with a time lag according to age group. The overall effect of the pertussis vaccination program as measured by the reduction in incidence in the 0 to 14 year olds between the first and third epidemic peak was $VE_{III} = (127.3 - 68.9)/127.3 = 0.46$ (Table 13.2). The most dramatic decline was for the children aged 6 to 23 months, where the reduction in incidence, or overall effectiveness of the program was $VE_{III} = (170.5 - 36.3)/170.5 = 0.79$. The indirect and total effects are not estimable from the data in Table 13.2 because the incidence rates by vaccine status are not given. The median age of pertussis cases rose steadily from 4.1 years in 1986 to 5.3 years in 1990 and 6.2 years in 1993 (Figure 13.2).

13.2.2.2 Pertussis in England and Wales

Miller and Gay (1997) discuss the effect of vaccination on pertussis epidemiology in England and Wales. Vaccine uptake dropped dramatically after 1974, followed by a resurgence of pertussis cases in 1978. Considerable discussion in the literature

Table 13.2 Pertussis case distribution and incidence per age, during epidemic years, Niakhar, Senegal, 1984–1996 (Préziosi et al 2002)

Age	First Outbreak (1986)				Second Outbreak (1990)				Third Outbreak (1993)			
	Cases		No. of	Incidence/	Cases		No. of	Incidence/	Cases		No. of	Incidence/
	No.	%	PYR	1000 PYR	No.	%	PYR	1000 PYR	No.	%	PYR	1000 PYR
0-5 mo	97	7	582	166.6	68	6	557	122.1	38	4	575	66.1
6-23 mo	246	18	1443	170.5	144	12	1700	84.7	58	7	1598	36.3
2-4 yr	492	35	2530	194.5	348	30	2850	122.1	241	27	2969	81.2
5-14 yr	570	40	6481	88.0	612	52	7422	82.5	555	62	7811	71.1
Total	1,405	100	11,036	127.3	1,172	100	12,529	93.5	892	100	12,953	68.9

has centered on whether pertussis vaccination actually alters the transmission of pertussis in a population (See Chapter 12). Although there had been speculation that the drop in cases before 1974 had been due to improved social conditions, the steep increase in pertussis cases with decreasing uptake is evidence that the drop in cases before 1974 was due to vaccination. Miller and Gay suggest that the decline in incidence is greater than would be expected given the low protective efficacy estimates of pertussis vaccination (see Chapter 10). Using other sources of evidence as well, they argue that the results are consistent with pertussis vaccination lowering transmission and therefore pertussis vaccination likely has indirect effects in the population.

13.2.3 Pneumococcal vaccine in Alaska

Hennessy et al (2005) evaluated invasive pneumococcal diseases (IPD), antimicrobial resistance, and nasopharyngeal colonization before and after introduction of heptavalent pneumococcal conjugate vaccine (PCV7) in Alaksa Natives. On January 1, 2001 PCV7 was introduced into the childhood vaccination schedule for all Alaskan children. Population-based surveillance for IPD among persons of all races throughout Alaska was conducted by the CDC Arctic Investigations Program. Hennessy et al (2005) used the statewide surveillance for IPD to compare rates of disease in the six years prior to routine use of PCV7 (1995–2000) with disease rates in the three years after PCV7 use (2001–2003).

From October 1, 2001 to September 30, 2003 the proportion of 3- to 15-months-old Alaska Native children who were age-appropriately vaccinated with PCV7 increased from 51.9% to 73.2%. The proportion of 16- to 27-months-old children with 4 or more PCV7 doses increased from 0 to 57.7%. By September 30, 2003, 95% of 19- to 35-months-old Alaska Native children had received at least one dose of PCV7. From 1995 to 2003 a total of 1113 cases of IPD were reported in Alaska. Isolates were available on 90% of the cases. Table 13.3 shows the before and after rates and number of cases of IPD. The overall effectiveness against all serotypes in Alaska Native children <2 years was $VE_{III} = (403 - 142)/403 = 0.65$ and in non-

Table 13.3 Rates (per 100,000) of invasive *Streptococcus pneumoniae* by time period, age group, race, and vaccine serotype, Alaska, 1995–2003 (Hennessy et al 2005)

Age	Alaska Natives			Non-Alaska Native		
Group (Years)	1995–2000 Rate (Number)	2001–2003 Rate (Number)	p-value	1995–2000 Rate (Number)	2001–2003 Rate (Number)	p-value
Conjugate vaccine serotypes (4, 6B, 9V, 14, 18C, 19F, 23F)						
<2	275.3 (84)	24.7 (4)	<.001	101.3 (86)	20.0 (9)	<.001
2–4	47.0 (21)	0 (0)	<.001	13.6 (17)	7.5 (5)	.247
5–17	5.9 (12)	0.9 (1)	.035	1.0 (6)	2.5 (8)	.095
18–44	6.1 (6)	5.7 (8)	.909	4.3 (52)	1.09 (7)	.792
≥45	15.1 (23)	13.6 (11)	.792	11.4 (102)	7.4 (35)	.023
Nonconjugate vaccine serotypes						
<2	95.1 (29)	105.0 (17)	.738	23.6 (20)	28.8 (13)	.568
2–4	13.4 (6)	8.4 (2)	.610	4.0 (5)	7.5 (5)	.333
5–17	7.8 (16)	5.5 (6)	.484	2.6 (16)	1.5 (5)	.307
18–44	16.6 (44)	17.8 (25)	.779	3.6 (43)	2.8 (18)	.403
≥45	32.9 (50)	54.6 (44)	.016	10.4 (93)	7.0 (33)	.043
All cases (including unknown serotypes)						
<2	403.2 (123)	142.0 (23)	<.001	133.1 (113)	51.0 (23)	<.001
2–4	73.9 (33)	12.7 (3)	<.001	18.4 (23)	16.6 (11)	.792
5–17	15.2 (31)	8.3 (9)	.103	3.9 (24)	4.6 (15)	.616
18–44	25.3 (67)	24.9 (35)	.947	9.2 (111)	4.7 (30)	<.001
≥45	57.9 (88)	75.7 (61)	.112	23.5 (210)	16.9 (80)	.010

Natives was $VE_{III} = (133 - 51)/133 = 0.62$, both of which were found to be statistically significant, ignoring that comparison is just before and after in one population. In children aged 2–4 years the overall effectiveness against all serotypes in Alaska Native children was $VE_{III} = (73.9 - 12.7)/73.9 = 0.83$ but was just 0.10 in non-Natives. Most of the dramatic decline was in the vaccine serotypes. Overall effectiveness against PCV7 serotypes among children <2 years for Alaska Natives was $VE_{III} = (275 - 25)/275 = 0.91$ and in non-Natives $VE_{III} = (101 - 20)/101 = 0.80$.

Colonization studies were also conducted from 1998 to 2003 community wide in eight rural Alaska villages and in urban clinics from 2000 to 2003 in children aged 3 to 59 months. The proportion of persons colonized with *S. pneumoniae* of PCV7 serotypes declined substantially after PCV7 introduction. Decreased vaccine-type colonization and invasive disease in adults demonstrate indirect effects. Although not all denominators are given, Hennessy et al (2005) estimated that in children ≥5 years old, who were not eligible to receive PCV7, 41 cases of vaccine type IPD (95% CI 20–64 cases) were indirectly prevented by PCV7 introduction.

Table 13.4 Attack rate (AR) of confirmed meningococcal serogroup C infection in unvaccinated children before and after the launch of the vaccination campaign (Ramsay et al 2003)

	July 1998–June 1999			July 2001–June 2002				
Cohort	Cases	Population	AR per 100,000 (95% CI)	Cases	Est coverage (%)	Est. pop	AR per 100,000 (95% CI)	Indirect effect, VE_{IIA} (95% CI)
Adolescent	96	1,818,034	5.28 (4.2, 6.3)	11	66	614,110	1.79 (0.7, 2.8)	66 (37, 82)
Grades 7–10	141	2,546,938	5.54 (4.6, 6.4)	4	86	359,118	1.11 (0.02, 2.2)	80 (46, 93)
Grades 1–6	76	3,911,606	1.94 (1.5, 2.4)	5	87	498,068	1.00 (0.1, 0.9)	48 (−28, 79)
Preschool	81	2,055,120	3.94 (3.1, 4.8)	6	76	501,449	1.20 (0.2, 2.2)	70 (30, 87)
Toddlers	41	601,045	6.82 (4.7, 8.9)	2	84	97,369	2.05 (−0.7, 4.9)	70 (−24, 93)
Infants	24	320,562	7.49 (1.5, 10.5)	1	80	64,112	1.56 (−1.5, 4.6)	79 (−54, 97)
Total	459	11,235,305	4.08 (3.7, 4.5)	29		2,134,226	1.36 (0.86, 1.85)	67 (52, 77)

13.2.4 Meningococcal vaccine in the United Kingdom

The United Kingdom introduced routine meningococcal serogroup C vaccination for infants in November 1999. The vaccine was also offered to all children and adolescents aged <18 years in a phased catch-up program. Adolescents were vaccinated first and the program was completed by the end of 2000. Ramsay et al (2003) compared cases in unvaccinated children from each age group in the period from July 1, 2001 to June 30, 2002 with those in the same age groups for the period from July 1, 1998 to June 30, 1999. The denominator was mid-1999 population estimates from the Office of National Statistics for the age group, adjusted for the proportion of each cohort vaccinated. The cases were identified at the Public Health Laboratory Service by confirmation of serogroup C disease. They investigated the vaccination history of all such identified cases. They computed vaccination coverage from data from immunization coordinators and departments of child health in England. They identified a total of 37 cases in the 2001–2002 period in the cohorts targeted for vaccination, 8 in vaccinated children and 29 in unvaccinated children.

Table 13.4 contains the number of cases in the unvaccinated children before and after launch of the vaccination campaign. The estimated indirect effect in children based on the attack rate over all age groups is $VE_{IIA} = (4.08 - 1.36)/4.08 = 0.67$ with a 95% CI (0.52–0.77) with a range of 0.48 to 0.80 in the different age groups. Using a denominator of 9,119,078 for the eight vaccinated cases for an attack rate of 0.09/100,0000, Ramsay et al (2003) computed the estimated direct protective efficacy of the vaccine to be $(1.36 - 0.09)/1.36 = 0.94$ (95% CI 0.86–0.97).

13.2.5 Cholera vaccine in Bangladesh

Ali et al (2005) reanalyzed data from a large-scale, double-masked, individually randomized field trial of killed whole cell cholera vaccines given orally, either with or without cholera toxin B subunit in Bangladesh to ascertain whether there was

Table 13.5 Risk of cholera in placebo and recipients of killed oral cholera vaccines, by level of coverage of the bari during the first year of follow-up (Ali et al 2005)

Level of Vaccine Coverage	Target Population	Vaccine Recipients N	Cases	Risk per 1000 population	Placebo Recipients N	Cases	Risk per 1000 Population	Protective Efficacy (95% CI)
<28%	24,954	5627	15	2.67	2852	20	7.01	62 (23 to 82)
28-35%	25,059	8883	22	2.48	4429	26	5.87	58 (23 to 77)
36-40%	24,583	10772	17	1.58	5503	26	4.72	67 (36 to 83)
41-50%	24,159	11513	26	2.26	5801	27	4.65	52(14 to 73)
>51%	22,394	12541	16	1.28	6082	9	1.48	14(-111 to 64)
Total	121,149	49,336	96	1.94	24,667	108	4.37	56(41 to 67)

evidence of indirect as well as direct vaccine protection of individuals. The trial was done in the Matlab field area of the International Centre for Diarrhoeal Disease Research, Bangladesh (ICDDR,B): Centre for Health and Population Research during the 1980s (Clemens et al 1990). All children aged 2 to 15 years and women older than 15 years were randomized to receive either one of the cholera vaccines or *Escherichia coli* K12 placebo. The main objective of the original trial was to assess whether receipt of three doses of vaccine was associated with lower incidence of cholera than that observed after receipt of three doses of placebo. At one year of follow-up, protective efficacy was 62% for B subunit-killed whole cell oral cholera vaccine and 53% for killed whole cell only oral cholera vaccine. The reanalysis to assess indirect effects was motivated by the lack of enthusiasm for introducing the vaccine in populations with endemic cholera because of the moderate direct protective effects.

A bari in Bangladesh is a patrilinearly-related household living in clusters. Ali et al (2005) chose the bari as the unit of analysis because baris are geographically discrete and because there may be transmission within these units. A total of 6423 baris were included in the analysis, with the median number of individuals in a bari eligible for the trial being 17 (interquartile range 7–26). The analysis was restricted to the first year of follow-up to have a more stable population and minimize the effects of migration. Level of vaccine coverage was defined as the number of vaccinated individuals divided by the number of people who were eligible for participation in the trial by age and sex criteria. Then because the coverage of nearby baris might affect the risk of cholera of bari residents, the vaccine coverage of the bari was defined as the coverage of bari residents and those living within a 500 meter radius according to a geographic information system mapping.

Table 13.5 presents a summary of the data divided into quintiles by level of coverage of the baris and the protective efficacy for each quintile. For the indirect and total effects, models based on generalized estimating equations with a logit link and exchangeable correlation matrix including potential confounding variables were used (see Section 13.7). The risk of cholera in recipients of two or more doses of either vaccine or placebo is inversely related to the level of vaccine coverage of the bari. The trend is statistically significant in placebo recipients (Spearman's correlation coefficient −1.00, $p = 0.02$), but not in vaccine recipients (−0.90, $p = 0.08$). Three analyses were done using the generalized estimating equations, one using all recipients with ≥2 doses of vaccine or placebo (overall effect), one for those with vaccine (total effect), and one for those with placebo (indirect effect). The odds ratios for the level of cholera vaccine coverage of the bari were 0.97 (95% CI 0.96–0.98), 0.98 (95% CI 0.96–1.00), 0.96 (95% CI 0.94–0.98). respectively. Thus, there was a significant gradient by level of coverage for the overall effect and the indirect effect, with a borderline significant gradient for the total effect.

13.2.6 Drawbacks of nonrandomized evaluation

Evaluation of indirect, total, or overall effects based on pre- and post-vaccination surveillance data can often provide good evidence, at least of the overall effects. However, if the change is to be attributed to the vaccination program, one must assume there are no major secular trends. A particular example of the difficulty of using nonrandomized studies or studies based on comparing just one or two populations is influenza (Halloran and Longini 2006). Attempts have been made before to demonstrate the community-wide effectiveness of vaccinating school children against influenza. Just before the epidemic in 1968, Arnold Monto and colleagues vaccinated 85% of the school-age children in Tecumseh, Michigan, against influenza, resulting in a 67% decrease in the influenza-like illness attack rate in Tecumseh compared with neighboring Adrian (Monto et al 1969). In an ongoing community vaccination study in Central Texas with LAIV, Paul Glezen and colleagues are attempting to demonstrate that vaccinating school children reduces incidence of influenza-like illness in adults (Piedra et al 2007). Although these studies are rigorous, they each have only one or two comparison communities and use influenza-like illness for the outcome. A study in several schools in the former Soviet Union used a nonspecific outcome as well, so the results are difficult to interpret (Monto et al 1993). The Japanese national vaccination strategy was targeted at school children for over two decades until 1987 with the intention to reduce epidemic influenza. A retrospective reassessment suggesting that the Japanese strategy reduced excess deaths among elderly adults (Reichert et al 2001) is open to criticism because it is based on non-specific mortality data over time. The time trends could result from factors not related to influenza vaccination. A review of 14 studies concluded that further evidence is needed of the indirect effects of influenza vaccination in children (Jordan 2005). King et al (2006) tried to demonstrate that school-based influenza vaccination reduced spread of influenza in households and communites, but used an influenza-like illness outcome, not influenza. The use of a non-specific case definition compounds the difficulty of evaluating the indirect effects of influenza vaccination strategies. A larger scale study with numerous comparison communities is needed to gather convincing data to counter remaining scepticism.

13.3 Group-Randomized Studies

To evaluate indirect, total, and overall effects of a vaccination strategy, ideally one would randomize several communities to receive the vaccination strategy of interest and several communities to serve as controls. Then the outcomes in the intervention communities would be compared with those of the control communities. Most commonly, the luxury of conducting a prospectively designed study of a vaccination strategy in multiple groups or populations to estimate indirect, total, and overall effects will not be an option. The more feasible approach will often be to plan well for a comparison of the pre- and post-implementation incidence in the relevant populations as the studies described in the previous section. Despite the increasing interest in using group-randomized studies to evaluate population-level effects of vaccination, few actual studies have been conducted up to now. However, prospectively designed community-randomized studies may become more common in the future.

Community-, group-, or cluster-randomized studies are those in which the intervention, or intervention strategy, is randomized to groups of individuals. With vaccines, one can in principle, have two levels of randomization. The vaccination strategy can be randomized at the group level, then individuals within the target populations in the group can be further randomized at the individual level. There is an extensive literature on group-randomized designs (Murray 1998; Hayes and Moulton 2009). Cluster-randomized studies are often conducted because it is not feasible to allocate the intervention individually, even though the effects on the individuals are of interest. Vaccination studies sometimes use a group-randomized design even when the direct protective effects are of interest because of practical or ethical consideration. An example was the original design of the large polio vaccine trials in the United States in the 1950s, although the design was changed to individual randomization midway through (Section 1.1). Group-randomized designs may be used in household-based studies of vaccination where the parents or other household members might be unwilling to do a discordant or individual randomization. We discuss group-randomized studies here primarily for our interest in measuring indirect, total, or overall effects.

One often distinguishes the unit of assignment, the unit of intervention, the unit of observation, and the unit of analysis (Murray 1998). The unit of assignment could be the unit that is assigned the allocation strategy, say a community is randomized to receive the vaccination strategy of interest, and another is assigned to receive a control vaccination strategy. With vaccines, the additional unit of assignment is the individual within the community. The assignment at the individual level within each community may be randomized or not. For a selected target group, such as children under two years of age, one might vaccinate whoever comes to a clinic to be vaccinated. Then the children who are vaccinated within a group randomized to the vaccination strategy are not a random sample, but subject to a selection mechanism as in an observational study, the rule of which is unknown to the investigator. The unit of intervention could be health clinics or physician's practices within a community, or the nurse practitioner's office within a school. The unit of observation for cases is generally the individual, whether it be individual cases picked up

Table 13.6 Design considerations in group-randomized studies to estimate indirect, total, or overall effects of vaccination strategies

Design Consideration
Primary and secondary questions of interest
Vaccination strategy
Clinical endpoints
Study population and subpopulations
Sources of transmission
Case ascertainment
Choice of randomization unit at the group level
Allocation mechanism at the individual level: randomization or observational

through surveillance systems or clinical studies. Individual covariates and outcomes are ascertained. In community studies, there will likely also be community-level covariates, such as prevalence or incidence levels, amount of rainfall, distance from roads, or distance from a health clinic. The community is the unit of observation for community-level covariates. Much discussion in the literature considers the appropriate unit of analysis. In general, the unit of analysis is determined by the study design. "A unit is a unit of analysis for an effect if and only if that effect is assessed against the variation among those units" (Murray 1998, page 105). Several design considerations in group-randomized studies to estimate the different types of effects are summarized in Table 13.6.

13.3.1 Scientific or public health question of interest

The scientific or public health question of interest will influence the choice of allocation strategy. There may be primary and secondary questions of interest. For example, the primary interest may be in evaluating the total effects of vaccination compared to no vaccination, as in the pneumococcal vaccine study designed by Moulton et al (2001) (Figure 13.3). In this case, one would want to vaccinate as many individuals in the target population as possible to maximize the total effects. The secondary interest may be in evaluating the indirect effects of vaccination on those not vaccinated.

If pure indirect effects were of primary interest, then the best approach would depend on which subgroups were receiving the vaccines and in which subgroups the indirect effects were to be measured. For example, if the indirect effects in the subgroup receiving the vaccine were of primary interest, then there would be a tradeoff to consider. If too many people in the intervention communities are vaccinated, there will be few people left unvaccinated and few events in the unvaccinated people in the intervention community. If too few people in the intervention communities

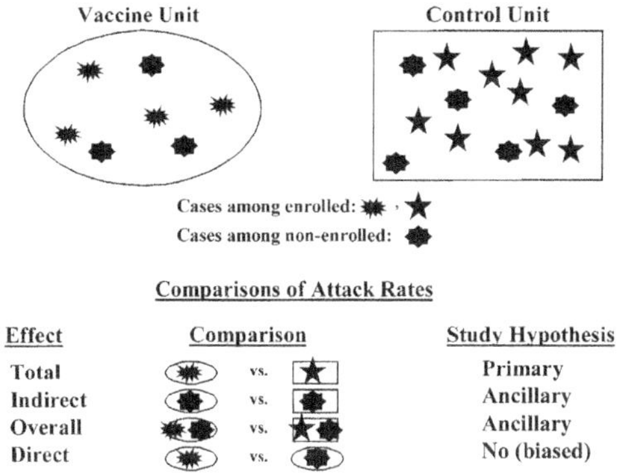

Fig. 13.3 Schematic of the questions of interest in the pneumococcal vaccine trial in Native Americans. Participants in each vaccine unit receive PCV7 vaccine, and those in each control unit receive MnCC vaccine (Moulton et al 2001, Contr Clin Trials 22:438–452. Reprinted with permission from Elsevier.)

are vaccinated, there may be no detectable indirect effect. On the other hand, if one were interested in estimating the indirect effects in adults of vaccinating children, then the goal would be to vaccinate as many children as possible in the intervention communities. Studies can be designed to evaluate direct as well as indirect, total, and overall effects. If in addition to indirect or total effects, one is also interested in evaluating the direct effects of vaccination, then one would want to vaccinate few enough people that sufficient transmission remains to produce the number of events necessary to estimate the direct effects.

13.3.2 Choice of group-level randomization unit

The choice of the group at the level of the group-randomization depends on both practical and theoretical considerations. One wants the groups to be transmission-dynamically separate. If communities receiving vaccine interact with communities not receiving vaccine, the contamination across groups could dilute the indirect, total, or overall effects of the vaccination program. Contiguity can occur through spatial proximity or social mixing patterns among units. Contamination across units will decrease the power of the study. The vaccination delivery system may determine the randomization units. Vaccination delivery could be through health care clinics or EPI vaccination team catchment areas. Political units such as towns or counties might be natural randomization units. One can also use smaller randomization units, such as schools (King et al 2006) or households, such as in the mini-community design (Chapter 12).

Given a study population, a trade-off exists between the size of the cluster with number of expected cases per cluster and the number of clusters. If incidence rates are relatively high, and the effect to be measured is also expected to be substantial, then one can divide the population into fewer clusters. However, there will be a loss of efficiency as the number of individuals per randomization unit increases. Care should be taken that the randomization units are not too small. The efficiency of a study also depends on the intragroup correlation which could be affected by the size of the community chosen as the unit of randomization (Hayes et al 2000). If small communities are chosen, then the intracommunity correlation might be quite high, whereas in large communities, the correlation might be smaller. Also, small randomization units might have considerable mixing among the groups, resulting in diminished indirect, total, and overall effects. In general, one would prefer to increase the number of communities to have more randomization units with fewer individuals if they are transmission-dynamically separate. The choice of the randomization unit for any particular study will depend on the local conditions.

13.3.3 Sources of transmission

Consideration of the likely transmission patterns and sources of exposure to infection in a population is required in anticipating possible detection of indirect effects. These transmission patterns will influence the magnitude of the indirect effects of an intervention strategy. For example, many influenza researchers believe that school children are the primary sources of transmission in the community. Widespread vaccination of school children could be expected to have considerable indirect effects on reducing influenza in a community (Halloran and Longini 2006; Piedra et al 2007). On the other hand, in the study aimed to evaluate the total effects of vaccinating children <2 year olds with pneumococcal vaccine (Moulton et al 2001, 2006), the contribution to transmission of school children or adults who are colonized with the bacteria is not understood well. If the older children who are unvaccinated are important sources of transmission, then the vaccination strategy, at least in the early years upon introduction, will have low indirect effects, and the total effects will be dominated by the direct protection.

13.3.4 Designs and randomization schemes

One consideration in group-randomized studies is the temporal order of randomizing to vaccination strategy or control. Another consideration is the randomization scheme (Table 13.7). Three general group-randomized study designs are parallel designs, stepped wedge designs, and crossover designs (Hughes 2003). Any of these three study types can be used when the randomization unit is either an individual or a group, but the focus here is the context of group-randomized studies to evaluate

Table 13.7 Community-randomized designs and randomization schemes

Design	Randomization Scheme	Covariate Constraints
Parallel	Completely randomized	Unconstrained
Stepped wedge	Stratified	Constrained
Crossover	Matched-pairs	

indirect, total, and overall effects of vaccination. In the parallel design, the groups are randomized to receive one or another of the interventions before the start of the study, and the intervention assignment does not change until the end of the study. In the stepped wedge design, the intervention is introduced in more and more groups over time. This allows the groups in which the intervention is not yet introduced to serve as control groups. In the crossover design, the groups are first randomized to receive one or another of the interventions at the beginning, then at some point, the interventions are switched. This latter design likely has no application in vaccine studies, because in general one cannot de-vaccinate people or populations. We do not consider it further here. Both the parallel design and the stepped wedge design can be used to evaluate direct, indirect, total, and overall effects of vaccination. That is, groups can be randomized to vaccination or control, then individuals within groups may or may not be randomized to receive vaccine or not.

Once either the parallel or stepped wedge design is chosen, then a randomization scheme is required. Three general randomization schemes are the completely randomized study, stratified randomization, and matched-pairs randomization. In a completely randomized parallel study, groups are randomized to intervention or control without any consideration of variability among the groups. In a completely randomized stepped wedge design, the order of introduction of the intervention is randomized without any consideration of variability among the groups.

Group-randomized trials often have only a limited number of identifiable groups to assign to the different interventions. Two key issues arise in choosing a randomization scheme when the number of groups is limited. First, in a completely randomized study, variability among communities could swamp out the estimates of the effects of the vaccination strategy. Second, generally there will not be enough groups to ensure that the potential sources of bias among the intervention conditions will be evenly distributed. Even if the groups or communities contain thousands of participants, if there is important variability of characteristics between groups, a study that is completely randomized at the group level could have imbalances in important covariates. If these characteristics are also related to the outcome of the study, an example would be the incidence rate of the disease of interest in the community, then the results of the study may be difficult to interpret. Even if it is possible to do some adjustment at the time of analysis, the results will be open to criticism. For example, consider a study to evaluate the total effectiveness of widespread vaccination, with five communities randomized to intervention and five to control. It could happen that the five communities with the lowest baseline incidence of the disease in question would be randomized to receive vaccination. If that were to happen, the results of the study could be criticized as being biased in favor of the vaccination strategy by the realized randomization.

Two main approaches are available to increase power and to reduce the chance of imbalance of covariates when there is considerable variability among communities. One is to stratify groups by pre-randomization group-level covariates of interest, including transmission characteristics, then randomize to vaccination intervention or control within strata. The other, an extreme version of stratification, is to match pairs of communities on the covariates of interest, so the strata contain only two communities, then randomize to intervention or control within the pairs. Groups rather than individuals are stratified/matched prior to randomization. Hayes et al (1995) matched on transmission characteristics in a community trial of the effect of improved sexually transmitted disease treatment on the HIV epidemic in rural Tanzania (Grosskurth et al 1995). Pre-randomization stratification or matching requires information on factors related to the primary endpoint used for the stratification/ matching prior to randomization.

Even in stratified or pair-matched designs, an unlucky randomization can result in the intervention always being assigned to the lower incidence groups. An appealing approach to randomizing groups that avoids gross imbalances on known and measured variables is covariate-based constrained randomization (Moulton 2004). In the constrained, or restricted, randomization, certain balancing criteria are determined before randomization that still retain validity of the design. Then the final randomization scheme is randomly chosen from among those that both satisfy the constraining criteria and are still valid. A completely randomized design is valid if each pair of randomization units has the same probability of being allocated the same treatment (Bailey 1983). A design is biased, if, across the randomization units, there is any difference in probability of assignment to a given treatment. Constrained randomization can be used in completely randomized, stratified, or pair-matched designs.

13.3.5 Other design considerations

13.3.5.1 Study population, vaccines, and vaccination strategy

The choice of study population will be determined by the vaccine and the ability to conduct a large-scale study in the population. The ability to administer the vaccine, keep records, and also to obtain data on the clinical outcomes is important. Exactly what the intervention program of interest is will depend on the vaccine, the vaccination schedule for that vaccine, and which subgroups suffer the greatest morbidity. The comparisons may be made between different levels of vaccination coverage, between allocation within different age groups, or between otherwise defined subgroups. In a parallel design, it might be necessary to consider using a different active vaccine as a control. This would help preserve masking and inactive placebos are often considered unethical for vaccine studies. The active vaccine as a control also provides a comparable group, in that those people who actually receive the vaccine in the two arms might be assumed the appropriate groups for comparison in estimating total effects. For example, in the pneumococcal vaccine study of total effects, the control vaccine was an investigational meningococcal C conjugate vacccine (Moulton et al 2001). In a phased implementation design (Section 13.4), an active control vaccine would generally not be used.

13.3.5.2 Case ascertainment and clinical endpoints

In large community studies, to evaluate indirect, total, or overall effects, whether randomized or observational, good methods for thorough case ascertainment is important. Examples include active population surveillance as in the Niakhar study, biological confirmation of suspected cases in reference laboratories, or general surveillance and reporting systems. Active population surveillance can demand a lot of resources. If considerable underreporting of cases is suspected, and two or more sources of surveillance or case reporting are available, capture–recapture methods can be considered to provide better estimates of the number of cases (Gjini et al 2004).

Clinical endpoints can be defined as a combination of clinical symptoms and/or by biological confirmation of the infectious agent targeted by the vaccination. The infectious agents can further be identified as being contained in the vaccine or not contained in the vaccine. For example, in pneumococcal vaccine studies, the cases can be categorized as being a vaccine serotype or a nonvaccine serotype. In influenza vaccine studies, the infections are classified either as homologous with the vaccine type or heterologous, indicating some degree of antigenic mismatch between the vaccine strains and the circulating strains.

Two possibly related problems may arise in large, group-randomized studies. First, if the disease is common, such as in influenza, the number of suspected cases in the large study may be too many for all cases to be confirmed biologically. Second, surveillance may not be specific for the illness of interest. For instance, influenza incidence in post-licensure vaccine studies is generally measured using nonspecific case definitions, such as influenza-like illness or medically attended acute respiratory illness, which include many diseases in addition to influenza. A nonspecific case definition can attenuate the estimates of indirect and overall effects. In Chapter 8 the concept of using validation sets to obtain more accurate efficacy estimates when the main case definition is nonspecific was discussed. Especially in studies to evaluate total or overall effects, validation sets might be helpful to improve the ability to detect a signal above the noise.

As an illustration, Figure 13.4 shows results of 100 stochastic simulated estimates of the indirect effects of vaccinating 50% of the children with an influenza vaccine in one community as compared with another community without vaccination (Halloran and Longini 2001). Each population has 10,000 people, half children and half adult. The indirect effects are set to 0.25. In each pair of populations, the population in which children were vaccinated had an influenza incidence rate reduced by a

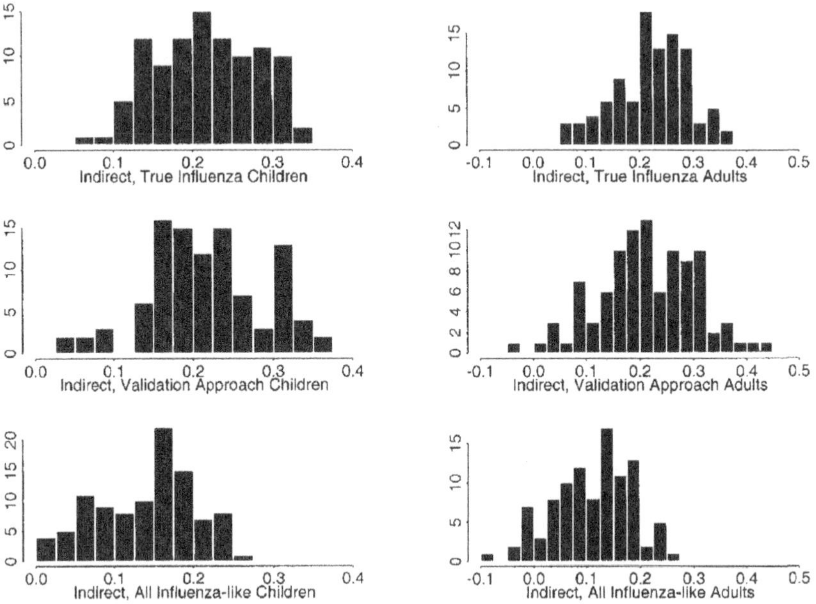

Fig. 13.4 Estimated indrect effects of vaccination of children among children (left) and among adults (right) when the indirect effects are set to 0.25. Estimates were based on true influenza cases (top), the validation set approach (middle), and all influenza-like illnesses. The expected incidence in children varied weekly over the 12-week epidemic period as (0.014, 0.024, 0.034, 0.05, 0.06, 0.055, 0.05, 0.044, 0.038, 0.024, 0.015, 0.01). The expected incidence of influenza in adults was half that. The expected incidence rate of noninfluenza in both children and adults was set to 0.02 per week. The baseline incidences of true influenza and background noninfluenza are multiplied by random numbers between 0.085 and 1.15 so the baseline incidences in each comparison pair are similar but not identical (Halloran and Longini 2001, Am J Epidemiol, 154:391–398. Reprinted with permission).

factor of 0.25. VE_S is assumed to be 0.90 (leaky). The top histograms of estimates based on ascertainment of all true influenza cases in children and adults are centered around 0.25. However, if we use all influenza-like illnesses, the estimates are much lower (bottom rows). The histogram is centered around 0.14 in children and 0.10 in adults. However, by incorporating a random sample of the influenza-like illnesses that are biologically confirmed, we can adjust the estimates based on the influenza-like illnesses (middle row). The histograms are once again centered around 0.25, although the histograms based on the validation set approach show more variability than the histograms based on confirming all true influenza cases.

Although it may not be feasible to confirm biologically every clinically determined case in a large study to evaluate indirect, total, or overall effects, a small random sample of confirmed cases could be quite useful. There are trade-offs in using a nonspecific outcome on more groups and reducing the number of groups and using validation sets. Given the variability and background noise among communities, schools, or other group, for a fixed budget, it is probably better to use fewer groups in general and get more specific outcomes on some of the participants. These potential trade-offs have yet to be studied rigorously.

13.4 Parallel and Stepped Wedge Designs

13.4.1 Parallel designs

The simplest parallel group-randomized design is one in which N groups are randomized to either the vaccination strategy or the control strategy, for a total of $2N$ groups. It would also be possible to have an unbalanced allocation in which N groups are randomized to the vaccination strategy, and $M \neq N$ groups are randomized to the control strategy.

13.4.2 Parallel pneumoccocal vaccine study

Moulton et al (2001) designed a group-randomized, double-masked Phase III trial of a seven-valent *Streptococcus pneumoniae* conjugate vaccine (PCV7) in American Indian populations in the United States. The study had a parallel design. An active control, a conjugate meningococcal group C vaccine (MnCC vaccine) was used in groups randomized to control. The primary goal of the trial was to evaluate the total effects of vaccination, with secondary interest in the indirect effects, and at the same time to serve as a pivotal vaccine study. At the time of the design of the study, another Phase III study with standard individual randomization was ongoing in northern California (Black et al 2000). However, the number of invasive pneumococcal cases occurring in that trial was small. The group-randomized study was designed to estimate the total efficacy, which takes the direct protective effects on the vaccinated individuals as well as the indirect effects into account, so that the effects could potentially be greater than the effects in the individually randomized study. The study was the first group-randomized vaccine trial in the United States designed to be a pivotal trial for licensure.

There were 4164 infants enrolled in the PCV7 communities and 3926 in the MnCC communities between April 1997 and December 1999. The study had 38 geographically defined randomization groups The choice of randomization unit was made in consultation with groups knowledgeable about the social and geographic aspects, including representatives from the Navajo Nation, to minimize mixing among the social and geographic units. Half the groups were randomized to study vaccine, PCV7, the other half to the active control, MnCC vaccine. The goal in each randomization group was to vaccinate as many children under two years of age as possible to achieve the highest total effects.

Originally the trial was designed to continue until 48 cases of invasive pneumococcal disease due to vaccine serotypes had accumulated. However, on February 17, 2000, the FDA approved the licensure of the PCV7 vaccine based on the results of the primary efficacy study in northern California (Black et al 2000). Ethically the study could not be continued, and PCV7 vaccine was offered in the MnCC communities. Only nine cases had accrued at that time.

Later, Moulton et al (2006) estimated the indirect effects on the unvaccinated children in the communities (Section 13.7.1). To estimate indirect effects they compared the incidence rate of invasive pneumococcal disease in vaccine units among nonenrolled children versus the incidence rate in control units in nonenrolled children. By using the nonenrolled children in both communities, they hoped to have comparable children in their analysis. By combining the information from the study with information from Indian Health Service User Population data and birth logs, they were able to obtain denominators for each of the 38 randomization units. They were also able to interpolate the number of nonenrolled children at any day between April 1997 and October 2000. The numerator for invasive disease was obtained from surveillance data that had been subject to a standard protocol during the study. There were 21 cases of invasive disease due to study vaccine serotypes among non-study children living in MnCC randomization units, and 27 cases among those in the PCV7 units.

13.4.3 Stepped wedge designs

Stepped wedge designs can be used when a parallel design is infeasible either for practical or for ethical reasons. For example, if a vaccine is already licensed, then it may be unethical to randomize some communities or individuals not to receive vaccine during the trial. Practical considerations may delay introducing the vaccine everywhere at once, either because insufficient vaccine is available or for logistical reasons of not being able to administer it everywhere or to everyone at once. By the end of a trial using a stepped wedge design, all randomization units will have received the vaccination strategy. Thus the clusters are not randomized to receive the vaccine intervention or not, but rather the time of the introduction of the vaccine intervention to each cluster is randomized (Figure 13.5). The stepped wedge design is also referred to as phased implementation (Gambia Hepatitis Study Group 1987).

The idea of the stepped wedge design is gaining in popularity (Moulton et al 2007; Hussey and Hughes 2007; Hughes 2008), although it has been slower to be used in randomized vaccine trials to estimate indirect, total, or overall effects. Not all outcomes of interest can be studied by a stepped wedge design. For example, if one is interested in the change in age of first infection, then one would possibly conduct the study over several years. If a vaccine is unlicensed, this may be infeasible, because one would not want to wait for years to license the vaccine on this outcome. If a vaccine is licensed, such a long-term study would likely not be ethical. Thus, the observational studies of pre- and post-vaccination will have to suffice (Section

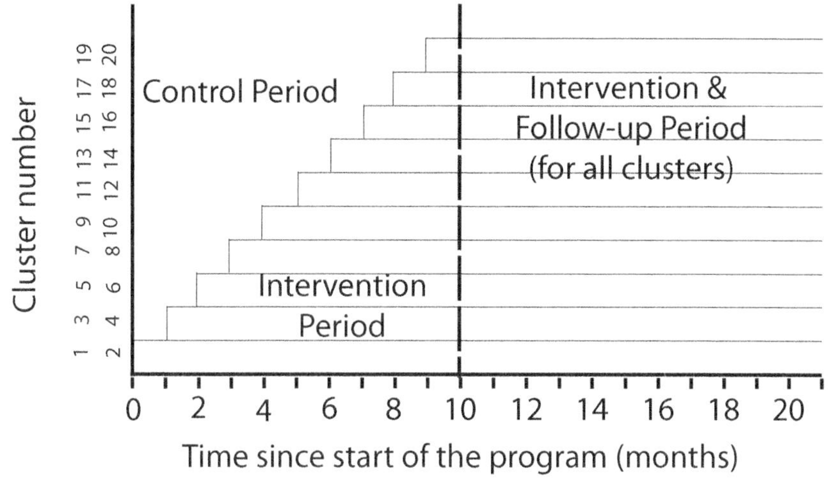

Fig. 13.5 Example of a stepped wedge design.

13.2.1) or mathematical models can be substituted as a means of experiment (Chapters 4 and 5).

13.4.4 The Gambia Hepatitis Intervention Study

One of the first studies using a stepped wedge design was a hepatitis B vaccine study in The Gambia (Gambia Hepatitis Study Group 1987). Although this study was not designed to evaluate indirect or overall effects of vaccination, we present it here because of its early use of the stepped wedge group-randomized design.

Chronic liver disease and liver cancer are thought to be partially caused by hepatitis B viral infection. In West Africa, including The Gambia, chronic liver disease and liver cancer are important public health problems. It used to be that nearly everyone in The Gambia was infected with HBV during childhood and between 10 to 20% became chronic carriers. The goal of the hepatitis B vaccination study was to evaluate the effect of infant vaccination on preventing chronic liver disease and liver cancer later in life. Thus, a long-term follow-up for over 30 years was planned. However, it was undesirable to do a parallel randomized study in which half of the children were followed for 30 to 40 years before initiating mass vaccination campaigns. Thus, a phased implementation, or stepped wedge design was proposed. Because at that time, four injections were required for full immunization, and the vaccine was to be administered along with the routine EPI vaccines, it was considered logistically infeasible to do an individually randomized trial, as well as potentially ethically questionable.

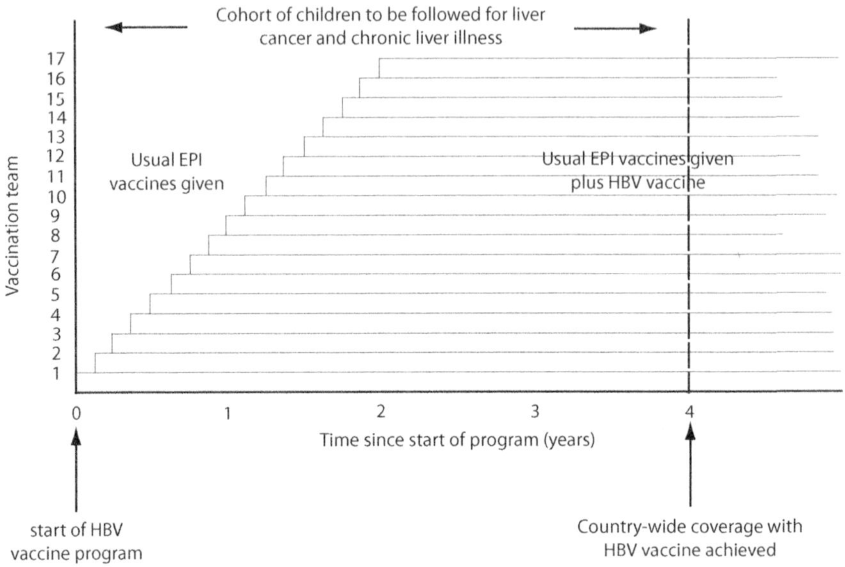

Fig. 13.6 Stepped wedge design in the Gambia hepatitis B vaccine study (adapted from the Gambia Hepatitis Study Group 1987).

The choice of study designs was further influenced by the expense of the vaccine and its limited availability prohibiting immediate universal hepatitis B vaccination. To avoid confounding by secular trends, the stepped wedge design provided the ability to have comparison groups available from the same time period. They also hoped that the hepatitis B vaccine would be widely available by the end of the study. Based on these considerations, phased introduction of hepatitis B vaccine to the EPI schedule was planned, with injections within one month of birth, and at 2, 4, and 9 months of age. There were 17 EPI vaccination teams each assigned a portion of 104 delivery points that were visited at least once every two weeks. The study plan randomized one of the teams every 10 to 12 weeks to introduce the hepatitis B vaccine to the EPI schedule by vaccinating all newborns who reported to the vaccination points served by the team. This was to continue for a period of about four years, when all teams would be giving the vaccine, so that countrywide coverage would be achieved (Figure 13.6). The alternative parallel design, in which EPI vaccination teams would have been randomized to give HBV or not for four years is statistically more powerful, but would have been less acceptable (Jaffar et al 1999).

Evaluation of the protective effect of HBV vaccination against liver cancer and chronic disease was planned through the long-term follow-up of those children born during the four-year period over which HBV vaccine was introduced. For children born in each three-month period, incidence of later liver cancer and chronic liver disease would be compared among those receiving HBV vaccine and those not. For example, those newborns entering in the first three months of the study would be compared later in life to those newborns reporting to the 16 other vaccination teams. This approach to comparison controls for secular trends that might affect the risk of developing liver cancer. Randomization of the order in which the EPI teams introduced the HBV vaccine minimizes the bias in the comparison of the vaccinated and unvaccinated groups. To further avoid bias, the plan was to restrict the analysis to comparison of those who attend the vaccination clinics at all four ages at which HBV would be given.

Considerable efforts were undertaken to enable identification of the persons enrolled 30 to 40 years after enrollment, which in The Gambia can be a challenge. For follow-up, a nationwide cancer registry and active surveillance were established. A number of studies to assess intermediate endpoints were built into the long-term follow-up. A subset was followed for serological data on a regular basis through childhood and adolescence. Cross-sectional studies were also performed to compare acquisition of HBV markers at different ages. The findings 20 years into the study were, among other things, that (i) protection against HBV infection was not dependent on the number of vaccine doses received, (ii) the HBV attributable risk of liver cancer at age >50 years was 70% to 80% lower than initially assumed, and (iii) hepatitis B vaccine coverage was 15% higher than originally assumed (Viviani et al 2008). This is an example of the need to plan for long-term studies and follow-up in vaccine studies.

13.5 Covariate-Constrained Randomization

13.5.1 Parallel design

We consider covariate-constrained randomization primarily in the context of a completely randomized parallel design. We then briefly consider using constrained randomization in the stepped wedge design. Different constraints can be used for different types of constraining variables (Moulton 2004). For continuous covariates such as incidence rates of the disease of interest, one can choose some measure based on the standard deviation or absolute mean difference. For dichotomous covariates, $\pm$ some percentage points might be appropriate. For example, suppose there was a difference in the incidence of disease between the north and south regions of the study area. Then one would not want all of the intervention sites in the north and control sites in the south. One could assign a 0,1 dummy variable for north and south and require that the difference between the intervention and control values be less than 10%. Other important aspects, such as sources of water, proportion of the population with a certain educational level, health clinics, or roads within geographic areas can also be balanced within some specified range. Composite scores or more than one covariate can be used for defining the constraints that need to be satisfied. The constraining criteria can vary among the covariates.

Once constraints are set, then one needs to identify all of the possible allocations that satisfy the constraints. To do this, one forms a list of all the possible allocations. For a design completely randomized at the group level, there will be $\binom{2N}{N}$ entries, where $2N$ is the total number of groups. For a pair-matched design, there will be 2^N entries, where N is the number of pairs. Making a pass through all of these entries, one selects those allocations that meet the specified criteria.

Once the allocations that meet the set of constraints have been identified, they need to be checked to see whether the possible allocations meet the requirement of validity of the randomization scheme (Moulton 2004). For example, some pairs of groups may always be in the same arm of the study, and others may never be in the same arm. To check the allocations, make a matrix whose elements are the number of times, from among those allocations satisifying the constraints, each pair is together. Examine the list for signs of over- or underrepresented pairs. If the allocations seem overly constrained, then relax one or more of the constraining criteria. Identify the allocations that satisfy the new constraints, and check them once again. Repeat the relaxation of the constraints until the allowable allocations seem appropriate. Then randomly select one of the allowable allocations. If there are too many possible allocations to enumerate, one can construct the matrix from a large number of acceptable designs, and choose one of them. A computational macro is available to perform this algorithm (Chaudhary and Moulton 2006).

13.5.1.1 Hypothetical dengue vaccine study

As a simple example, suppose that we are designing a dengue vaccine study in four communities where interest is in the overall effects of vaccination. Two of the villages will be randomized to receive vaccine and two not. This small number of communities is chosen only for illustrative purposes. Generally more communities would be required. The expected annual incidence of dengue in each community is correlated with the outcome of interest, thus there is concern about the balance of the dengue incidence in the two vaccination strategy communities and the two control communities. With four communities, there are six possible unique allocations of vaccination and control (Table 13.8). Baseline surveillance over the three previous years yielded estimates of average annual incidence 3, 5, 11, 13% in the four communities. If no constraints were placed on the randomization, then one of the six allocations would result. However, in allocation A, the two communities with the lowest incidences receive the vaccination strategy, and in allocation F, the two communities with the highest incidences receive the vaccination strategy. The mean absolute difference in baseline incidence is 8%, higher than the overall average incidence. There is a one in three chance of selecting one of these randomizations. Alternatively, one could say that only those allocations are acceptable that yield exact balance on the average annual incidence. In this example, allocations C and D satisfy this constraint, although generally one could not expect that any allocation would yield an exact balance.

Table 13.8 Baseline average annual dengue incidence rate (percent) over the past three years in each of four communities to be included in the dengue vaccine trial. The balance of the randomization is measured by the mean difference in average annual incidence between the communities to receive vaccine and the control communities (adapted from Moulton (2004))

	Communities				
Allocation	Vaccine		Control		Mean Difference
A	3	5	11	13	−8
B	3	11	5	13	−2
C	3	13	5	11	0
D	5	11	3	13	0
E	5	13	3	11	2
F	11	13	3	5	8

However, the problem now is that in allocations C and D, the two communities with incidence rates of 3% and 13% and the two communities with 5% and 11% are always together. This violates the validity principle stated above, because, for example, the pair 5 and 13 do not have a chance of being randomized together. In essence, each pair of communities in allocations C and D is acting as a single community. To alleviate this problem, the constraint could be relaxed, so that the mean difference in annual incidence is less than 3%. Then allocations B, C, D, and E would satisfy the contraint. Although the communities with 3% and 5% and those with 11% and 13% could never be together, this is the same as would happen if it were a pair-matched design (3% and 5%, 11% and 13%) with randomization within pairs. More details are in Moulton (2004).

13.5.1.2 Hypothetical influenza vaccine study

A hypothetical study to evaluate the indirect effects of vaccinating children against influenza illustrates the use of a stratified randomization with constrained randomization. The study region is divided into 20 natural villages of varying sizes based around community centers. The study is a parallel design with half of the units receiving killed influenza vaccine, and the other half receiving inactivated polio vaccine. Two of the villages contain large markets, so one stratification will be villages with or without markets. The nonmarket villages fall into two natural regions, with 6 villages north and 12 villages south of the markets. No baseline data are available on influenza incidence, but there is no evidence suggesting that there is a high variability in incidence among the villages. However, it seems reasonable to stratify the randomization in the nonmarket villages by north and south. So, there are three strata pre-randomization.

The funding agency has provided an equal number of doses of influenza and polio vaccine, so it is of interest to constrain the randomization so that approximately equal numbers of eligible children are in the influenza and the control arms of the study. The constraint could be defined such that the relative difference in the number of eligible children in the two arms is less than some proportion. Different levels of constraints could be checked for whether they meet the requirement of the randomization scheme. This example illustrates that the pre-randomization stratification covariates can be different from the constraining covariates.

13.5.2 *Stepped wedge design*

One would also like to achieve balance in group-level covariates when randomizing the sequence of groups converting from control to vaccination intervention in a stepped wedge design. For example, it would be undesirable for all of the low-incidence communities to be randomized to introduce the vaccination strategy early in the stepped wedge study. One might want to aim for a balance on group-time spent in the control and vaccination program status with respect to the group-level covariates of interest. Moulton et al (2007) developed a method for constrained randomization in the stepped wedge design of a study introducing screening for tuberculosis in HIV clinics in Rio de Janeiro. The general idea in designing the stepped wedge constrained randomization is that for each possible sequence of introduction of the vaccination strategies, the constraints are checked to see whether they are satisfied. If the number of groups is too large to enumerate all possible sequences, then sequences are sampled randomly from all possible ones by random permutations of the group labels. For each permutation, the constraints are checked to see whether they are satisfied. Then when a large number of acceptable sequences have been identified, one is randomly selected from it.

Moulton et al (2007) suggested the following ad hoc approach to check the constraints. For each jth covariate of the ith group, $i = 1,\ldots,N$, x_{ij}, and for a given time of entry t_i of group i into the vaccination strategy, $t = 1,\ldots,T$, let c_j be a proportional covariate-specific tolerance. The constraint can be expressed as

$$\frac{1}{1+c_j} < \frac{\sum_{i=1,t_i \neq T}^{N}(T-1-(t_i-1))x_{ij}}{\sum_{i=1,t_i \neq T}^{N}(t_i-1)x_{ij}} < (1+c_j). \tag{13.1}$$

Then the sum of the covariate values weighted by the number of time units in the vaccine intervention must be within $c_j \times 100\%$ of that for the control status. A similar approach to that described in Section 13.5 is followed. One tries to avoid constraints that always pair two groups to enter simultaneously, as this would effectively reduce them to a single randomization unit.

13.6 Power and Number of Communities

In group-randomized studies, the sample size calculation needs to take into account that randomization is by group rather than by individual. In general, group-randomized designs are less efficient than individually randomized studies due to the related factors of intragroup correlation and intergroup variability. That is, the more similar the individuals within each group are to each other and the more different the groups are from one another, the greater the group design effect on sample size will be. For a given sample size, a stepped wedge design will generally be less efficient than a parallel design, so further allowance needs to be made when planning a stepped wedge design study.

Two different measures are used in calculating sample size for group-randomized studies. One is the coefficient of variation k, the standard deviation divided by the mean of the incidence rate, or other outcome measure of interest such as proportions (attack rates) or mean of a continuous variable in the groups in the study. Another approach uses the design effect D, or variance inflation factor σ. For trials with equal numbers of individuals in each community,

$$D = \sigma = 1 + (n-1)\rho, \tag{13.2}$$

where n is the number of individuals per community, ρ is the intracluster correlation coefficient, and D is the factor by which the sample size needs to be increased above that required for an individually randomized trial to make up for randomization by cluster (Donner and Klar 1994).

We consider sample size calculations based on incidence rates, proportions (attack rates), and means of continuous outcomes. For clarity, the following discussion is just about rates, but could apply to proportions (attack rates) and means as well. The sample size calculations require estimates or assumptions about the baseline incidence rate λ_0, and an assumption of the effect of the vaccination intervention strategy, or equivalently, the rate in the vaccination intervention group λ_1. Exactly what the λ_0 and λ_1 of interest are will depend on whether the primary interest is on estimating indirect, total, or overall effects, or possibly even direct effects. For example, if the total effect of a vaccination strategy is of interest, then λ_0 might be the incidence rate in the children receiving a control vaccine in the control groups, and λ_1 the incidence rate in children receiving the vaccine of interest in groups randomized to receive the vaccination strategy. If overall effects were of interest, λ_0 and λ_1 could be the incidence rates in all age-appropriate children (or all children) in the control and the vaccination intervention groups. If the indirect effects of vaccinating schoolchildren against influenza on the incidence rates in adults were of interest, then λ_0 and λ_1 could be the rates in the adults in the control and intervention groups. If more than one effect is of interest, then sample size calculations can be made for more than one effect.

Hayes and Bennett (1999) provide simple formulae to determine sample size for parallel design group-randomized studies. The next section is based primarily on their paper, where further details, references, and examples are available. Many group-randomized studies of vaccination strategies may require more complex computations than these. In some cases, stochastic simulations of the populations with the planned intervention strategies can be used to estimate expected effects, power, and sample sizes for the studies (Halloran et al 2002a). Sample size requirements under randomization tests are similar to those for model-based inference procedures (Murray 1998, page 117).

13.6.1 Sample size for parallel design

Assuming equal numbers of groups in the vaccine intervention arm and the control arm, let N be the number of groups in each study arm. Then the total number of groups in the study is $2N$. Let k be the coefficient of variation. Let $z_{\alpha/2}$ and z_{β} be the standard normal distribution values corresponding to upper tail probabilities of $\alpha/2$ and β. The corresponding sample size will give a power of $100(1-\beta)\%$ of obtaining a significant difference ($P < \alpha$ on a two-sided test), assuming that the true population rates in the intervention and control groups are λ_1 and λ_0. If the outcome is based on person-time, let y denote the person-time of follow-up in each group. Then the number of groups required in each arm is

$$N = 1 + (z_{\alpha/2} + z_{\beta})^2 \frac{(\lambda_0 + \lambda_1)/y + k^2(\lambda_0^2 + \lambda_1^2)}{(\lambda_0 - \lambda_1)^2}. \tag{13.3}$$

If the outcome is based on proportions (attack rates), let π_0 and π_1 be the true population proportions (attack rates) in the vaccine intervention and control groups. Let n be the number of individuals in each group. Then the number of groups required in each arm is

$$N = 1 + (z_{\alpha/2} + z_{\beta})^2 \frac{\pi_0(1-\pi_0)/n + \pi_1(1-\pi_1)/n + k^2(\pi_0^2 + \pi_1^2)}{(\pi_0 - \pi_1)^2}. \tag{13.4}$$

If the outcome is based on a continuous reponse, such as parasite density, then the objective is to compare the mean of that variable in the vaccine intervention and control groups. Let μ_1 and μ_0 be the true population means and σ_1 and σ_0 be the within-group standard deviations of the outcome variable in the vaccine intervention and control groups. Let n be the number of individuals in each group. Then the number of groups required in each arm is

$$N = 1 + (z_{\alpha/2} + z_{\beta})^2 \frac{(\sigma_0^2 + \sigma_1^2)/y + k^2(\mu_0^2 + \mu_1^2)}{(\mu_0 - \mu_1)^2}. \tag{13.5}$$

If one is interested in direct protective effects, these equations are analogous to those for individually randomized trials in equations (6.13)–(6.15). The design effect on the sample size associated with the group-randomization can be estimated by dividing the equation in this chapter by the corresponding equation in Chapter 6.

When pairs of groups are matched before randomization on the basis of factors expected to be correlated with the main study outcomes, the hope is the matching will minimize the degree of between-group variation within matched pairs. However, there is a trade-off between the increase in power and precision by increasing the comparability of the vaccine intervention and control groups and the loss of power due to the reduced degrees of freedom that is well discussed in the literature (Martin et al 1993; Hayes et al 1995). Much has been written on characteristics of the general size and correlation between the endpoint of interest and matching covariates and power in cluster-randomized trials (see, for instance, Murray 1998). Hughes (2005) more generally considers using baseline data in designing a group-randomized trial to choose between an unmatched or pair-matched design, choice of effect measure, and the power to be expected from the various strategies. Equations (13.3)–(13.5) can be adjusted to take account of matching with two changes. First, to adjust for the required number of degrees of freedom, add 2 instead of 1 to the required number of groups in each arm (Snedecor and Cochran 1967). Second, the coefficient of variation k is replaced by k_m, the coefficient of variation in true rates (or means or proportions) between groups within the matched pairs prior to intervention.

13.6.2 Coefficient of variation

A value for the coefficient of variation k is needed for the sample size calculations, thus in the absence of any empirical data, an assumption about the value must be made. In this case, one can compute power curves and examine the number of clusters required for plausible values of k. Sometimes data may be available from baseline surveillance studies. Alternatively, data may be available from a pilot study conducted to check the implementation plan that is also used to collect data to estimate the intergroup variability of the main outcome of the trial. A subset of the groups can be selected and data on a small fraction of the population of interest be recorded. Alternatively, data might be available on similar groups in different areas of the country. Hayes and Bennet (1999) provide formulae for estimating the coefficient of variation for unmatched (k) and matched (k_m) studies. Generally k will be larger than k_m. The coefficient of variation is for the variation in the true rates between groups, not the variation in the estimated rates which contains an element of within-group random variation. The general idea is to compute the empirical variance of the group-specific results, then substract the component of the variance due to sampling error. See Moulton et al (2007) for an example.

In another approach to sample size calculation for a group-randomized study, one might compute the number of events needed under individual randomization to achieve a certain power, possibly for the lower bound of a 95% confidence interval to lie about a certain pre-determined efficacy if, in fact, the true efficacy is some other higher efficacy. Then, to account for intragroup correlation, multiply the number of events by the usual design effect in equation (13.2). One can possibly get an initial estimate of the overdispersion σ^2 directly from some baseline data from a sample of the communities (Moulton et al 2001).

13.6.3 Sample size for stepped wedge design

Considerations of design and power in the stepped wedge design revolve around the timing of the individual observations, the interval at which the intervention is introduced into groups, and the number of groups switched from control to intervention at any given time. Observation of individuals could occur continuously, or somehow be aligned with the timing of switching the groups from control to intervention. The number of time points chosen to introduce a given number of clusters into a trial influences the power of the study. The higher the number of time points, the higher the power is, especially if the number of observations on individuals is correlated with the number of time points (Hussey and Hughes 2007). However, if individuals are observed continuously, then there is less effect on power. In vaccine studies in which cases are reported as they occur, the effect on power would be lower.

To take account of the stepped wedge design in the sample size, Moulton et al (2007) suggest a modification to equations (13.3)–(13.5). Essentially the standard deviates $z_{\alpha/2}$ and z_β used in equations (13.3)–(13.5) are multiplied by a factor >1 that accounts for the lower efficiency of the stepped wedge design. In addition, if the variability between groups is large, they suggest substituting the harmonic mean for the simple mean.

The multiplicative factor can be computed in various ways. As an example, consider a stepped wedge design study in which the analysis was based on a comparison of the incidence in groups receiving the vaccination intervention to those not yet receiving the vaccination intervention within the time interval between converting the next groups to intervention. This is a slight simplification of the problem compared to the analysis based on a conditional likelihood as in equation (13.9). Following Moulton et al (2007), one weights the hazard function within the time unit of interest (week, month) by the log-rank to estimate the effect of the stepped wedge design. Let T be the last time unit at which control groups begin the intervention. Let d_{T_i} be the number of incident cases in the ith time unit in the vaccination intervention groups, Y_{T_i} be the number of persons at risk in those groups, and d_i and Y_i be the cases and persons in both vaccination intervention and control groups in the ith time unit. The log-rank test statistic is

$$Z = \frac{\sum_{i=1}^{T-1}[d_{T_i} - Y_{T_i}(d_i/Y_i)]}{\{\sum_{i=1}^{T-1}(Y_{T_i}/Y_i)(1-(Y_{T_i}/Y_i))(Y_i-d_i)/(Y_i-1)\}^{1/2}d_i} \tag{13.6}$$

The statistic (13.6) can be computed by generating data sets under two different assumptions. First generate data assuming that the number of persons at risk in the vaccination intervention and control groups is equal and constant over the course of the study. This simulates a time-uniform equal allocation parallel design study, yielding Z_E to denote equal allocation. Second, generate data so that the persons at risk in each month in the vaccination intervention groups increase in each time unit according to the plan of the phased implementation to yield Z_{SW}. In general, for such hypothetical studies, given the same sample size, incidence, and effectiveness, the stepped wedge study's test statistic will be smaller than that for a parallel study by a factor of Z_{SW}/Z_E, where Z_{SW} is always smaller than Z_E (Moulton et al 2007). To account for a stepped wedge allocation, multiply the standard normal deviates in equation (13.3) by a factor of Z_E/Z_{SW}. Finally, one should vary the values of the coefficient of variation, the assumed incidence rates, and the assumed effectiveness of the intervention to determine the range in which one would have the desired power and Type I error, and then examine whether these conditions are feasible under the conditions of the proposed study.

13.7 Analysis

The key issue in analyzing group-randomized studies is to account for the clustering or group-randomization. The variability of the estimates is determined not only by the number of individuals in the study, but the amount of intra- and intergroup variability. There are two general approaches to analysis that account for potential within-cluster correlation (Donner et al 1994). One approach is to reduce the data for each cluster to a single observation and to perform a standard two-sample analysis. Another approach is to do the analysis at the individual level but account for correlation somehow. Correlation within the units could be taken into account by doing a bootstrap (Efron and Tibshirani 1993) at the level of the entire community (Halloran et al 2003; Moulton et al 2006) (see Section 12.3.2). One could fit a marginal model, such as using generalized estimating equations or a random effects model. As discussed in Section 12.3.2, in marginal models, inference about population averages is the focus. In considering vaccine effects, the primary scientific question is about the population average, or marginal, vaccine effect measures. Thus, the marginal model would likely be the model of choice. Another approach is to use a robust variance estimator (Moulton et al 2006).

The stepped wedge design trials present additional complications. Each randomization unit spends time in both the control and intervention conditions. There could be substantial secular trends in the incidence of the disease of interest, confounding the treatment effect. Moulton et al (2006) take an approach that compares the outcomes at any point in time across all groups, then combines the results over time at the same time accounting for within-cluster correlation (see below). They accomplish this by conditioning on each time unit of the study and comparing incidences in those groups that have not introduced the intervention with those that have. The analysis is carried out by maximizing a partial likelihood function that is similar to a Cox proportional hazards model.

13.7.1 Pneumococcal vaccine study

One approach to analysis is to use a model based on a nonhomogeneous Poisson process in time and space (Moulton et al 2006). Let λ_{it} be the rate of disease among the individuals of interest in randomization unit i on day t. Let n_{it} be the person-days of exposure in the ith group on day t, α_t be the effect of the tth day, and γ be the log rate ratio comparing those in the vaccine intervention communities ($z_i = 1$) to those in the control unit ($z_i = 0$). A simple model for λ_{it} is given by

$$\lambda_{it} = n_{it}\exp(\alpha_t + \gamma z_i). \tag{13.7}$$

The parameter α_t is a nuisance parameter that captures any secular trends specific to day t, such as seasonal or weekend effects.

If living in the intervention community confers protection on the individuals of interest, then γ will be negative. One can imagine a number of different comparisons, depending on whether one is trying to estimate indirect, total, or overall effects. Moulton et al (2006) were interested in estimating the protective indirect effects on invasive pneumococcal disease for nonenrolled children under two years of age.

The problem with model (13.7) is that it does not allow for different levels of coverage among the randomization units. One option is to group the coverage levels or enrollment levels, and to use dummy variables in the model that are crossed with the dummy variable for three treatment arm. Let Mnc_{it}^{25-49} be one for the ith unit on the tth day if it is a community randomized to MnCC vaccine, and if 25–49% of the children under age two on that day have received at least one immunization, otherwise it is zero. Moulton et al (2006) fit the model

$$\begin{aligned}\lambda_{it} = n_{it}\exp(\alpha_t &+ \beta_1 Mnc_{it}^{25-49} + \beta_2 Mnc_{it}^{50+} \\ &+ \beta_3 Pnc_{it}^{0-24} + \beta_4 Pnc_{it}^{25-49} + \beta_5 Pnc_{it}^{50+}).\end{aligned} \tag{13.8}$$

Because the communities were not randomized to different coverage levels, there may be unmeasured confounders associated with the coverage levels. So then one can compare across treatment arms within coverage levels. For example, if the difference $\beta_4 - \beta_1$ is negative, then it suggests presence of indirect effects at that level of coverage 25–49%. The rate ratio comparing the two treatment arms at above 50% coverage is given by $\exp(\beta_5 - \beta_2)$.

To eliminate the nuisance parameter α_t, Moulton et al (2006) suggest an analytic strategy that conditions on each day of the study. Similar to a Cox regression model, each day delineates a risk set, similar to a stratum in a case-control study. The characteristics of those randomization units that experienced a case on that day are compared to those that did not have any cases on that day. The comparison is done for each day, and then the probabilities are multiplied together to get the conditional likelihood function. Let T be the number of days in the study. Let δ_t be one if there is a case on the tth day and zero otherwise. Define $R(t)$ as the set of indices of those units at risk on day t. Let x_{jt} be the row vector of dummy variables for the jth unit on day t, with $j = i$ representing the community with a case on that day. The conditional likelihood function is

$$\prod_{t=1}^{t=T}\left[n_{it}\exp(x_{it}\beta)/\sum_{j\in R(t)} n_{jt}\exp(x_{jt}\beta)\right]^{\delta_t}. \tag{13.9}$$

Table 13.9 Analysis results from fitting conditional logistic models with five dummy variables to represent six vaccine arm/percentage vaccine coverage combinations. Conditional maximum likelihood estimates (CMLE), standard errors (SE), robust 95% confidence intervals, and 95% bootstrap percentile intervals. The reference category is units that received MnCC vaccine which on a given day had less than 25% of children enrolled in the study. The CMLEs are the log rate ratios comparing incidence in nonenrolled childrein in the given category in the reference category (from Moulton et al (2006))

Dummy Variable (Arm/ % Coverage)	CMLE	Robust SE	Bootstrap SE	Robust CI	Bootstrap Percentile Interval
MnCC 0–24%	0				
MnCC 25–49%	1.18	0.51	0.62	0.18, 2.17	0.12, 2.74
MnCC 50+%	1.93	0.66	0.81	0.64, 3.23	0.46, 4.25
PCV7 0–24%	1.09	0.49	0.60	0.14, 2.04	−0.07, 2.58
PCV7 25–49%	0.98	0.62	0.75	−0.24, 2.19	−1.05, 2.59
PCV7 50+%	1.96	0.71	0.85	0.56, 3.37	0.68, 4.37

Estimates of β are obtained by maximizing the conditional likelihood function. Software for conditional logistic regression can be used for computation with an offset term of $\ln(n_{it})$.

Table 13.9 contains the results of fitting the conditional logistic model with a linear predictor as in equation (13.8). The analysis did not yield significant indirect effects on nonenrolled children. One can compare the units with similar coverage levels. For example, at the coverage levels >50%, $\exp(\hat{\beta}_5 - \hat{\beta}_2) = \exp(1.96 - 193) = 1.03$. Using the naive covariance matrix for the parameter estimates yields a 95% Wald interval for the ratio 1.03 of (0.31, 3.45). The issue may be that the proportion of the population vaccinated was quite small, and that carriage from older siblings could have been important. The number of cases was also quite small. There were 27 cases during the PCV7 phase in communities and 21 cases during the MnCC phase in communities. Eighteen of the 38 units had no cases at all.

13.7.2 Other approaches

Ali et al (2005) entered coverage level as a continuous variable in the cholera study. In a community-randomized study, one would also add a variable for the treatment arm. One could deal with a secular trend by examining rate changes for groups and months when the treatment status is the same, then adjust for the estimated trend. This approach might produce results that are difficult to interpret if there is no smooth trend. The model of α_t assumes that the secular trends represented by α_t are the same for all randomization units. This might not be the case if a study such as for a meningococcal vaccine were being done on different continents. However, then a more complex model that allowed for some continent- or geographic-specific secular trends might be possible. One might also consider a combination of matched-pair design and analysis, even in the case of a stepped wedge design. Certain other aspects, for example, that immunization might not begin simultaneously in all units, can be taken into account by entering the randomization unit into the analysis on the day of the first immunization in the unit.

13.8 Causal Inference for Indirect, Total, and Overall Effects

13.8.1 General approach

In Section 13.1.1 we informally define direct, indirect, total, and overall effects using concepts from the potential outcome approach to causal inference. In Chapters 9 and 15 we use causal inference to define estimands of interest. Defining causal estimands for indirect, total, and overall effects using potential outcomes is not straightforward. The approach assumes that individuals could potentially receive each of the treatments under study and that each of those treatments could be enumerated. Generally the assumption is made that the outcome in one individual is independent of the treatment assignment in the other individuals in the study population. This is called the assumption of no interference (Cox 1958) and is an essential aspect of the stable unit treatment value assumption (SUTVA) (Rubin 1978). Under the assumption of no interference, if there are two treatments, such as vaccine and control, then a person has two potential outcomes, one for each treatment.

The general approach in causal inference using potential outcomes is to define causal estimands and the conditions under which they can be identified from the data. One has a population of individuals. The individual causal effect can be defined, but it is not identifiable. An average causal effect estimand for the population is defined that is also not identifiable. Under the assumption of no interference and a posited assignment mechanism, such as randomization of individuals to either treatment, then the average causal effect in the population is estimable from the observed outcomes.

In the dependent happenings in infectious diseases, the assumption of no interference does not hold and indeed is the source of the indirect, total, and overall effects of interest in this chapter. The vaccine status of other individuals in the population can affect the potential outcomes of an individual, so a person can have many more than two potential outcomes, depending on the vaccine assignment to the other individuals. Rubin (1990) suggested a general notation in which the potential outcome of a person was defined as a function of the vector of treatment assignment to the person of interest as well as the treatment assignments to other individuals in the population. Let $Z = (Z_1, \ldots, Z_n)$ be the vector of treatment assignments in the population of size n, where $Z = 1$ denotes vaccine and $Z = 0$ denotes control. Then the potential outcome of individual i if the population receives treatment assignment Z is denoted by $Y_i(Z)$. Halloran and Struchiner (1995) defined the individual direct causal effect of being vaccinated compared with not being vaccinated in an individual i when the rest of the population $j \neq i$ receives treatment assignment $Z_{j \neq i}$ as

$$Y_i(Z_{j \neq i}, Z_i = 1) - Y_i(Z_{j \neq i}, Z_i = 0). \tag{13.10}$$

The direct causal effect is a family of values that depends on the treatment assignment vector Z in the population.

To define the indirect, total, and overall effects of one vaccination strategy compared with another, one needs to consider a second strategy, denoted Z'. They define the individual indirect causal effect of intervention program Z compared with Z' as

$$Y_i(Z_{j \neq i}, Z_i = 0) - Y_i(Z'_{j \neq i}, Z_i = 0), \tag{13.11}$$

where now the individual of interest has not received the vaccine under either intervention program. Halloran and Struchiner (1995) defined the individual total and overall causal effects analogously. However, they found problems with taking the usual approach in causal inference to average over the potential outcomes to arrive at causal estimands of direct, indirect, total, and overall effects.

Hudgens and Halloran (2008) defined causal estimands of direct, indirect, total, and overall effects in the presence of interference by positing a population of groups, blocks, or clusters composed of individuals with interference within the groups but not between the groups as in the study designs described in this chapter. Taking as their point of departure the individual causal effects proposed by Halloran and Struchiner (1995), Hudgens and Halloran (2008) define average individual, group, and population outcomes over all possible treatment assignments for a particular allocation strategy or strategies of interest within and across groups (Sobel 2006). They define causal estimands of the direct, indirect, total, and overall effects that are also averages within the groups and across the population of groups. By specifying an assignment mechanism at two levels, that is, randomization of groups to allocation strategies, and then randomization of individuals within groups to treatment by the allocation strategy assigned to the group, the average causal direct, indirect, total, and overall effects are estimable from the observed outcomes.

The development of the causal estimands is not specific to infectious diseases, and the causal effects are defined based on differences, not relative risks as efficacy measures. For example, consider the data from Ali et al (2005) in Table 13.5. Suppose that the groups with >51% and <28% coverage are thought of as groups A and B. Effects of vaccination can be estimated based on differences in the incidence of cholera during the first year of follow-up of the trial. The direct effects are estimated by comparing the incidence (risk per 1000 population) between vaccinated individuals and unvaccinated individuals within each group. For example, the estimated direct effect in group B is $7.01 - 2.66 = 4.35$, suggesting vaccination results in 4.35 fewer cases of cholera per 1000 individuals per year. The estimated direct effect in group A is $1.47 - 1.27 = 0.20$, considerably lower than in group B. The estimated indirect effect in the unvaccinated (B − A) is $7.01 - 1.47 = 5.54$. The estimated total effect (B − A) is $7.01 - 1.27 = 5.74$. Note the total effect (B−A) estimate equals the direct effect estimate in group A plus the indirect effect estimate in the unvaccinated (B − A). The overall effect can be estimated by the difference in incidence between the two groups, ie, $35/8479 - 25/18,623 = 2.79/1000$.

13.8.2 Formalization

The chapter finishes with a brief summary of the formal approach in Hudgens and Halloran (2008) to defining causal estimands and estimators for direct, indirect, total, and overall effects. Suppose there are $N > 1$ groups of individuals. For $i = 1,\ldots,N$, let n_i denote the number of individuals in group i and let $Z_i \equiv (Z_{i1},\ldots,Z_{in_i})$ denote the treatments those n_i individuals receive. Assume Z_{ij} is a dichotomous random variable having values 0 or 1 such that Z_i can take on 2^{n_i} possible values. Let $Z_{i(j)}$ denote the $n_i - 1$ subvector of Z_i with the jth entry deleted. The vector Z_i is referred to as an intervention or treatment *program*, to distinguish it from the individual treatment Z_{ij}. Let z_i and z_{ij} denote possible values of Z_i and Z_{ij}. Define R^j to be the set of vectors of possible treatment programs of length j, for $j = 1,2,\ldots$; eg, $R^2 \equiv \{(0,0),(0,1),(1,0),(1,1)\}$. Possible values z_i of Z_i are elements of R^{n_i}. For positive integer n and $k \in \{0,\ldots,n\}$, define R^n_k to be the subset of R^n wherein exactly k individuals receive treatment 1. For example, $\sum_{j=1}^{n_i} z_{ij} = k$ for all $z_i \in R^{n_i}_k$.

Denote the potential outcome of individual j in group i under treatment z_i as $Y_{ij}(z_i)$. The notation $Y_{ij}(z_i)$ allows for the possibility that the potential outcome for individual j may depend on another individual's treatment assignment in group i, but the potential outcomes for individuals in group i do not depend on treatment assignments of individuals in group i' for $i' \neq i$.

13.8.2.1 Treatment Assignment Mechanisms

Let ψ and ϕ denote parameterizations that govern the distribution of Z_i for $i = 1,\ldots,N$. For example, ψ might correspond to randomly assigning half of individuals in a group to treatment 1 and the other half to treatment 0, whereas ϕ might correspond to assigning all individuals in a group to treatment 0. The goal is to assess the causal effects of assigning groups to the individual treatment assignment strategy ψ compared to ϕ.

The experimental design is a two-stage randomization procedure. In the first stage, each of the N groups is randomly assigned to either ϕ or ψ. In the second stage, individuals are randomly assigned treatment conditional on their group's assignment in the first stage. For example, in the first stage half of the N groups might be assigned to an allocation strategy ϕ and the other half ψ; in the second stage, 2/3 of the individuals within a group are randomly assigned treatment 1 for groups assigned ϕ, and 1/3 of the individuals within a group are randomly assigned treatment 1 for groups assigned ψ.

Corresponding to the first stage of randomization, let $S \equiv (S_1, \ldots, S_N)$ denote the group assignments with $S_i = 1$ if the ith group is assigned to ψ and 0 otherwise. Let ν denote the parameterization that governs the distribution of S and let $C \equiv \sum_i S_i$ denote the number of groups assigned ψ.

13.8.2.2 Average potential outcomes

Similar to Halloran and Struchiner (1995), Hudgens and Halloran (2008) begin by writing the potential outcomes for individual j in group i under $z_{ij} = z$ as

$$Y_{ij}(z_{i(j)}, z_{ij} = z), \tag{13.12}$$

for $z = 0, 1$. They then proceed to define the *individual average potential outcome* under treatment assignment z by

$$\overline{Y}_{ij}(z; \psi) \equiv \sum_{\omega \in R^{n_i - 1}} Y_{ij}(z_{i(j)} = \omega, z_{ij} = z)\Pr_\psi(Z_{i(j)} = \omega | Z_{ij} = z).$$

In other words, the individual average potential outcome is the conditional expectation of $Y_{ij}(Z_i)$ given $Z_{ij} = z$ under assignment strategy ψ. Averaging over individuals, they define the *group average potential outcome* under treatment assignment z as $\overline{Y}_i(z; \psi) \equiv \sum_{j=1}^{n_i} \overline{Y}_{ij}(z; \psi)/n_i$. Finally, averaging over groups, they define the *population average potential outcome* under treatment assignment z as $\overline{Y}(z; \psi) \equiv \sum_{i=1}^{N} \overline{Y}_i(z; \psi)/N$.

The *marginal* individual average potential outcome is defined by $\overline{Y}_{ij}(\psi) \equiv \sum_{z \in R^{n_i}} Y_{ij}(z) \Pr_\psi(Z_i = z)$, ie, the average potential outcome for individual j in group i when group i is assigned ψ. Similarly, the marginal group and population average potential outcomes are defined by $\overline{Y}_i(\psi) \equiv \sum_{j=1}^{n_i} \overline{Y}_{ij}(\psi)/n_i$ and $\overline{Y}(\psi) \equiv \sum_{i=1}^{N} \overline{Y}_i(\psi)/N$.

13.8.2.3 Causal estimands

Define the *individual direct causal effect* of treatment 0 compared to treatment 1 for individual j in group i by

$$CE_{ij}^{D}(z_{i(j)}) \equiv Y_{ij}(z_{i(j)}, z_{ij} = 0) - Y_{ij}(z_{i(j)}, z_{ij} = 1). \tag{13.13}$$

The causal estimands are then defined in terms of average potential outcomes. Hudgens and Halloran (2008) define the *individual average direct causal effect* for individual j in group i by

$$\overline{CE}_{ij}^{D}(\psi) \equiv \overline{Y}_{ij}(0; \psi) - \overline{Y}_{ij}(1; \psi), \tag{13.14}$$

ie, the difference in individual average potential outcomes when $z_{ij} = 0$ and when $z_{ij} = 1$ under ψ. Finally, define the *group average direct causal effect* by $\overline{CE}_i^D(\psi) \equiv \overline{Y}_i(0;\psi) - \overline{Y}_i(1;\psi) = \sum_{j=1}^{n_i} \overline{CE}_{ij}^D(\psi)/n_i$ and the *population average direct causal effect* by $\overline{CE}^D(\psi) \equiv \overline{Y}(0;\psi) - \overline{Y}(1;\psi) = \sum_{i=1}^{N} \overline{CE}_i^D(\psi)/N$.

The *individual indirect causal effect* of treatment program z_i compared with z_i' on individual j in group i is defined by

$$CE_{ij}^I(z_{i(j)}, z_{i(j)}') \equiv Y_i(z_{i(j)}, z_{ij} = 0) - Y_i(z_{i(j)}', z_{ij}' = 0), \tag{13.15}$$

where z_i' is another n_i dimensional vector of individual treatment assignments. (Note z_i' does not denote the transpose of z_i.)

Similar to direct effects, the *individual average indirect causal effect* is defined by $\overline{CE}_{ij}^I(\phi,\psi) \equiv \overline{Y}_{ij}(0;\phi) - \overline{Y}_{ij}(0;\psi)$. Clearly if $\psi = \phi$, then $\overline{CE}_{ij}^I(\phi,\psi) = 0$; ie, there are no individual average indirect causal effects. Finally, define the *group average indirect causal effect* as $\overline{CE}_i^I(\phi,\psi) \equiv \overline{Y}_i(0;\phi) - \overline{Y}_i(0;\psi) = \sum_{j=1}^{n_i} \overline{CE}_{ij}^I(\phi,\psi)/n_i$ and the *population average indirect causal effect* as $\overline{CE}^I(\phi,\psi) \equiv \overline{Y}(0;\phi) - \overline{Y}(0;\psi) = \sum_{i=1}^{N} \overline{CE}_i^I(\phi,\psi)/N$.

Define the *individual total causal effects* for individual j in group i as

$$CE_{ij}^T(z_{i(j)}, z_{i(j)}') \equiv Y_{ij}(z_{i(j)}, z_{ij} = 0) - Y_{ij}(z_{i(j)}', z_{ij}' = 1). \tag{13.16}$$

Then define the individual average, group average, and population average total causal effect similar to the indirect causal estimands.

Hudgens and Halloran (2008) define the *individual overall causal effect* of treatment z_i compared to treatment z_i' for individual j in group i by $CE_{ij}^O(z_i, z_i') \equiv Y_{ij}(z_i) - Y_{ij}(z_i')$. Similarly, for the comparison of ϕ to ψ, define the *individual average overall causal effect* by $\overline{CE}_{ij}^O(\phi,\psi) \equiv \overline{Y}_{ij}(\phi) - \overline{Y}_{ij}(\psi)$, the *group average overall causal effect* by $\overline{CE}_i^O(\phi,\psi) \equiv \overline{Y}_i(\phi) - \overline{Y}_i(\psi)$, and the *population average overall causal effect* by $\overline{CE}^O(\phi,\psi) \equiv \overline{Y}(\phi) - \overline{Y}(\psi)$.

13.8.2.4 Estimation and inference

Assuming the randomized assignment strategies at both levels of randomization in which the number of groups randomized to a strategy is fixed, and the number of individuals within each group randomized to received treatment is fixed, Hudgens and Halloran (2008) show that the observed data yield unbiased estimators of the causal estimands. Suppose $S_i = 1$. Let $\widehat{Y}_i(z;\psi)$ the average of observed outcomes for individuals in group i receiving treatment z under treatment program Z_i. They show that

$$\widehat{Y}_i(z;\psi) \equiv \frac{\sum_{j=1}^{n_i} Y_{ij}(Z_i) I[Z_{ij} = z]}{\sum_{j=1}^{n_i} I[Z_{ij} = z]} \quad \text{for } z = 0, 1, \tag{13.17}$$

is an unbiased estimator of $\overline{Y}_i(z;\psi)$. Also $\widehat{CE}_i^D(\psi) \equiv \widehat{Y}_i(0;\psi) - \widehat{Y}_i(1;\psi)$ is a conditionally unbiased estimator of $\overline{CE}_i^D(\psi)$ given $S_i = 1$. Finally, they show $\widehat{Y}(z;\psi) \equiv \sum_{i=1}^N \widehat{Y}_i(z;\psi)I[S_i = 1]/\sum_{i=1}^N I[S_i = 1]$ is an unbiased estimator of $\overline{Y}(z;\psi)$ for $z = 0, 1$. Thus, unbiased estimators for the population average direct, indirect, and total causal effects are given by $\widehat{CE}^D(\psi) \equiv \widehat{Y}(0;\psi) - \widehat{Y}(1;\psi)$, $\widehat{CE}^I(\phi,\psi) \equiv \widehat{Y}(0;\phi) - \widehat{Y}(0;\psi)$, and $\widehat{CE}^T(\phi,\psi) \equiv \widehat{Y}(0;\phi) - \widehat{Y}(1;\psi)$ where $\widehat{Y}(z;\phi)$ is defined analogously to $\widehat{Y}(z;\psi)$ for $z = 0, 1$.

Let $\widehat{Y}_i(\psi) \equiv \sum_{j=1}^{n_i} Y_{ij}(Z_i)/n_i$ and $\widehat{Y}(\psi) \equiv \sum_{i=1}^N \widehat{Y}_i(\psi)I[S_i = 1]/\sum_{i=1}^N I[S_i = 1]$. The unbiased estimator of the overall effect causal estimand $\overline{CE}^O(\phi,\psi)$ is given by $\widehat{CE}^O(\phi,\psi) \equiv \widehat{Y}(\phi) - \widehat{Y}(\psi)$ where $\widehat{Y}(\phi)$ is defined analogously to $\widehat{Y}(\psi)$.

Under the further assumption of stratified interference, that is, that the potential outcomes depend on the number of individuals within a group that receive a treatment, but not exactly who receives the treatment, Hudgens and Halloran (2008) derive variance estimators. A one-to-one mapping of the causal estimands of direct, indirect, total, and overall effects of Hudgens and Halloran (2008) to the group-randomized studies presented in this chapter is the subject of future research.

Problems

13.1. Constrained randomization

(a) Consider designing a community-randomized trial of a cholera vaccine in eight communities. The average annual incidence of cholera in the eight communities is 1, 3, 4, 7, 9, 10, 11, 12%. How many different allocations of the vaccine and control are there for a pair-matched design? For a completely randomized (at the group level) design?

(b) What would be a reasonable constraint to ensure a fairly balanced allocation under complete randomization?

13.2. Overall effectiveness in Alaska of PCV7

Compute the overall effectiveness of PCV7 vaccination against all serotypes in the 2–4 year age group in Alaska natives and and Non-Alaska natives.

13.3. Randomization for stepped wedge design

Assume there are 24 communities that will be randomized to introduction of rotavirus vaccine into the Expanded Program of Immunization in a stepped wedge design. Two teams will introduce the vaccine every two months, so that it will take two years to complete introduction of the vaccination strategy. How many possible distinct orderings of the introduction of the vaccination strategy are there?

13.4. Computing sample size in stepped wedge design (Moulton et al 2007)

(a) Assume $Z_E/Z_{SW} = 1.2$ Suppose one wants to have power of 80% and Type I error of 5% in a study. What values of z-score does one need to use in in expression 13.3?

(b) By what factor would the sample size in expression 13.3 be multiplied? (see Moulton et al 2007, p. 195)

(c) Suppose one decided to change the entry of groups into the intervention arm at every three months instead of every two months, at the same time increasing the duration of the study by a factor of 1.5. What would be the approximate increase in effective sample size barring any substantial secular trends?

Chapter 14
Randomization and Baseline Transmission

14.1 Interpreting Efficacy Estimates

Vaccination could interact with population characteristics such as pre-existing immunity, genetic composition, intensity of transmission, or nutritional status, so that estimates of efficacy of a given vaccine in different populations could differ considerably. The biologic efficacy could be the same in the different populations, but the composition of the population would result in the differing efficacy estimates based on the epidemiological outcome of interest. Considerations along these lines demonstrate the role and limitations of randomization. Randomization is one assignment mechanism under which treatment is assigned independent of the potential outcome of interest. The treatment assignment is also independent of other covariates under randomization. Randomization also allows, on average, for a balanced distribution of any covariates, observed or not, in the vaccine and placebo groups. Thus, the treatment groups are seen as comparable. Baseline transmission, pre-existing immunity, and individual responsiveness are examples of possibly relevant factors. For these reasons, randomization, in addition to double-masking, are usually proposed as good research practices for valid clinical trials (Efron 1971).

Randomization, however, does not guarantee that the estimated effect is an unbiased estimate of the biologic effect of interest. Statistical validity does not necessarily guarantee epidemiological validity. That is, there is a distinction between statistical bias and epidemiological confounding. The ability of randomization to control for confounding has been challenged from at least two perspectives. Greenland and Robins (1986), Greenland (1987), and Greenland et al (1999) state the problem from the perspective of potential outcomes and show that effect measures can be confounded even if the treatment assignment mechanism is random. Gail (1986, 1988) and Gail et al. (1984, 1988) examine the effects of omitting a covariate that has the same distribution among exposed and unexposed subjects from regression analyses of cohort data. They describe the conditions under which a balanced covariate can be omitted without biasing the estimates.

M.E. Halloran et al., *Design and Analysis of Vaccine Studies*, Statistics for Biology and Health, DOI 10.1007/978-0-387-68636-3_14,

These results hold as well in randomized Phase III vaccine efficacy field trials. A new dimension is added when the covariate being considered is the natural challenge to infection, such as an infectious mosquito bite or a sexual contact, which is assigned by nature to the study participants. As discussed in Chapter 2, although the efficacy estimate can be based on parameters such as the transmission probability that condition on exposure to infection, most vaccine studies do not collect information on the number of infectious challenges. Thus, many efficacy estimates are based on unconditional parameters such as incidence density, hazard rates, or cumulative incidence (Chapter 2. Measures of vaccine efficacy expressed as functions of the cumulative incidence (Halloran et al 1991) or hazard rates (Struchiner et al 1994) depend on the level of transmission. In this chapter, we consider the limitations of randomization in interpreting results within and across populations. We distinguish biologic efficacy from outcome efficacy.

14.1.1 Malaria vaccine trials

Malaria is the most important parasitic disease in humans. Four main species of human malaria have influenced human evolution over the ages. The most lethal species is *Plasmodium falciparum* which is prevalent in warm tropical climates. *P. vivax* is also quite prevalent in milder climates as well. *P. malariae* and *P. ovale* are the other two forms. A fifth species, *P. knowlesi*, was recognized as having made the jump to humans in 2008.

Development of a vaccine against *P. falciparum* is a public health priority. In the late 1980s, the vaccine candidate SPf66 was produced in Colombia (Patarroyo et al 1988). SPf66 is a synthetic peptide polymer malaria vaccine containing four different peptides, one from a pre-erythrocytic stage protein and three from asexual stage proteins. Community-based studies to evaluate the efficacy of SPf66 in Colombia (Amador et al 1992; Valero et al 1993), Ecuador (Sempertegui et al 1994), and Venezuela (Noya et al 1994) were suggestive of protection against clinical attacks of malaria. Another South American study was conducted in Brazil (Urdaneta et al 1998). In one study in Colombia (Valero et al 1993), where transmission was relatively low, vaccine efficacy was estimated to be 34% (95% CI 19 to 46%), suggesting a beneficial effect of the vaccine.

There was some concern about the design and conduct of the studies in South America. The international community decided to conduct further studies of the SPf66 vaccine candidate in other regions. Double-blind randomized controlled trials were conducted in Tanzania (Alonso et al 1994), The Gambia (D'Alessandro et al 1995), and finally Thailand (Ballou et al 1995; Nosten et al 1996). The estimated efficacy against clinical malaria in the Tanzanian trial, conducted under conditions of intense malaria transmission in children aged 1–5 years, was 31% (95% CI 0 to 52%). The estimated efficacy in the trial in The Gambia, conducted under lower transmission conditions in infants aged 6–11 months, was 8% (95% CI -18 to 29%). The estimated vaccine efficacy in the Thai trial, where transmission intensity was between that of Africa and South America conducted in children aged 2–15 years, was −9% (95% CI −33 to 14). The report of the trial in Thailand concludes that SPf66 does not protect against clinical falciparum malaria and that no further efficacy trials should be conducted (Nosten et al 1996).

Malaria raises particularly difficult design issues. The definition of a case of malaria varies from place to place depending on the malaria transmission conditions. In some places, it would be fever with detection of any parasites. In the trial in Tanzania, the case definition required fever and a *P. falciparum* parasite density over 20,000/μL. In the Gambian trial, the primary case definition was fever and a parasite density over 6000/μL. Due to evolutionary pressure, some populations have a high prevalence of genetic traits that have advantages in the presence of malaria. The genetic composition relevant for protection against malaria varies from place to place. For example, it is difficult for *P. falciparum* to replicate in red blood cells in people who have the sickle cell trait. Having one allele for sickle cell hemoglobin and one healthy allele allows the person to survive but limits the ability of the falciparum malaria parasite to replicate, conferring some protection on the individual. In the Gambian SPf66 study, 19.4% of the infants were heterozygous for sickle cell trait. Studies in different sites can vary in other important aspects. In the SPf66 studies, the age-eligibility differed substantially across sites as illustrated in the previous paragraph.

These considerations motivated Struchiner et al (1994) and Struchiner and Halloran (2007) to explore the interplay of the immune mechanisms in malaria, their implications for protection at the population level, and the disease transmission cycle mediated by the mosquito vectors with the efficacy of vaccination. The interaction of these factors poses challenges for interpreting the epidemiological effects of vaccination.

New generations of malaria vaccines have been under development and field evaluation since SPf66. The design and interpretation issues raised by these earlier malaria vaccine studies remain current. Of particular interest is the problem of interpreting efficacy estimates in different epidemiological settings even if the biologic effect would be the same. Dengue vaccine trials pose similar problems of design and interpretation across populations with different pre-exposure to dengue virus.

14.2 Biologic Versus Outcome Efficacy

Figure 14.1 provides a convenient framework for organizing the discussion of general principles of validity in vaccine evaluation (Struchiner et al 1994). It merges a very simple description of the sequence of pathogenic processes leading to the endpoint of interest that a vaccine is supposed to prevent (represented by boxes and arrows in continuous lines) and the relevant issues on the use of statistical models and selection of parameters (Gail 1991) descriptive of the various concepts of vaccine efficacy (represented by boxes and arrows in dashed lines).

program

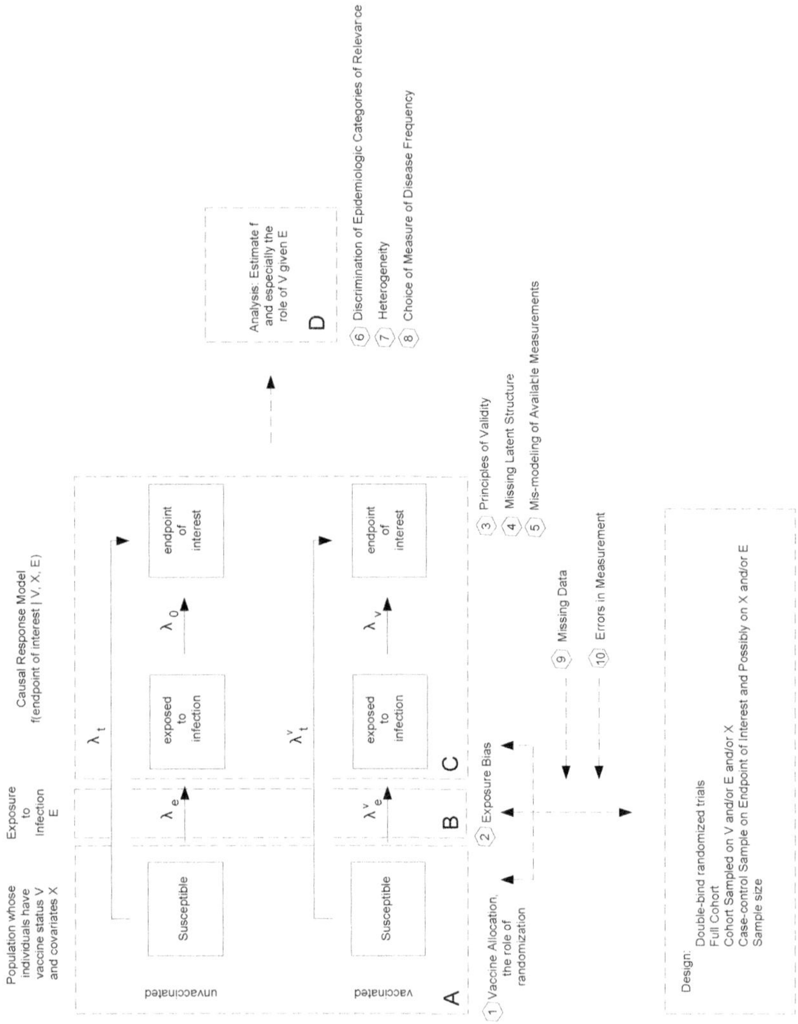

Fig. 14.1 Epidemiological framework for the discussion of general principles of validity in vaccine trials (from Struchiner et al 1994).

In this schematic representation of various aspects of the design and analysis of vaccine field trials, the first dashed rectangle (A) represents vaccine status (V) and covariate levels (X) for each individual in the trial population. Vaccine status and covariate levels can both be either constant or time-dependent. Vaccine allocation and the role of randomization are important design considerations at this point.

Moving to the right in the diagram is the dashed rectangle (B) labeled "Exposure to Infection (E)." In field trials, vaccinated and unvaccinated individuals are exposed to infection, for example, bitten by infected mosquitos, by natural means. Thus, in practice status E is not known or difficult to assess. The rates λ_e and λ_e^v denote the instantaneous probability of being bitten and are functions of time and other environmental factors. Good study design practices recommend that both rates be equal (Greenwood and Yule 1915). Lack of compliance with this is known as exposure bias (Halloran et al 1994b).

Once exposed to infection, vaccinated and unvaccinated individuals might progress up to the endpoint of interest at rates λ_v and λ_0 (dashed rectangle C). Both rates depend on time and covariates X. The main point of the trial is then to infer on the causal response model $f(\text{endpoint of interest}|\text{V,X,E})$. This task can be difficult because one does not have data on the rates λ_v and λ_0 directly, but instead on total or compound rates λ_t^v and λ_t, which denote the transition from the susceptible vaccinated and unvaccinated states to the endpoint of interest. It would be desirable in a valid study to be able to reconstitute the desirable comparison λ_v to λ_0 from the observable comparison λ_t^v to λ_t. This is hampered by missing latent structures (lack of knowledge of λ_e^v and λ_e) or mismodeling of available measurements (selection of the wrong functional form $f(\cdot)$).

14.2.1 Principles of validity in vaccine studies

One of the conditions for valid inference in vaccine studies is exchangeability of the vaccinated and unvaccinated groups. Exchangeability generally assures that it would be possible to describe the occurrence of the outcome of interest among the treated individuals, had they not been treated, from the observed data on the untreated (Greenland and Robins 1986). In Figure 14.1, comparison of rates λ_t and λ_t^v requires that the epidemiological compartments (susceptible unvaccinated and susceptible vaccinated) in dashed rectangle A be exchangeable. Yet, comparison of rates λ_0 and λ_t require exchangeability between the vaccinated and unvaccinated individuals who were actually exposed to infection as depicted in the dashed rectangle C in Figure 14.1. As shown in other parts of this book, the concept of vaccine efficacy is not unique, but depends on many choices of outcome measures. Because exchangeability within both pairs of comparison groups does not necessarily hold simultaneously, field trials that yield valid measures of vaccine efficacy of one kind can potentially lead to biased estimates of efficacy of a different kind. The lack of exchangeability is considered in the particular example of post-infection selection bias in Chapter 9.

The principle of exchangeability in actual vaccine field trials involves at least two dimensions. The first is where in the sequence of pathogenic processes comparisons between vaccinated and unvaccinated groups is being sought, which leads to the concept of biologic efficacy. The second is at what level exchangeability is of interest, whether across individuals or across populations to estimate either direct effects within one population or across several populations, or indirect effects comparing across several populations. In several other chapters, we have considered these different levels of comparisons.

If we were interested in comparing the estimates from the SPf66 malaria vaccine trials, then we would raise the question of the exchangeability of the various study sites. Suppose the set of parameters $(\theta_1, \ldots, \theta_n)$ represents the vaccine efficacies of the n SPf66 malaria vaccine sites. If no information other than the data on efficacy is available to distinguish any of the θ_js from any of the others, then in a Bayesian hierarchical model, one would assume symmetry among the parameters in their prior distribution. This symmetry is called exchangeability in the Bayesian context (DeFinetti 1974). To compare the estimates from the different sites or to combine them in a meta-analysis without accounting for the pre-existing immunity, genetic differences, or transmission conditions, we need to assume exchangeability of the sites. However, given what we know about the different sites, this assumption is likely not valid.

A second condition for valid inference is that the treatment assignment is independent of the potential outcomes of interest. Actual study populations are often heterogeneous in biological, social, or environmental characteristics relevant to the validity of vaccine field trials. These heterogeneities result in differences in susceptibility, exposure to infection, outcome assessment, and propensity to loss to follow-up. Sometimes a few of these factors can be identified and measured and are represented by the covariates X in Figure 14.1. Most sources of heterogeneity, however, remain unknown. Randomization and double-blinding are two strategies designed to distribute these unmeasured heterogeneities approximately equally across groups. Randomization prevents statistical bias because trials conducted this way yield estimates that do not deviate on average from the expected probability distribution describing possible results of the trial.

Randomization, however, does not necessarily ensure that the statistical benefits of randomization propagate to further steps in the sequence of pathogenic processes. Thus, if study subjects are randomly assigned to the two epidemiological compartments in the dashed rectangle A of Figure 14.1, this does not necessarily imply that the same statistical benefits will be preserved when comparing rates λ_0 and λ_v between the epidemiological compartments in dashed rectangle C.

More generally, consider a sequence of pathogenic processes denoted by states

$$S_0 \rightarrow S_1 \rightarrow \cdots \rightarrow S_p \rightarrow S_{p+1} \rightarrow \cdots \rightarrow S_n \, .$$

Under pathogenic processes, we might also consider transmission of infection to mosquito vectors. Let, in addition, I_v and I_0 denote the transition rates from pathogenic state S_p to S_{p+1} in the vaccinated and unvaccinated groups. Hence, the biologic efficacy can be defined as $1 - I_r$, where $I_r = I_v/I_0$. Precise knowledge of the states S_p and S_{p+1} where the vaccine is affecting the sequence of pathogenic effects might be unavailable either because it is impossible to measure them or because practical considerations dictate that data be collected on other states. The overall rate for multiple stages is less than the lowest component transition rates. Thus, for any given biological protection, different measures of efficacy can be estimated depending on the baseline point of departure and the outcome picked by the investigator. The outcome measures could have different, possibly nonlinear, relationships to the underlying biologic efficacy.

A third condition for valid inference is equal exposure to infection in the vaccinated and unvaccinated groups. Exposure to infection in the two groups is presumed to be equal under randomization. However, the level of transmission can influence the estimates of vaccine efficacy, as discussed in more detail in Section 14.3.

These three criteria were stated as early as 1915 by Greenwood and Yule as three conditions necessary for valid inference:

1. The persons must be, *in all material respects,* alike.
2. The effective exposure to the disease must be identical in the case of inoculated and uninoculated persons.
3. The criteria of the fact of inoculation and of the fact of the disease having occurred must be independent.

The first condition corresponds to exchangeability, the third to the treatment assignment being independent of the potential outcome, with randomization being an example, and the second to equal exposure to disease in the vaccinated and unvaccinated groups. Although these three conditions are necessary for statistically valid inference, they do not guarantee lack of confounding or easily interpretable vaccine efficacy estimates.

14.3 Randomization and Baseline Transmission

In this section we focus on the role and limits of randomization in studies based on unconditional estimators of vaccine efficacy that do not explicitly take into account the number of exposures to infection that each person has (Halloran and Struchiner 1995). Based on a simple model of the biologic efficacy of interest, Struchiner and Halloran (2007) extended Greenland's (1987) and Gail's (1986, 1988) arguments on comparability and collapsibility, respectively, to examine the limits of randomization to control for unmeasured covariates in vaccine field studies. They showed that randomization does not guarantee easily interpretable estimates of vaccine efficacy within trials or across sites. A series of examples illustrates the extent of the bias possible under a number of plausible biologic assumptions. Estimates from randomized, placebo-controlled Phase III field trials that differ in baseline transmission may not be comparable unless baseline transmission and pre-existing immunity are taken into account.

14.3.1 Stochastic risk model

Consider a double blinded vaccine trial of N subjects from the study population with vaccine randomly assigned to N_1 subjects and placebo to N_0 subjects. For simplicity, we consider estimating the effect of vaccine compared to placebo on the binary outcome of either becoming infected or not. To begin with, we set infection equal to disease. The prevaccination covariates represent the values of variables describing the individuals in the population, such as age, gender, genetic composition, and pre-existing immunity. The values of any particular covariate may or may not be measured and recorded, depending on the design of the study. For example, we might not measure and record the antibody titer for each person before we begin the study.

For simplicity, consider a binary covariate, C, where a portion of the population has $\mathrm{C} = \mathrm{c}$ and the rest has $\mathrm{C} = \bar{\mathrm{c}}$. Let N_{1c} and N_{0c} be the number of individuals in the vaccinated and unvaccinated groups with covariate value $\mathrm{C} = \mathrm{c}$, and $\mathrm{N}_{1\bar{c}}$ and $\mathrm{N}_{0\bar{c}}$ be the number of individuals in the vaccinated and unvaccinated groups with $\mathrm{C} = \bar{\mathrm{c}}$ (Table 14.1).

14.3.1.1 Individual measures

Under a stochastic risk model, let the probability of being infected per potentially infective contact for an unvaccinated person i be p_{0i} and the probability of not being infected after one contact be $1 - p_{0i}$. This is similar to the stochastic risk model of Greenland (1987), except here the risk conditions on a potentially infective contact. All individuals in whom the infection was not successful at the time of the infective contact return to the pool of individuals at risk to become infected. Analogously, let the probability that a vaccinated individual becomes infected after one exposure to infection be p_{1i} and of not being infected be $1 - p_{1i}$. The unknown probabilities p_{0i} and p_{1i} are called the individual transmission probabilities per potentially infectious contact. An individual thus has two different potential transmission probabilities, one with and one without the vaccine. Which of these potential transmission probabilities determines the stochastic risk for an individual depends on whether the individual is assigned to vaccine or placebo.

Assume that the vaccine has the effect of reducing the transmission probability in an individual i by a multiplicative factor θ_i from p_{0i} to $p_{1i} = \theta_i p_{0i}$, where θ_i could be specific to each individual. The effect of vaccination compared to no vaccination on infection outcome given one specified exposure to infection may be measured in terms of one minus the individual transmission probability ratio or the individual transmission probability difference:

$$\mathrm{VE}_{S,p_i} = 1 - \frac{p_{1i}}{p_{0i}} = 1 - \theta_i,$$
$$\mathrm{D}_i = p_{0i} - p_{1i} = p_{0i}(1 - \theta_i).$$

The vaccine efficacy based on the ratio will be undefined if the transmission probability with no vaccine is zero. Under the multiplicative model, the risk difference depends on p_{0i} whereas VE_{S,p_i} does not. Below, we also use the notation $p_{0i} = TP_{0i}$, $p_{1i} = TP_{1i}$, and $\theta_i = TPR_i$, as equivalent for the transmission probabilities in the unvaccinated and vaccinated individual i, and the individual transmission probability ratio.

14.3.1.2 Special role of exposure to infection

The infection outcomes in an individual would generally depend on whether a person is exposed to infection at all, the size of the inoculum, and how often the person is challenged. The probability of not being infected after the first contact, but then being infected after the second contact is $(1 - p_{0i})p_{0i}$, and so forth for any number of potentially infective contacts, so that the probability an individual becomes infected during a study depends on the number of exposures during the study. We assume that all exposures to infection are equivalent and independent (Section 4.3.1). We assume that the susceptibility remains the same after being exposed to infection post-randomization.

If infection or disease is an outcome of interest, the individual must receive an infectious challenge to contribute information to the study. In controlled settings with a curable disease, following vaccine and placebo allocation, individuals are sometimes challenged with a known amount of inoculum. In this case, treatment consists of both the vaccine allocation and the infectious challenge. In field trials, often individuals are not exposed to infection. These individuals are recipients of incomplete treatment and are uninformative with respect to the effect of the vaccine on infection and disease. That is, in evaluating prophylactic vaccines, there are actually two levels of treatment. The first is to give either the vaccine or placebo, which we can assign randomly to people. The second is the exposure to infection, which in field trials is assigned by nature (Halloran and Struchiner 1995).

14.3.1.3 Population measures

The fundamental problem of causal inference (Holland 1986) is that we cannot observe the individual i both with the vaccine and with the placebo, not to mention at a specified exposure to infection (Halloran and Struchiner 1995; Rubin 1978), so that we cannot observe the effect of the vaccine compared to placebo in the individual. What we can observe is the difference in the average observable outcomes in those who actually received placebo and the average observable outcomes in those who actually received the vaccine. Because we cannot estimate the θ_i for each person, we do a study in a population to estimate the average effect of the vaccine compared to the placebo. The parameter of interest is the average multiplicative effect, $\overline{\theta}$, or the average difference in the transmission probabilities, $\overline{p_0(1 - \theta)}$, of the vaccine in the population if the people were vaccinated compared to if they were unvaccinated.

Let a_1 and a_0 denote the expected number of cases in the vaccinated and unvaccinated groups, respectively, at the end of the study. The proportion expected to develop the infection if each individual in the group receives one exposure to infection is the average transmission probability, $\overline{TP}_1$ and $\overline{TP}_0$, which is the expected number of infections divided by the number of exposures to infection:

$$\overline{TP}_1 = \frac{\sum_1 p_{1i}}{N_1} = \frac{a_1}{N_1}, \quad \overline{TP}_0 = \frac{\sum_0 p_{0i}}{N_0} = \frac{a_0}{N_0},$$

where $\sum_1$ and $\sum_0$ denote summation over the vaccinated and unvaccinated groups, respectively. The proportion of the population expected to develop infection by the end of the study is the attack rate or cumulative incidence, denoted CI_1 and CI_0, respectively:

$$CI_1 = \frac{a_1}{N_1}, \quad CI_0 = \frac{a_0}{N_0}.$$

The cumulative incidences are interpreted as the average unconditional risks in the vaccinated and unvaccinated groups, respectively.

Vaccine efficacy estimated from the relative average transmission probability is

$$\widehat{\mathrm{VE}}_{S,TP} = 1 - \mathrm{TPR} = 1 - \frac{\overline{\mathrm{TP}}_1}{\overline{\mathrm{TP}}_0}.$$

Denote by a_{1c} and b_{1c} the number of vaccinated people with covariate value $\mathrm{C} = \mathrm{c}$ at the end of the study who develop infection or not, respectively, $a_{1c} + b_{1c} = N_{1c}$, and by a_{0c} and b_{0c} the number of unvaccinated people with covariate value $\mathrm{C} = \mathrm{c}$ who develop infection or not, respectively, $a_{0c} + b_{0c} = N_{0c}$. The analogous notation is used in the stratum with $\mathrm{C} = \bar{\mathrm{c}}$ (Table 14.1). Let $R = CI_1/CI_0$. The crude measurable $\mathrm{VE}_{S,CI}$ estimated from the ratio of the cumulative incidences in the vaccinated group compared to the unvaccinated group is (Table 14.1)

$$\mathrm{VE}_{S,CI} = 1 - \mathrm{R} = 1 - \frac{CI_1}{CI_0} = 1 - \frac{\mathrm{a}_1/\mathrm{N}_1}{\mathrm{a}_0/\mathrm{N}_0} = 1 - \left(\frac{a_{1c} + a_{1\bar{c}}}{N_1} \Big/ \frac{a_{0c} + a_{0\bar{c}}}{N_0}\right).$$

The crude risk difference measured by the difference in the cumulative incidence in the vaccinated group compared to the unvaccinated group is (Table 14.1)

$$\mathrm{CI}_D = \frac{a_0}{N_0} - \frac{a_1}{N_1} = \frac{a_{0c} + a_{0\bar{c}}}{N_0} - \frac{a_{1c} + a_{1\bar{c}}}{N_1}.$$

Greenwood and Yule (1915) discuss the different interpretation of the ratio and difference measures for vaccines based on the cumulative incidence.

Vaccine efficacy based on the odds ratio, OR, in which the controls are those that remain free of disease is

$$\mathrm{VE}_{S,OR} = 1 - \mathrm{OR} = 1 - \frac{(a_{1c} + a_{1\bar{c}})(b_{0c} + b_{0\bar{c}})}{(a_{0c} + a_{0\bar{c}})(b_{1c} + b_{1\bar{c}})}. \tag{14.1}$$

Table 14.1 Example tables template for Tables 14.2 to 14.9: TP, transmission probability; TPR, transmission probability ratio; $C = c, \bar{c}$, binary covariate; VE_c, $\text{VE}_{\bar{c}}$, vaccine efficacy in those with c, $\bar{c}$; a_{ij}, number of cases; b_{ij}, number of noncases; $a_{ij} + b_{ij} = N_{ij}$. (Struchiner and Halloran 2007)

Site		TP_c	C = c; VE_c = 1-TPR_c	$\text{TP}_{\bar{c}}$	C = $\bar{c}$; $\text{VE}_{\bar{c}}$ = 1-$\text{TPR}_{\bar{c}}$	$\text{VE}_{S,CI}$	CI_D	$\text{VE}_{S,\text{OR}}$
A	Vac	TP_{1c}	a_{1c} b_{1c} N_{1c}	$\text{TP}_{1\bar{c}}$	$a_{1\bar{c}}$ $b_{1\bar{c}}$ $N_{1\bar{c}}$	$1-\frac{\frac{a_{1c}+a_{1\bar{c}}}{N_{1c}+N_{1\bar{c}}}}{\frac{a_{0c}+a_{0\bar{c}}}{N_{0c}+N_{0\bar{c}}}}$	$\frac{a_{0c}+a_{0\bar{c}}}{N_{0c}+N_{0\bar{c}}} - \frac{a_{1c}+a_{1\bar{c}}}{N_{1c}+N_{1\bar{c}}}$	$1-\frac{(a_{1c}+a_{1\bar{c}})(b_{0c}+b_{0\bar{c}})}{(a_{0c}+a_{0\bar{c}})(b_{1c}+b_{1\bar{c}})}$
	Unv	TP_{0c}	a_{0c} b_{0c} N_{0c}	$\text{TP}_{0\bar{c}}$	$a_{0\bar{c}}$ $b_{0\bar{c}}$ $N_{0\bar{c}}$			

This odds ratio is based on the cumulative or epidemic case-control design (Rothman et al 2008), and depends on the rare disease assumption to be a close approximation of the relative risk based on cumulative incidence. Other odds ratios not dependent on the rare disease assumption are discussed in Section 8.1.

The columns at the far right in Table 14.1 give the vaccine efficacy based on the crude cumulative incidence ratio, the crude cumulative incidence difference, and the crude odds ratios. The question of interest is to what extent, even under randomization, does the estimated efficacy measure the effect of interest? In particular, if no information on actual exposure to infection is gathered, to what extent does $\text{VE}_{S,CI}$ estimate $1-\overline{\theta}$ or CI_D estimate $\overline{p_0(1-\theta)}$?

14.3.2 Randomization and comparability of treatment groups

Randomization is supposed to ensure that the vaccine and placebo groups are comparable in that the experience of the group with the vaccine would have been the same as the group that did not receive the vaccine had the vaccinated group in fact received the placebo, and vice versa. Randomization coupled with blinding is also supposed to ensure that post-randomization exposure to infection is balanced.

Under randomization, it should not matter which of the groups receives the vaccine or placebo. Following Greenland and Robins (1986), we say there is no confounding due to lack of comparability if, in the absence of vaccination, the average risk would have been the same among the people who in fact were vaccinated and those who were not vaccinated. Under the assumption of comparability of the two groups, we can replace the experience of the unvaccinated group with the experience of the vaccinated group if it had not been vaccinated, so that $\sum_0 p_{0i}/N_0 = \sum_1 p_{0i}/N_1$. Here $\sum_1 p_{0i}$ denotes the experience that the vaccinated group would have had if they had not been vaccinated and exposed just once to infection. By balancing the distribution of observed and unobserved covariates in a study, randomization is supposed to ensure that the vaccinated and unvaccinated groups are comparable. The expected proportion of the unvaccinated and vaccinated groups in either level of a binary covariate should be the same in both groups,

$$\frac{N_{1c}}{N_1} = \frac{N_{0c}}{N_0}, \quad \frac{N_{1\bar{c}}}{N_1} = \frac{N_{0\bar{c}}}{N_0}.$$

The conditions for comparability rely on the assumption that the outcome in each individual is independent of the outcomes and treatment assignments in the other individuals. The independence is part of the stable unit treatment value assumption (SUTVA) (Rubin 1980). Halloran and Struchiner (1995) and Hudgens and Halloran (2008) (Section 13.8) consider consequences of the violation of SUTVA in more detail. If we imagine that a small proportion of the population is vaccinated in the trial, then the violations would be minimal.

14.3.2.1 Limits of comparability with one homogeneous exposure to infection

In this section, we assume that everyone is exposed exactly once to infection during the study. If the trial participants were each to receive a single infectious challenge (infected mosquito bite), the expected cumulative incidence ratio would equal the expected average transmission probability ratio:

$$\mathrm{R} = \frac{\mathrm{a}_1/\mathrm{N}_1}{\mathrm{a}_0/\mathrm{N}_0} = \frac{\sum_1 p_{1i}/\mathrm{N}_1}{\sum_0 p_{0i}/\mathrm{N}_0} = \mathrm{TPR}.$$

Following the arguments of Greenland (1987), even under the assumption of comparability, and exactly one exposure to infection per person, the ratio of the cumulative incidences (average transmission probabilities) is not equal to the average of the individual ratios of the transmission probabilities, $\overline{\theta}$. Formally, assuming comparability, the expected cumulative incidence ratio (ratio of the average transmission probabilities) is

$$\mathrm{R} = \frac{\overline{\mathrm{TP}}_1}{\overline{\mathrm{TP}}_0} = \frac{\frac{a_1}{N_1}}{\frac{a_0}{N_0}} = \frac{\frac{\sum_1 p_{1i}}{N_1}}{\frac{\sum_0 p_{0i}}{N_0}} = \frac{\frac{\sum_1 \theta_i p_{0i}}{N_1}}{\frac{\sum_0 p_{0i}}{N_0}} = \frac{\frac{\sum_1 \theta_i p_{0i}}{N_1}}{\frac{\sum_1 p_{0i}}{N_1}}$$

$$= \frac{\sum_1 \theta_i p_{0i}}{\sum_1 p_{0i}} \neq \frac{\sum_1 \frac{p_{1i}}{p_{0i}}}{N_1} = \frac{\sum_1 \theta_i}{N_1} = \overline{\theta}.$$

The inequality is true in general, unless the $p_{1i}/p_{0i} = \theta$ are the same for all i in the vaccinated group, a strong assumption. In words, the previous expressions indicate that the population-level measure of efficacy based on either the transmission probability or the incidence proportion cannot be interpreted as the average, among the study population, of the individual effect of the vaccine, except in the unlikely case that $\theta = p_{1i}/p_{0i}$ for each individual i in the population. In general, the expected value of R is biased for the average effect of the vaccine in the vaccinated group, $\sum_1 \theta_i/N_1$, in randomized, double-blinded Phase III vaccine trials.

In contrast, under the assumption of comparability, the difference CI_D of the cumulative incidences (or average transmission probabilities) in the unvaccinated and vaccinated groups is equal to the average of the individual differences in the transmission probabilities, even when individuals have different vaccine responses θ_i:

$$\mathrm{CI}_D = \frac{a_0}{N_0} - \frac{a_1}{N_1} = \frac{\sum_0 p_{0i}}{N_0} - \frac{\sum_1 p_{1i}}{N_1} = \frac{\sum_1 p_{0i}}{N_1} - \frac{\sum_1 \theta_i p_{0i}}{N_1}$$
$$= \frac{\sum_1 p_{0i}(1-\theta_i)}{N_1} = \overline{p_0(1-\theta)}.$$

14.3.2.2 Comparability-based confounding: Homogeneous effect; two or more exposures to infection

To illustrate confounding due to unmeasured postvaccination exposure to infection, we assume for simplicity that the effect of the vaccine on susceptibility is the same in everyone, that is, $\theta_i = \theta$ for each individual i, but that everyone receives two challenges to infection (see also Halloran et al (1991)). Assume that the first contact with the infective agent does not leave an immune memory. If everyone is challenged twice, then the expected number of cases in the unvaccinated group is the number of people expected to get infected from the first challenge plus the number of people expected to get infected from the second challenge, $a_0 = \sum_0[p_{0i}(1-p_{0i}) + p_{0i}]$. The number of cases in the vaccinated group is $a_1 = \sum_1[p_{1i}(1-p_{1i}) + p_{1i}]$. Under the assumption of comparability of the vaccinated and unvaccinated groups:

$$\mathrm{R} = \frac{\frac{a_1}{N_1}}{\frac{a_0}{N_0}} = \frac{\frac{\sum_1[p_{1i}(1-p_{1i})+p_{1i}]}{N_1}}{\frac{\sum_0[p_{0i}(1-p_{0i})+p_{0i}]}{N_0}} = \frac{\frac{\sum_1[\theta p_{0i}(1-\theta p_{0i})+\theta p_{0i}]}{N_1}}{\frac{\sum_1[p_{0i}(1-p_{0i})+p_{0i}]}{N_1}} \neq \theta.$$

If we had information on the number of exposures to infection and knew after which exposure each person becomes infected, we could use the transmission probability ratios to estimate the effect of the vaccine, although even the ratio $\overline{\mathrm{TP}}_1/\overline{\mathrm{TP}}_0 \neq \overline{\theta}$ unless $\theta_i = \theta$.

If the investigator did not have access to information on exposure to infection, as in field trials based on unconditional parameters such as cumulative incidence, he or she would report vaccine efficacy as $1-(\mathrm{a}_1/\mathrm{N}_1)/(\mathrm{a}_0/\mathrm{N}_0) \neq 1-\theta$. Thus, exposure to infection can be a confounder even in a double-blinded placebo-controlled trial in which randomization ensures comparability, and in particular, when the exposure to infection is not only comparable in the two groups, but homogeneous within groups. This result holds even if the transmission probability is homogeneous for everyone.

As a corollary to this result, because the number of challenges to infection, assigned by nature in field trials, depends on the baseline transmission level, two different randomized, double-blinded, placebo-controlled studies taking place in sites that differ by the level of transmission would report different estimates of vaccine efficacy even if the level of protection conferred by the vaccine to a specified challenge to infection is the same in both studies.

The previous result is easily extended to the more realistic situation that in field conditions, nature provides the infection challenge and, thus, some individuals are not challenged at all, some are challenged just once, and some are challenged two or more times. In the general case, the inequality holds even if $p_{0i} = p_0$, and $p_{1i} = p_1$. A similar argument could be constructed to show that the difference of $\mathrm{CI}_0 - \mathrm{CI}_1$ does not equal the average difference in susceptibility in the vaccinated compared to the unvaccinated, $(1-\theta)(\sum_1 p_{0i})/N_1$. In summary, the population measure of R does not estimate θ, and there can be confounding even when

1. the study is randomized;
2. the multiplicative effect of the vaccine is the same for all individuals, ie, there is no heterogeneity in vaccine efficacy;
3. comparability is preserved, ie, controls describe what would have happened to the vaccinated group if they had not been vaccinated;
4. the amount of infectious challenge is the same among vaccinated and unvaccinated; and
5. SUTVA is not violated.

14.3.2.3 Collapsibility with balance of unmeasured covariates

Because on average, randomization achieves balance of prevaccination covariates, under certain conditions, a covariate can be omitted from the analysis without changing the value of the regression parameter of interest (Gail 1986, 1988; Gail et al. 1984, 1988). In this case, the analysis is said to be collapsible with respect to the covariates, and such covariates are called nonconfounders. The discussions related to collapsibility and omitting a balanced covariate from regression models are concerned with statistical bias and are model-dependent (Greenland 1996). Greenland (1989) argues against the identification of effects with regression model coefficients, because that results in model dependence of causal concepts such as "effect" and "confounder" which is undesirable and unnecessary. Randomized clinical trials analyzed with linear or multiplicative models yield unbiased estimates of regression coefficients which, however, are not necessarily appropriate estimates of the individual biologic effect of a vaccine.

14.3.2.4 Collapsibility-based confounding

Suppose that the stratum-specific cumulative incidence ratio for the jth stratum is $\mathrm{R}_j = \mathrm{CI}_{0j}/\mathrm{CI}_{1j}$, where the jth stratum is defined in terms of the number j of exposures to infection, $j = 0,\ldots,J$, where J is the maximum number of exposures possible in the study, and,

$$\mathrm{k} = \mathrm{R}_1 = \cdots = \mathrm{R}_j = \cdots = \mathrm{R}_J.$$

As already shown, this assumption cannot be true even if there is a common multiplicative effect of the vaccine, $\theta = p_{1i}/p_{0i}$, for all i, because then the R_j would differ. Thus, neither the crude measure of effect, nor the adjusted measure of effect once baseline transmission level is controlled for, are easily interpretable.

Interpretation of a multiplicative measure of efficacy, even in the absence of confounding defined in terms of collapsibility (Greenland 1996), is problematic unless one makes the very unlikely assumptions that the biologic effect is the same for all individuals and that study participants could be challenged at most once, in which case all people in the study would share the same value of the covariate defined by the number of exposures to infection.

14.3.2.5 Heterogeneity of effect: Effect modification

We now consider the special case that there are strata within which the effect of the vaccine is homogeneous, but that it varies among subgroups. This heterogeneity of effect is called effect modification in the epidemiological literature. Of actual interest would be to estimate the different efficacies in each stratum. If it is not possible to stratify on the relevant variable, then the efficacy measure will be a summary measure under heterogeneity (Greenland 1982; Halloran et al 1992). The estimated crude efficacy will depend on the proportional composition of the population of each subgroup in which the vaccine has a different effect.

14.3.3 Examples

Struchiner and Halloran (2007) present several examples of how unmeasured covariates, and in particular, unmeasured pre-vaccination or post-vaccination exposure to infection, could alter the estimates of vaccine efficacy even if the field trial were randomized. In every case considered, the vaccine trial is a randomized, double-blind, placebo-controlled trial. In developing these examples, we had in mind an infection like malaria, although the results are quite general. For those readers who know the malaria literature, the transmission probability, TP_0, or p_0, corresponds to the b in the usual malaria models, the probability that a sporozoite-positive mosquito bite results in successful infection.

In the examples, the covariate C can play several different roles. If C is related to a pre-vaccination covariate that affects susceptibility, then the risk of infection per potentially infective contact in the unvaccinated group with C = c is TP_{0c} and in the unvaccinated group with covariate value C = $\bar{c}$ is $\mathrm{TP}_{0\bar{c}}$. If the vaccine effect is the same at both covariate levels, then $\theta = \theta_c = \mathrm{TPR}_c = \theta_{\bar{c}} = \mathrm{TPR}_{\bar{c}}$. Table 14.1 is a template for the examples.

If the vaccine effect is related to C, then $\mathrm{TPR}_c = \theta_c = \mathrm{TP}_{1c}/\mathrm{TP}_{0c}$. The effect of the vaccine in the stratum with C = $\bar{c}$ is $\mathrm{TPR}_{\bar{c}} = \theta_{\bar{c}} = \mathrm{TP}_{1\bar{c}}/\mathrm{TP}_{0\bar{c}}$. In this case, there would be two measures of effect of interest that would be measurable if it were possible to stratify on the covariate C. The covariate C could also be related only to

Table 14.2 Homogeneous pre-vaccination susceptibility among sites, homogeneity of vaccine effect within sites, no boosting, and increasing N_c; infectious challenge as a confounder, one exposure to infection in stratum C = c and 0 otherwise; $VE_c = VE_{\bar{c}} = 0.5$; $TP_{c0} = TP_{\bar{c}0}$; $N_c \neq N_{\bar{c}}$. (Struchiner and Halloran 2007)

Site		TP_c	C = c; VE_c = .5			$TP_{\bar{c}}$	C = $\bar{c}$; $VE_{\bar{c}}$ = .5			$VE_{S,CI}$	CI_D	$VE_{S,OR}$
A	Vac	1/4	**1**	**3**	4	1/4	**0**	**496**	496	0.5	0.002	0.501
	Unv	1/2	**2**	**2**	4	1/2	**0**	**496**	496			
B	Vac	1/4	**62**	**186**	248	1/4	**0**	**252**	252	0.5	0.124	0.571
	Unv	1/2	**124**	**124**	248	1/2	**0**	**252**	252			
F	Vac	1/4	**124**	**372**	496	1/4	**0**	**4**	4	0.5	0.248	0.665
	Unv	1/2	**248**	**248**	496	1/2	**0**	**4**	4			

the number of post-vaccination exposures to infection with a homogeneous effect of vaccination, so that $TP_{0\bar{c}} = TP_{0c}$, and $\theta_c = \theta_{\bar{c}}$.

14.3.3.1 C is post-vaccination challenge; homogeneous VE; infectious challenge as a confounder

Consider a vaccine candidate that is being evaluated in different trials, possibly on different continents (Table 14.2). Let the trial sites be designated by capital letters, such as A, B, and F. In Table 14.2, we consider a situation in which the response to the vaccine is actually homogeneous within each trial site and across each trial site, but that not everyone gets exposed to infection. Thus, C = c denotes being exposed to infection just once, and C = $\bar{c}$ denotes not being exposed to infection. The transmission probability in the unvaccinated susceptibles, $TP_0 = 0.5$, and the effect of the vaccine in reducing the transmission probability, $TPR = TP_1/TP_0 = 0.5$, are the same for all study participants in all three sites. Thus, $VE_c = VE_{\bar{c}}$. In Table 14.2, the proportion receiving exactly one exposure to infection (C = c) increases from 3% in site A to 97% in site F. In Site A, $\widehat{VE}_{S,CI} = 2/500 - 1/500 = 0.5$, and in Site F, $\widehat{VE}_{S,CI} = 124/500 - 248/500 = 0.5$. The estimated efficacy based on $VE_{S,CI}$ is 0.5 regardless of the proportion exposed to infection during the trial, so that under this multiplicative effect model, heterogeneous exposure to infection does not act as a confounder if the maximum number of exposures to infection is 1. The CI_D increases from 0.002 at site A to 0.248 in site F, reflecting that the vaccine is more important as a public health tool when more people are exposed to infection.

In Table 14.3, those people who are exposed to infection (C = c) are exposed twice, compared to only once in Table 14.2. Otherwise the situations in Tables 14.2 and 14.3 are the same. This situation illustrates exposure to infection as a confounder, because the expected $VE_{S,CI}$ decreases from 0.5 in Table 14.2 to 0.417 in Table 14.3 at all sites, but allowing for the small sample size and integer infections,

Table 14.3 Homogeneous pre-vaccination susceptibility among sites, homogeneity of vaccine effect within sites, no boosting, and increasing N_c; infectious challenge as a confounder, two exposure to infection in stratum C = c and 0 otherwise; $VE_c = VE_{\bar{c}} = 0.5$; $TP_{c0} = TP_{\bar{c}0}$; $N_c \neq N_{\bar{c}}$. (Struchiner and Halloran 2007)

Site		TP	C = c; VE = .5			TP	C = c̄; VE = .5			$VE_{S,CI}$	CI_D	$VE_{S,OR}$
A	Vac	1/4	**2**	**2**	4	1/4	**0**	**496**	496	0.333	0.002	0.335
	Unv	1/2	**3**	**1**	4	1/2	**0**	**496**	496			
B	Vac	1/4	**109**	**139**	248	1/4	**0**	**252**	252	0.414	0.154	0.529
	Unv	1/2	**186**	**62**	248	1/2	**0**	**252**	252			
F	Vac	1/4	**217**	**279**	496	1/4	**0**	**4**	4	0.417	0.310	0.736
	Unv	1/2	**372**	**124**	496	1/2	**0**	**4**	4			

it is 0.333 in site A. In Table 14.3, the change in CI_D from site A to site F is greater than in the situation of lower transmission in Table 14.2.

14.3.3.2 C is related to heterogeneous VE; effect modification

In Table 14.4, we assume that in all sites, an immunologically naive susceptible person has a probability of $p_{0i} = p_0 = TP_0 = 1.0$ of becoming infected after one exposure to infection. The vaccine effect is heterogeneous. The heterogeneous response could be due to a covariate unrelated to history of exposure to infection, such as genetic composition, nutritional status, or gender. One half of the population has C = c and the vaccine reduces the transmission probability by 0.5, so that $TPR_c = 0.5$, and $VE_c = 0.5$. One half of the population has C = c̄ and the vaccine has no effect in this group, so that $VE_{\bar{c}} = 0$. The average efficacy of the vaccine on the transmission probability is 0.25. The average transmission probability difference is also 0.25.

In Table 14.4, the number of exposures to infection per person increases from top to bottom, with equal probability of being exposed in the vaccinated and unvaccinated groups and at the different levels of C. That is, exposure to infection is independent of both vaccine status and C. In site A, only 1 in 125 are exposed to infection once, and the others not at all. In site B, one-half are exposed once, and one-half not at all. In site F, everyone is exposed once. In sites G through M, the number of exposures to infection per person increases from two to eight. When the number of exposures to infection is less than or equal to one (sites A, B, F), vaccine efficacy measured by $VE_{S,CI}$ does not change for different proportions of the population exposed to infection and equals the average of the effect of the vaccine in the two strata. Efficacy measured by the CI_D increases until both measures based on ratio and difference are equal when the whole population is exposed just once (site F). Under these conditions, the expected crude cumulative incidence ratio equals the average effect in the population, and the same for the differences of the two. Effi-

Table 14.4 Heterogeneous pre-vaccination susceptibility among sites; heterogeneity of vaccine effect within sites and confounding from exposure to infection; no boosting; increasing proportion exposed to infection in trial (A: 1/125, once; B: 1/2, once; F: 1/1, once; G: 2; H: 3; I: 4; J: 5; K: 6; L: 7; M: 8); $VE_c = 0.5$; $VE_{\bar{c}} = 0$; $TP_{c0} = TP_{\bar{c}0} = 1$; $N_c = N_{\bar{c}} = 500$. (Struchiner and Halloran 2007)

Site		TP_c	$C = c$; $VE_c = 0.5$	$TP_{\bar{c}}$	$C = \bar{c}$; $VE_{\bar{c}} = 0$	$VE_{S,CI}$	CI_D	$VE_{S,OR}$
A	Vac	1/2	**1 249** 250	1	**2 248** 250	0.250	0.002	0.25
	Unv	1	**2 248** 250	1	**2 248** 250			
B	Vac	1/2	**62 188** 250	1	**124 126** 250	0.250	0.124	0.40
	Unv	1	**124 126** 250	1	**124 126** 250			
F	Vac	1/2	**125 125** 250	1	**250 0** 250	0.250	0.250	1.00
	Unv	1	**250 0** 250	1	**250 0** 250			
G	Vac	1/2	**188 62** 250	1	**250 0** 250	0.124	0.124	1.00
	Unv	1	**250 0** 250	1	**250 0** 250			
H	Vac	1/2	**219 31** 250	1	**250 0** 250	0.062	0.062	1.00
	Unv	1	**250 0** 250	1	**250 0** 250			
I	Vac	1/2	**235 15** 250	1	**250 0** 250	0.030	0.030	1.00
	Unv	1	**250 0** 250	1	**250 0** 250			
J	Vac	1/2	**243 7** 250	1	**250 0** 250	0.014	0.014	1.00
	Unv	1	**250 0** 250	1	**250 0** 250			
K	Vac	1/2	**247 3** 250	1	**250 0** 250	0.006	0.006	1.00
	Unv	1	**250 0** 250	1	**250 0** 250			
L	Vac	1/2	**249 1** 250	1	**250 0** 250	0.002	0.002	1.00
	Unv	1	**250 0** 250	1	**250 0** 250			
M	Vac	1/2	**250 0** 250	1	**250 0** 250	0.000	0.000	—
	Unv	1	**250 0** 250	1	**250 0** 250			

cacy measured as $1 - OR$ decreases as the level of exposure to an infective contact increases. As expected, it approaches the measure based on the cumulative incidence ratio when the disease is rare, because of the (not recommended) cumulative case-control design.

Proceeding down Table 14.4, after all individuals were exposed to an infective contact once, we mimic a second round of contacts assuming that the first round leaves no immune memory. This is represented at site G in Table 14.4, in which from the 125 subjects that had not yet shown the outcome of interest, half of them (to the nearest integer) succumb to the infection. Successive rounds of contacts follow until after eight exposures to infection (M), all study participants present the outcome of interest. All three measures of efficacy progress towards the null when transmission

Table 14.5 Heterogeneous pre-vaccination susceptibility among sites, heterogeneity of vaccine effect within sites, and boosting, all modulated by infection history; everyone exposed once to infection; $VE_c = 0.5$; $VE_{\bar{c}} = 0$; $TP_{c0} \neq TP_{\bar{c}0}$; $N_c = N_{\bar{c}} = 500$. (Struchiner and Halloran 2007)

Site		TP_c	$C = c$; $VE_c = .5$	$TP_{\bar{c}}$	$C = \bar{c}$; $VE_{\bar{c}} = 0$	$VE_{S,CI}$	CI_D	$VE_{S,OR}$
A	Vac	1/4	**62 188** 250	1/2	**125 125** 250	0.249	0.124	0.40
	Unv	1/2	**125 125** 250	1/2	**125 125** 250			
B	Vac	1/8	**31 219** 250	1/2	**125 125** 250	0.166	0.062	0.24
	Unv	1/4	**62 188** 250	1/2	**125 125** 250			
F	Vac	1/250	**1 249** 250	1/2	**125 125** 250	0.008	0.002	0.01
	Unv	1/125	**2 248** 250	1/2	**125 125** 250			

increases. The decrease in estimated efficacy would also occur if the vaccine effect were homogeneous.

If we conducted a study of the vaccine in three different sites, say in sites A, G, and L, and estimated vaccine efficacy from $VE_{S,CI}$, we would expect three different estimates of the efficacy of the vaccine, namely 0.25, 0.124, and 0.002, even though the vaccine had exactly the same effect in each population, and the study is randomized and balanced. The difference among sites would be due to differences in post-vaccination exposure to infection in the three sites, not due to differences in the immune protection conferred by the vaccine.

14.3.3.3 C related to infection history: Pre-vaccination heterogeneity, heterogeneity of effect, boosting

In the example in Table 14.5, the covariate C is related both to pre-vaccination susceptibility and to the heterogeneous response of the vaccine. We let c and $\bar{c}$ denote previous exposure to infection and no previous exposure to infection, respectively, whereby we assume that half of each population has the covariate value C = c and half has C = c̄. Suppose that in the three trial sites A, B, and F, the susceptibility of immunologically naive unvaccinated susceptibles is the same, with $TP_{0\bar{c}} = 0.5$. That is, if we took the naive susceptibles from A, B, and F and challenged them with infection, then the transmission probability for each of the three groups would be the same, namely 0.5.

In the people with previous exposure to infection, however, the transmission probability ranges from 0.5 (no change over naive) in site A, to 0.25 at site B to $1/125$ at site F. Now assume that the vaccine has an effect only in people who were previously exposed to infection. That is, perhaps the vaccine boosts pre-existing immunity, but has no effect on naive susceptibles. The effect of the vaccine in the previously exposed groups is assumed to be the same in each of the three trial sites, and to have no effect in the naive susceptibles. That is, the biologic efficacy of the vaccine in the three trial sites is identical, with $TPR_{\bar{c}} = p_{1i}/p_{0i} = 1$ and

Table 14.6 Heterogeneous pre-vaccination susceptibility among sites, heterogeneity of vaccine effect within sites, all modulated by infection history, and no boosting; everyone exposed once to infection; $VE_c = 0.5$; $VE_{\bar{c}} = 0$; $TP_{c0} \neq TP_{\bar{c}0}$; $N_c = N_{\bar{c}} = 500$. (Struchiner and Halloran 2007)

Site		TP_c	C = c; $VE_c = 0$			$TP_{\bar{c}}$	C = $\bar{c}$; $VE_{\bar{c}} = .5$			$VE_{S,CI}$	CI_D	$VE_{S,OR}$
A	Vac	1/2	**125**	**125**	250	1/4	**62**	**188**	250	0.249	0.124	0.398
	Unv	1/2	**125**	**125**	250	1/2	**125**	**125**	250			
B	Vac	1/4	**62**	**188**	250	1/4	**62**	**188**	250	0.333	0.124	0.443
	Unv	1/4	**62**	**188**	250	1/2	**125**	**125**	250			
F	Vac	1/125	**2**	**248**	250	1/4	**62**	**188**	250	0.496	0.124	0.568
	Unv	1/125	**2**	**248**	250	1/2	**125**	**125**	250			

$TPR_c = p_{1i}/p_{0i} = 0.5$ at each site, and the proportion with each covariate is exactly half at each site. At site B, the multiplicative protection conferred by previous exposure to infection is the same as the protection conferred by vaccine in those people in whom it has an effect. In Table 14.5, we further assume that each person is exposed exactly once to infection. The number of cases among the unvaccinated individuals in the C = c stratum, that is, those with decreased susceptibility before being vaccinated, decreases from site A to site F. Despite the effect of the vaccine actually being the same in sites A, B, and F of Table 14.5, the exposure to infection being exactly the same, and the distribution of C being exactly the same, the estimated efficacy of the vaccine decreases from 0.249 at site A to 0.008 at site F, depending on how susceptible those with pre-vaccination immunity are.

14.3.3.4 C related to infection history: prevaccination heterogeneity, heterogeneity of effect, no boosting

In Table 14.6, we find exactly the same pre-vaccination baseline situations in sites A, B, and F as described in Table 14.5. Assume, however, that the vaccine provides no additional protection to people who were previously exposed, C = c, but that it has an effect in naive susceptible people. In Table 14.6, the effect of pre-existing exposure to infection on $VE_{S,CI}$ is opposite to that in Table 14.5, and $VE_{S,CI}$ increases from 0.249 at site A to 0.496 at site F. Once again the biologic effect of the vaccine is the same in the different sites, but if we do not stratify on pre-existing immunity, we get very different efficacy estimates. How the efficacy estimates vary depends on whether the vaccine has greater or lesser effect in the people who had previous exposure. Vaccine efficacy measured as the risk difference, CI_D, however, is constant as long as exposure to infection is the same at all sites.

Table 14.7 Homogeneous pre-vaccination susceptibility among sites, heterogeneity of vaccine effect within sites, boosting, and increasing N_c, all modulated by infection history; everyone exposed once to infection; $VE_c = 0.5$; $VE_{\bar{c}} = 0$; $TP_{c0} \neq TP_{\bar{c}0}$; $N_c \neq N_{\bar{c}}$. (Struchiner and Halloran 2007)

Site		TP_c	$C = c$; $VE_c = .5$			$TP_{\bar{c}}$	$C = \bar{c}$; $VE_{\bar{c}} = 0$			$VE_{S,CI}$	CI_D	$VE_{S,CI}$
A	Vac	1/8	**1**	**7**	8	1/2	**246**	**246**	492	0.004	0.002	0.008
	Unv	1/4	**2**	**6**	8	1/2	**246**	**246**	492			
B	Vac	1/8	**31**	**217**	248	1/2	**126**	**126**	252	0.165	0.062	0.240
	Unv	1/4	**62**	**186**	248	1/2	**126**	**126**	252			
F	Vac	1/8	**62**	**434**	496	1/2	**2**	**2**	4	0.492	0.124	0.564
	Unv	1/4	**124**	**372**	496	1/2	**2**	**2**	4			

Table 14.8 Homogeneous pre-vaccination susceptibility among sites, heterogeneity of vaccine effect within sites, and increasing N_c, all modulated by infection history, and no boosting; everyone exposed once to infection; $VE_c = 0$; $VE_{\bar{c}} = 0.5$; $TP_{c0} \neq TP_{\bar{c}0}$; $N_c \neq N_{\bar{c}}$. (Struchiner and Halloran 2007)

Site		TP_c	$C = c$; $VE_c = 0$			$TP_{\bar{c}}$	$C = \bar{c}$; $VE_{\bar{c}} = .5$			$VE_{S,CI}$	CI_D	$VE_{S,OR}$
A	Vac	1/4	**1**	**3**	4	1/4	**124**	**372**	496	0.498	0.248	0.664
	Unv	1/4	**1**	**3**	4	1/2	**248**	**248**	496			
B	Vac	1/4	**62**	**186**	248	1/4	**63**	**189**	252	0.335	0.126	0.447
	Unv	1/4	**62**	**186**	248	1/2	**126**	**126**	252			
F	Vac	1/4	**124**	**372**	496	1/4	**1**	**3**	4	0.008	0.002	0.011
	Unv	1/4	**124**	**372**	496	1/2	**2**	**2**	4			

14.3.3.5 Varying the proportion with covariate C, boosting or no boosting

Tables 14.7 and 14.8 represent a comparison analogous to that between Tables 14.5 and 14.6, respectively. However, in Tables 14.7 and 14.8, the relative pre-vaccination susceptibilities are the same in all three sites, but the fraction of the population with the low prevaccination susceptibility varies among the different trial sites A, B, and F. Again, we can imagine that the low prevaccination susceptibility in the group with C = c comes from immunity acquired due to exposure to infection prior to the vaccine trial. For simplicity, we assume that protection conferred by naturally acquired immunity is the same as that conferred by the vaccine in groups where the vaccine has an effect, so $TP_{0c} = 0.5\ TP_{0\bar{c}}$ prior to vaccination. The proportion of the population with pre-vaccination immunity (C = c) varies from 1–2% in trial site A to 50% in trial site B to 97–98% in trial site F.

In Table 14.7, we assume that the vaccine has no effect in the naive susceptibles, but reduces susceptibility by 50% in those with previous immunity. In Table 14.8, the vaccine has no additional effect in those with previous immunity, but reduces susceptibility by 50% in the naive susceptibles. Because the distribution of the covariate C in the populations A, B, and F varies, the population average biologic

Table 14.9 Homogeneous prevaccination susceptibility among sites, heterogeneity of vaccine effect within sites, boosting, and increasing N_c, all modulated by infection history; everyone exposed once to infection; $VE_c = 0.75$; $VE_{\bar{c}} = 0.5$; $TP_{c0} \neq TP_{\bar{c}0}$; $N_c \neq N_{\bar{c}}$. (Struchiner and Halloran 2007)

Site		TP_c	$C = c$; $VE_c = .75$			$TP_{\bar{c}}$	$C = \bar{c}$; $VE_{\bar{c}} = .5$			$VE_{S,CI}$	CI_D	$VE_{S,OR}$
A	Vac	1/16	**1**	**15**	16	1/4	**121**	**363**	484	0.504	0.248	0.667
	Unv	1/4	**4**	**12**	16	1/2	**242**	**242**	484			
B	Vac	1/16	**16**	**244**	260	1/4	**60**	**180**	240	0.589	0.218	0.695
	Unv	1/4	**65**	**195**	260	1/2	**120**	**120**	240			
F	Vac	1/16	**30**	**454**	484	1/4	**4**	**12**	16	0.736	0.190	0.790
	Unv	1/4	**121**	**363**	484	1/2	**8**	**8**	16			

effect varies. In Table 14.7, it varies from about 0.01 at site A to 0.48 at site F, and vice versa in Table 14.8. This is reflected in the crude $VE_{S,CI}$ when each person is exposed once to infection. Thus, how the estimate of the vaccine efficacy varies will depend on the proportion with pre-existing immunity and how the vaccine interacts with this.

14.3.3.6 Effect in naive susceptibles and boosting

In Table 14.9, we consider a different biologically plausible situation. Suppose that the vaccine has an effect both in naive susceptibles and in people with previous exposure to infection, but due to immune boosting, the efficacy in those with previous immunity is greater. Assume that the vaccine reduces susceptibility by $TPR_{\bar{c}} = 0.5$ in the immunologically naive, and $TPR_c = 0.25$ in those people with previous immunity. We assume that previous exposure reduces susceptibility by 0.5, so $TP_{0c} = 0.5$ $TP_{0\bar{c}}$. The proportion in each of the three trial sites with previous immunity ($C = c$) varies from about 3% in site A to 50% in site B to 97% in site F. With exactly one infectious exposure to infection, the estimated vaccine effect based on $VE_{S,CI}$ varies correspondingly from 0.504, close to the biologic efficacy in the immunologically naive group, to 0.736, close to the biologic efficacy in the previously exposed group. Once again, at the individual level, the efficacy is the same in all three trial sites given the previous immune status of the individual. If no one had had previous exposure to infection, the biologic efficacy would have been exactly the same for everyone. The previous exposure acts as an effect modifier of the vaccine, and the final estimate of efficacy depends on the proportion of previously exposed people in the population.

14.3.3.7 Varying susceptibility, vaccine response and exposure to infection

As a final example we consider the situation described in Table 14.6 for the three vaccine trial sites, but now let the number of exposures per person vary from 1 up to 16 (Figure 14.2). The situation in which everyone is exposed once corresponds to that in Table 14.6. As the number of exposures per person increases, all the estimates of $VE_{S,CI}$ go towards 0. Suppose that site F with a low pre-vaccination susceptibility (pre-existing immunity) also has the higher transmission with a higher number of exposures, say 5, during the trial compared with just one in sites A and B. The estimated efficacy will be only 0.25 in site F, and it will be 0.25 in site A and 0.35 in site B. Thus, the difference in transmission level will make the crude efficacy in the three sites seem more similar than it would have been if everyone had had just one exposure to infection. If, on the other hand, transmission is higher in sites A and B than at site F, say 5 in A and B and 1 at F, then the difference in transmission will accentuate the differences between the sites. The estimates of $VE_{S,CI}$ at sites A and B would both be less than 0.20, and at site F it would be about 0.50. Of course, none of the expected efficacy estimates takes into account the underlying heterogeneity or gives an estimate of the actual biologic efficacy of the vaccine in the two strata at each site, which is exactly the same for all three sites. This could be part of the explanation for the difference between the South American SPf66 (Noya et al 1994; Valero et al 1993) vaccine trials and the trials in The Gambia (D'Alessandro et al 1995).

14.3.4 Interpretation

The results on the role and limits of randomization for estimates of effect in clinical trials in noninfectious disease are generally applicable to vaccine field trials. Randomization generally ensures that the treatment assignment mechanism is independent of the outcome of interest and of covariates relevant in determining this outcome. It is a good way to prevent additional problems of interpretation being introduced by the researcher and thus adding to the credibility of the study. Struchiner and Halloran (2007) showed that randomization in vaccine field trials does not guarantee that the estimated parameters are biologically meaningful. Nor does randomization guarantee that the estimates are unbiased, unconfounded, or insensitive to baseline transmission. The special role of exposure to infection and the availability of the additional conditional parameters such as the transmission probability in infectious diseases adds another layer of complexity to choice and interpretation of efficacy estimates.

We have not considered here the role of randomization under Bayesian inference. Lindley and Novick (1981) argue that randomization is not necessary, because inference is conditional on the observed data. From a subjective Bayesian standpoint, however, they add that randomization is good so that the treatment assignment should appear to be unconnected with any relevant factor and that other

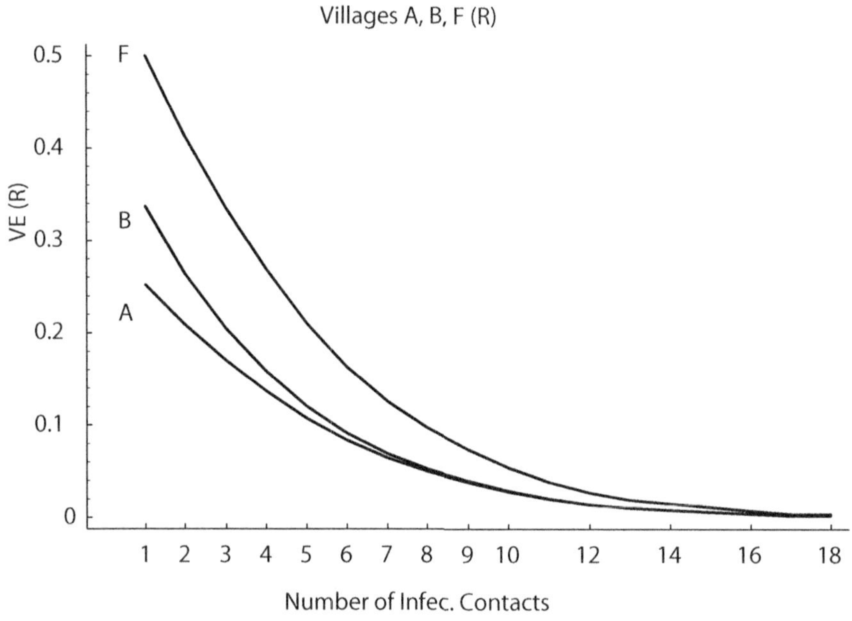

Fig. 14.2 Vaccine efficacy estimates based on the cumulative incidence cross over (Struchiner and Halloran 2007, Epidemiology and Infection, 135:181–194. Reprinted with permission).

people will believe the results. Rubin (1978, 1991) argues that randomization is good because it simplifies the analysis for Bayesian inference by making the ignorability of the treatment assignment mechanism explicit. However, even under Bayesian inference, randomization does not guarantee that an estimate has a biologically meaningful interpretation.

The examples presented here assumed a very simple multiplicative model of protective effects and did not differentiate between infection and disease. The relation between the possibly unobservable biologic efficacy of the vaccine and the efficacy as measured by the observable outcome may be much more complex and can depend on many factors (Breslow and Storer 1985; Struchiner et al 1994). Comparing efficacy estimates across populations could be more than a methodological problem. The differing apparent efficacy of vaccines across populations is one argument for testing vaccines in different populations, but it does not make comparison across populations easier.

Meaningful interpretation of vaccine efficacy estimates, even in randomized, double-blinded, placebo-controlled field trials, remains a challenge. As Savage (1962) wrote, "...whether one is a Bayesian or not, there is still a good deal to clarify about randomization."

Chapter 15
Surrogates of Protection

15.1 Replacing Clinical Outcomes

A holy grail of vaccine research is to identify a vaccine-induced immune response that predicts protection from infection and disease. If a measurable immune response to vaccination predictive of protection from infection and disease were available, it would help to avoid new large trials and facilitate getting new products and formulations approved. An immunological surrogate of protection could reduce the sample size or shorten the duration of a trial. If a good vaccine is already licensed and recommended, a trial with a new vaccine compared to placebo would be unethical. When both vaccines are highly efficacious or the clinical outcome of interest is rare, a relative efficacy trial comparing the two vaccines would be prohibitively large. Thus, identifying a good immunological surrogate of protection could make a trial much less expensive or indeed feasible.

If the interest is in evaluating new vaccine candidates in different populations, the primary goal is to predict how well the vaccine will do in new situations. Another use of immunological surrogates of protection is in designing vaccines for future emerging pathogens such as pandemic influenza or anthrax in which clinical outcome data are not available. These latter two types of studies are sometimes called bridge studies.

Much of this book has considered the effects of vaccination on clinical and infection outcomes and on transmission measured by clinical and infection outcomes. The era of using clinical outcomes in most primary vaccine efficacy trials may slowly be coming to an end, although clinical outcomes will still be useful in observational studies. In 1993, a Hib conjugate vaccine was approved for licensure in the United States based on immunological data (Frasch 1994) following the licensure of two others based on Phase III efficacy trials (Black et al 1992; Santosham et al 1991). Meningococcal C conjugate vaccines were licensed in England on the basis of serological correlates of protection without Phase III efficacy data (Andrews et al 2003). Identifying immunological correlates of protection is one of original topics of the Gates Grand Challenges. In this chapter, we present methods to assess

M.E. Halloran et al., *Design and Analysis of Vaccine Studies*, Statistics for Biology and Health, DOI 10.1007/978-0-387-68636-3_15,

correlates and surrogates of vaccine protection. The main focus is on immunological surrogates of protection, but we also briefly consider carriage as an endpoint in pneumococcal vaccine studies, the subject of ongoing research.

The primary clinical outcome of interest could be clinical disease, infection, or a post-infection outcome. For the discussion here we use VE_S to denote the clinical vaccine efficacy measure of interest and assume it is based on a binary clinical outcome, either infection or disease.

15.1.1 Biological versus statistical issues

In fields other than vaccine research, considerable interest developed in what were called surrogate endpoints as replacements for a primary clinical endpoint (Prentice 1989). Over the years, much methodological discussion has revolved around what constitutes a close relationship between the true endpoint and the potential surrogate endpoint. In the vaccine literature, traditionally the term correlate of protection has been used to describe the relation of a vaccine-induced response to protection against the clinical infection or disease outcome. Several different concepts were covered by the term correlate of protection. In establishing immunological correlates or surrogates of protection, part of the problem is biological and part of the problem is methodological.

The biological problem has several different aspects. The main scientific problem is to identify a candidate immunological measure or several measures likely associated with clinical protection. A statistical approach cannot validate an immunological measure as related to protection if a candidate has not been identified. Identification of a candidate immunological correlate requires precise specification of the measure of the immune response. The time of the assay after vaccination, and in the case of multiple doses, the timing after which dose, needs to be decided. The choice of assay can be important. Some assays are more sensitive than others, resulting in different response profiles. As knowledge of cell-mediated immunity grows, T-cell responses may be identified as important determinants of protection. The type of antibody measure can play a role. Assays can measure either the antibody concentration, the antibody avidity, or the concentration of functional antibodies. The avidity measures the total strength of the binding of the antibody with the antigen. The avidity can be high for bacteria that can have multiple identical sites. Antibodies with higher avidity can eliminate an antigen at lower concentrations than antibodies with low avidity. Another issue is whether an assay measures short-term protection or long-term protection from immunological memory. Maturation of antibody avidity is a sign of the presence of immunological memory. Functional antibodies may demonstrate bactericidal activity in assays using whole blood. Assay values may be titers or concentrations. The assays could measure antibodies, some aspect of cellular immunity, or immunological memory. In this development, we refer simply to antibody titers for simplicity.

As an example, the serum bactericidal assay (SBA) titer was established by Goldschneider et al (1969) as a correlate of protection for meningococcal C disease using a human complement assay. More recently, however, the rabbit complement assay has been recommended. Because the two assays have different sensitivities, the protective titers needed to be re-evaluated (Andrews et al 2003). Serological correlates of protection for meningococcal serogroup C can also be measured using avidity, which may be indicative of successful priming of the memory responses by vaccination. The SBA titer may be a correlate of short-term protection and the avidity, as a measure of immunological memory, may be a measure of long-term protection (Balmer and Borrow 2004). These issues are relevant for the planned licensing of the meningococcal A vaccine using immunological measures alone.

The correlates of protection may be based on individual measurements or population-level measures. Siber (1997) proposed that protective levels be estimated by a population-based analysis that identifies a level of antibody achieved by most of the protected population, such as an immunized group, and not achieved by most of a susceptible population, such as the nonimmunized group.

The methodological problem is to validate the identified potential correlates and surrogates of protection. There are two distinct but related problems. One is to identify immunological markers predictive of protection. The second is to identify immunological markers predictive of vaccine-induced protection. Most approaches to correlates and surrogates of protection assume that the protection conferred by titers produced by natural exposure and vaccination are equivalent.

15.1.2 Exposure to infection

One of the problems in evaluating correlates of protection is that not everyone in the group under observation is exposed to infection. Thus, a person might not develop disease because of not being exposed, not necessarily because of being protected. Models can capture the observed relation between immunological assay and protection from disease at high assay values (Dunning 2006). At high assay values very few people develop disease. However, at low assay values, whether a person develops disease could be associated with whether the person is exposed. Thus the probability of developing disease in individuals with low assay values could depend on the prevalence of the disease through the dependent happening relation or other factors not directly associated with the immunological measures.

A simple general approach assumes the probability of disease is a function of the probability of disease and the probability of being protected or not:

$$\begin{aligned}\Pr[\text{disease}] = {} & \Pr[\text{disease}|\text{not protected}] \times \Pr[\text{not protected}] \\ & + \Pr[\text{disease}|\text{protected}] \times \Pr[\text{protected}]. \qquad (15.1)\end{aligned}$$

Most of these models make an explicit assumption of an all-or-none model of vaccine protection. That is, a person is either completely protected or not protected, whether a threshold or continuous model is assumed. In the all-or-none model, the $\Pr[\text{disease}|\text{protected}] = 0$, so the second term in equation (15.1) is 0.

In a study, the probability of disease can be estimated by the attack rate or cumulative incidence. Thus, vaccine efficacy based on the attack rate or cumulative incidence can be written

$$\begin{aligned} VE_{S,CI} &= 1 - \frac{\Pr[\text{disease (vac)}]}{\Pr[\text{disease (controls)}]} \\ &= 1 - \frac{\Pr[\text{disease}|\text{not protected (vac)}]\Pr[\text{not protected (vac)}]}{\Pr[\text{disease}|\text{not protected (control)}]\Pr[\text{not protected (control)}]}. \end{aligned} \tag{15.2}$$

Under the assumption that exposure to infection is equal in the vaccinated and control groups, and that the probability of disease is equal in the two groups if exposed and not protected, the terms for the probability of disease if not protected cancel, leaving

$$VE_{S,CI} = 1 - \frac{\Pr[\text{not protected (vac)}]}{\Pr[\text{not protected (control)}]}. \tag{15.3}$$

The probability of not being protected can be based on a threshold level of antibody above which everyone is protected. Then the probability of being protected in equation (15.3) is estimated by the proportion of people with an immune response above the threshold. Alternatively, one can estimate the probability of protection as a continuous function of the level of antibody. In the continuous model, at a given antibody titer, a person is either protected or not with an antibody-specific probability. The probability of being protected increases with increasing antibody titer, but the level of protection does not increase, as would be the case if a leaky model were assumed. The probability of not being protected in equation (15.3) is replaced by the population average probability of being protected over the predicted probabilities of protection at the individual antibody titers.

A special case occurs if everyone is exposed to infection, as in challenge studies. Household exposure to infection has been used as a natural challenge. Then the probability of developing disease is modeled directly as a continuous function of the antibody titers (Storsaeter et al 1998). The threshold and regression approaches are presented in Sections 15.2 and 15.3.

15.1.3 Statistical versus principal surrogates

In a groundbreaking paper, Prentice (1989) proposed four criteria for a biomarker to be a surrogate endpoint for the primary clinical outcome of interest. In the context of vaccines (Kohberger et al 2008), the four can be stated as

1. Protection is significantly related to the vaccine.

2. The surrogate is significantly related to the vaccine.
3. The surrogate is significantly related to the clinical endpoint.
4. The surrogate explains all of the clinical endpoints.

The third criterion requires a correlation between the surrogate and the clinical endpoint of interest. Fleming and DeMets (1996) wrote, however, that "a correlate does not a surrogate make."

The fourth condition requires that the surrogate fully capture the vaccine's net effect on the clinical endpoint of interest. If one had the appropriate immune or other biological markers, knowledge of the vaccine status would provide no additional information for predicting the clinical outcome. The fourth criterion can be checked by a statistical regression model that has both the treatment indicator and the value or model for the surrogate in the model. Different approaches can be taken. One could say that if the regression coefficient for the treatment indicator is not significantly different from 0, then the criterion is met. In another approach, one could require that the regression coefficient actually be 0, which will generally not happen. The fourth condition is quite restrictive, making it difficult to validate correlates as surrogates (Degruttola et al 1997). Kohberger et al (2008) take an alternative approach to the fourth criterion based on estimation of the proportion of the clinical endpoint explained (PE) by the surrogate (Burzykowski, et al 2005).

Frangakis and Rubin (2002) criticized the Prentice approach because it is subject to post-randomization selection bias. In the vaccine context, under the Prentice approach, the risk of the clinical endpoints is compared in individuals with the observed values of the immunological markers. However, we observe only the immunological value and the clinical endpoint that the person has under the actual vaccine assignment. We do not observe the value of the immune marker value that the person would have had under the other vaccine assignment. However, similar to the discussion of VE_P in Chapter 9, comparisons based on the Prentice criteria are subject to a post-randomization selection bias and do not have a causal interpretation. Frangakis and Rubin (2002) call the surrogates evaluated by the Prentice criteria statistical surrogates. Using the framework of potential outcomes in causal inference (Section 1.4), they propose a definition of a principal surrogate based on comparison of individuals with the same pair of potential values of the candidate surrogate under the two treatment assignments. Sections 15.4 and 15.5 present levels of confidence in the immunological markers as correlates and surrogates of protection and how to evaluate them based on these ideas. These approaches, however, thus far have not taken the role of exposure to infection into account.

15.2 Thresholds for Protection

In a threshold model, let C be the threshold or cutoff value level of antibody assumed to be protective. Let $\Pr(Ab_v < C)$ and $\Pr(Ab_c < C)$ be the probabilities that vaccinated and control individuals have titers less than the protective threshold or cutoff. If $VE_{S,CI}$ based on the clinical outcome is known, the antibody level is measured in everyone, and exposure is assumed equal in the two groups, then using equations (15.2) and (15.3), we can simply solve the following equations for the level of antibody C that is protective:

$$\begin{aligned}\mathrm{VE}_{S,CI} &= 1 - \frac{\Pr[Y=1|\text{vaccinated}]}{\Pr[Y=1|\text{control}]}\\ &= 1 - \frac{\Pr[\text{not protected (vac)}]}{\Pr[\text{not protected (control)}]} = 1 - \frac{\Pr(\mathrm{Ab}_v < C)}{\Pr(\mathrm{Ab}_c < C)}. \qquad (15.4)\end{aligned}$$

In contrast, given a threshold C, from the observed titers in the vaccinated and control individuals, $\Pr(\mathrm{Ab}_v < C)$ and $\Pr(\mathrm{Ab}_c < C)$ can be estimated from the observed proportion with titers less than the protective threshold C. We can predict the vaccine efficacy based on the proportion of people in the vaccinated and control groups who are above that threshold.

$$\widehat{\mathrm{VE}}_{S,CI} = 1 - \frac{\%\text{ of vaccinated with }\mathrm{Ab}_v < C}{\%\text{ of controls with }\mathrm{Ab}_c < C}. \qquad (15.5)$$

Andrews et al (2003) used post-licensure surveillance of meningococcal C to validate the serological correlates of protection that were the basis to license the conjugate vaccine in England. Starting with equation (15.2), they assumed that exposure to infection was the same in the vaccinated and unvaccinated group, and that the protection conferred by titers produced by natural exposure or by vaccination is equivalent. They explored the efficacy predicted using equation (15.5) by different cutoff thresholds for protection (Table 15.1). The screening method (Section 8.1.4) was used to estimate the observed post-licensure efficacy (direct effectiveness). Cases of confirmed meningitis C infection that occurred in vaccinated and unvaccinated individuals in England from January 2000 to the end of 2001 and coverage levels of vaccination were used for the computation.

In preschool children, 27 cases occurred, all in unvaccinated children for an observed efficacy estimate of 100% (95% CI, 93.3–100%). Coverage levels were not given in the paper. From Table 15.1, in preschool children, the predicted efficacy from titers one month after vaccination is consistent with the observed efficacy at all of the cutoffs except 1:128. The predicted efficacy is most consistent with the observed efficacy at the cutoffs 1:4 and 1:8. Similar results were obtained for the infant and toddler age groups. However, using titers seven and nine months post-vaccination, the predicted vaccine efficacy significantly underestimated the observed efficacy in infants and toddlers (preschool children were not included). This finding suggests that when the post-vaccination titers have declined, immunologic memory and a rapid booster response may be responsible for efficacy, which would be better measured by antibody avidity.

Jódar et al (2003) use the threshold approach in equations (15.4) and (15.5) in the context of multivalent pneumococcal conjugate vaccines. The problem is complicated because of the lack of a serological correlate of protection and multiplicity of antigens in the pneumococcal conjugate vaccines. For several of the serotypes,

Table 15.1 Predicted vaccine efficacy and 95% CIs estimated for unvaccinated and vaccinated preschool children with titers below the different serum bactericidal assay (SBA) cutoffs one month after vaccination with the meningococcal C conjugate vaccine measured by SBA (from Andrews et al 2003)

	% Individual with Titers Below Cutoff		Predicted % Vaccine
Cutoff	Vaccinated	Unvaccinated	Efficacy (95% CI)
1:4	0.0	90.4	100 (95–100)
1:8	0.0	93.3	100 (95–100)
1:16	2.5	94.3	97 (92–99)
1:32	4.1	95.2	96 (90-98)
1:64	4.9	97.1	95 (89–98)
1:128	9.8	97.6	90 (83–94)

clinical efficacy has not been established, making type-specific thresholds difficult to define. Antigens against particular serotypes may be added to new formulations to take account of the serotypes responsible for invasive disease in different countries. With several antigens, comparison of antibody response of new formulations with previous formulations are subject to additional problems associated with multiple statistical comparsions. Jódar et al (2003) assumed IgG after three doses of vaccine predicts protection. They also assumed the relation of risk of disease and antibody is a stepwise function, although they acknowledged that it is continuous. Because it was unlikely that type-specific thresholds could be defined for additional serotypes that had not undergone efficacy trials, they used aggregate antibody titers for all serotypes rather than antibody titers for individual serotypes.

Jódar et al (2003) plotted the reverse cumulative distribution of pooled antibody titer above a certain level in the vaccinated and unvaccinated groups against the pooled antibody concentration. The threshold of 0.18 antibody concentration yielded the observed vaccine efficacy of 97.6 from the California pneumococcal conjugate vaccine trial study (Black et al 2000). At concentration 0.18, the proportion 0.979 of the vaccinated group and 0.129 of the unvaccinated group had antibody titers above this level, yielding the estimated $\widehat{\mathrm{VE}}_{S,CI} = 0.976 = 1-(1-0.979)/(1-0.129)$. Ignoring the antibody concentration in the unvaccinated individuals, they suggested a protective concentration of 0.20 as a preliminary threshold for protection. Several issues remain to be solved with the pneumococcal vaccine correlates, including the use of nasopharyngeal carriage as an endpoint (Section 15.6).

15.3 Regression Models for Correlates

Several issues limit the potential of threshold models. The threshold may not discriminate immune response in vaccinees and controls. Small changes in point estimate of efficacy may significantly change threshold antibody concentrations that predict efficacy. The relation between protection and antibody level is likely continuous, not discrete. An alternative is the use of continuous regression models.

To be used in the regression models, the immunological measurement must have a source of variability If the individuals in the study population have no previous exposure to the infection, they would generally have zero or near-zero immune measurements for the infectious agent of interest. Then the immunological correlate can only be evaluated in the vaccinated people. In some diseases in which repeated exposure occurs with the development of partial immunity, such as malaria, or repeated exposure with similar strains, such as influenza, an immunological measurement could be positive and have variability in the unvaccinated people as well as the vaccinated people. For such infectious diseases, the immunological correlate can be evaluated in both the unvaccinated people and the vaccinated people. That is, the clinical outcome of interest can be regressed on the immunological measurements in both the unvaccinated and the vaccinated groups. However, in most vaccine studies, the correlation between immune measure and outcome can be established only in the vaccinated group.

15.3.1 Regression models separating level of exposure

Dunning (2006) proposed a regression model that separates the effect of the assay values from such factors as level of exposure and disease prevalence. In fitting the data from individual-based measurements with clinical outcome and titers, the model estimates a parameter that represents levels of exposure to infection and other factors not included in the measured immune responses. The initial model does not include the vaccination status of the individuals. In the second step, when predicting vaccine efficacy from the estimated regression parameters, the estimated factor is assumed to cancel out as in equations (15.2) and (15.3).

Assume there are data from n participants, $i = 1, \ldots, n$. Let s_i be the assay value for participant i, and $y_i = 1$ if participant i develops disease, and $y_i = 0$ if not. It is assumed that s is log transformed so that it can have positive and negative values. The model has two main components. The first is the probability $\alpha(s)$ that a person with titer s is protected. The second is the probability ω that a susceptible individual develops disease. The probability ω can depend on prevalence of disease, as in the dependent happening relation, the probability of exposure, and other aspects specific to the particular study that are independent of the assay value. The probability $\alpha(s)$ is essentially an all-or-none model of protection where the probability of being completely protected is a function of the immunological assay value. The protected individuals are assumed completely immune from disease, and the proportion $(1 - \alpha(s))$ of susceptible individuals with assay value s are assumed to be homogeneously susceptible.

The probability that an individual develops disease is the product of the probability that the individual is susceptible and the probability that a susceptible individual will develop disease:

$$\Pr(Y_i = 1) = \omega(1 - \alpha(s_i)). \tag{15.6}$$

If an inverse logit function is used to model a relation of S, $f(S)$, to $\alpha(S)$, then the probability of being protected is modeled

$$\alpha(S) = \frac{1}{1 + \exp(-f(S))}. \tag{15.7}$$

The model $f(S)$ in Dunning (2006) is the two-parameter model $f(S) = a + bS$. For small assay values, the probability of being protected $\alpha(s)$ approaches 0, and as s gets large, the probability of being protected $\alpha(s)$ approaches 1.

Combining (15.6) and (15.7) gives a model for the probability that an individual with assay value S develops disease:

$$\Pr(Y_i = 1) = \frac{\omega}{1 + \exp(f(s_i))}. \tag{15.8}$$

The parameters ω, a, and b can be estimated by standard likelihood methods.

Given estimates of $\hat{a}$ and $\hat{b}$, suppose that in a trial of a new vaccine candidate in a similar setting, the immunological assays are performed but no clinical outcomes are measured. Let the vaccinated group be denoted by V and the control group by U. Let ω' be the unknown probability of developing disease in the susceptible individuals in the trial. From (15.8), the number of individuals expected to develop disease in the vaccinated group is

$$\sum_{i \in V} \Pr(Y_i = 1) = \sum_{i \in V} \frac{\omega'}{1 + \exp(\hat{a} + \hat{b} s_i)}. \tag{15.9}$$

A similar computation would yield the expected number of cases in the unvaccinated group. In the computation of vaccine efficacy, the value of ω' would cancel in the ratio of expected number of vaccinated and unvaccinated cases. The efficacy of the new vaccine formulation would be predicted by (Dunning 2006)

$$VE_{S,new} = 1 - \frac{1/n_v \sum_{i \in V} 1/(1 + \exp(\hat{a} + \hat{b} s_i))}{1/n_c \sum_{i \in U} 1/(1 + \exp(\hat{a} + \hat{b} s_i))}. \tag{15.10}$$

This model assumes the protective effect at a given titer is the same in the vaccinated and the unvaccinated group. Dunning (2006) used this model to estimate the probability of protection as a function of assay value for six pertussis assays. Forrest et al (2008) used this model to analyze a randomized efficacy study of live attenuated influenza vaccine in young children in the Philippines and Thailand. They had both an assay for cell-mediated immunity as measured by an IFN-γ ELISPOT and antibodies as measured by HAI.

15.3.2 Household exposure as natural challenge

One of the problems in evaluating correlates of protection is that possibly many of the participants in the study are not exposed to infection. Examining children with household exposure to pertussis was proposed as a natural challenge experiment (Storsaeter et al 1998). Under this design, the assumption is that everyone is exposed to infection. The model does not estimate the probability of disease separately as in equation (15.8) or assume that the probability of disease in the unprotected cancels as in (15.3).

Let the outcome Y be 1 if diseased and 0 if not diseased. Let (S,X) represent the values of the immunological assays S and possibly vaccination status and other covariates X. Let $g(S,X)$ be a function of (S,X), for example, a linear combination of (S,X), with unknown parameters to be estimated. The probability of disease is expressed as a function of (S,X) in the logistic model as

$$\Pr(Y = 1|S,X) = \frac{1}{1+\exp(-g(S,X))} \tag{15.11}$$

Although model (15.7) looks similar to model (15.11), the interpretation is very different. Model (15.11) is an expression for the probability of developing disease at certain assay and other covariate values, but model (15.7) is an expression for the probability of being protected at a certain assay value. Storsaeter et al (1998) used this approach to analyze a household study nested in a placebo-controlled vaccine efficacy trial. The trial evaluated an acellular five-component pertussis vaccine, an acellular two-component vaccine, and a whole cell vaccine all combined with diphtheria–tetanus toxoid compared with diptheria-tetanus toxoid alone (Gustafsson et al 1996). Using the method for household exposure to infection as a natural challenge is not feasible in meningococcal vaccine studies because of the low secondary attack rate (Andrews et al 2003).

The objectives of the pertussis vaccine study were (1) to estimate absolute efficacy after household exposure to *B. pertussis* for children with three doses of one of the three study vaccines compared to placebo recipients; (2) to evaluate possible serological correlates of protection by relating the clinical outcome after household exposure to the antibody levels against pertussis toxin (PT), pertactin (PRN), filamentous hemagglutinin (FHA), and fimbrial agglutinogens (FIM) at the time of exposure; and (3) to explore the possible use of post-vaccination anti-pertussis antibody levels as surrogate markers to predict protective efficacy of the whole cell or multicomponent acellular pertussis vaccines (Storsaeter et al 1998).

Of the 329 exposed study participants, 36 had fewer than three trial doses. The remaining 293 children were used in computing vaccine efficacy. Of those, 59 lacked a pre-exposure blood sample and 25 did not have a valid serum sample. Thus, 209 children fulfilled the general rules for a valid blood sample for being included in the primary analysis of serologic correlates of protection. The guidelines were (1) a pre-exposure sample taken within four months of exposure given that it was taken at least six months after the third trial dose, or (2) an acute blood sample was accepted

Table 15.2 Pertussis cases and vaccine efficacy after household exposure to culture-confirmed *B. pertussis* infection. Only the DTaP5 and DT groups are shown here (from Storsaeter et al 1998)

Clinical Definition	Exposed in DTaP5 Group $N = 86$ Cases (Cult Pos)	Exposed in DT Group $N = 74$ Cases (Cult Pos)	Vaccine Efficacy (95% CI)
Cough 1 day or more and positive lab criteria	28 (13)	63 (43)	61.8 (47.4 –72.2)
Cough 21 days or more and positive lab criteria	21 (11)	60 (43)	69.9 (55.6 – 79.6)
Spasmodic cough 21 days or more (WHO)	14 (10)	49 (36)	75.4 (59.2 – 85.2)

if there were no antibody titer rises against either PT, FHA, PRN, or FIM compared to earlier samples. An acute sample was chosen in 125 of the 209 children.

In the nested household study (Table 15.2), the efficacy of the five-valent DTaP5 against typical WHO pertussis was estimated at 75.4% (95% CI 59.1–85.2) and against any pertussis at 61.8% (95% CI 47.4–72.2). In the main trial, the unconditional vaccine efficacy was estimated at 85.6% and at 77.9% for the two case definitions. Fine et al (1988) suggest that the more intense and longer exposure in households could result in the commonly observed lower efficacy of pertussis vaccines measured in household-based studies.

Storsaeter et al (1998) analyzed the data using the arbitrary units obtained in the IgG ELISAs. They also dichotomized the IgG ELISA units in "Low" (0 to <5 units) and "High" (≥ 5 units). The results in the paper focus on the dichotomized analysis. In the analysis, "Low" was coded as 0 and "High" as 1. The logistic regression model using the WHO definition and the dichotomized titers was

$$g(x) = 0.675 - 1.12\text{PT} - 1.992\text{FIM} - 1.589\text{PRN} + 1.993(\text{PT} \times \text{FIM}). \tag{15.12}$$

The vaccine group of the child and anti-FHA titer were not statistically significant and not included in the final models. That the vaccine group was not statistically significant suggests that the immunological measures in the model might be considered as fulfilling the Prentice criteria for a surrogate. Based on the WHO definition, the model predicts an attack rate in those with all three values Low as 66.3%. For those with all three values High, the model predicts an attack rate of 11.0%.

Kohberger et al (2008) evaluated the validity of the Storsaeter et al (1998) model (15.12) based on the study in terms of the statistical criteria for the validity of surrogate endpoints. They also examined the predictive ability of the model using clinical efficacy data from a different pertussis vaccine efficacy study conducted in Sweden (Olin et al 1997). Using the values $g(S,X)$ in the estimated regression model (15.12) for the individuals in the vaccinated and unvaccinated groups, one can estimate the probability of disease for a person with immune measure s_i, $\Pr(Y = 1|s_i)$. In a vaccinated group of size n_v, the probability of disease is estimated from the

$$\text{probability of disease(vaccinated)} = \frac{\sum \widehat{\Pr}(Y = 1|s_i)}{n_v}.$$

Kohberger et al (2008) suggests that the probability of disease in the unvaccinated could be estimated from historical estimates or the probability estimated when antibody levels are negligible. Similar to equation (15.10), for a new vaccine, then

$$VE_{S,new} = 1 - \frac{\text{probability of disease(vaccinated)}}{\text{probability of disease(unvaccinated)}}.$$

15.4 Framework for Confidence in a Biomarker

In a series of papers, Gilbert and Hudgens (2008), Gilbert et al (2008), Qin et al (2007), and Qin et al (2008) propose a framework for assessing immunological correlates of protection in vaccine trials (Table 15.3). The framework is based on the methods of Prentice (1989) and Frangakis and Rubin (2002). The framework delineates different levels of confidence in immunological markers. They in particular distinguish correlates of risk and surrogates of protection. In contrast to the approaches in the first part of this chapter, they are not concerned with taking into account differences in exposure to infection in different settings. Rather, the approach is concerned with the problem of potential bias in using post-randomization immunological measures to determine causally related surrogates of protection for vaccine-induced immunity.

15.4.1 Correlates of risk

The first, and lowest, level of confidence is a correlate of risk. An immunological measurement that predicts a clinical endpoint in a particular population is a correlate of risk (CoR). To validate an immunological measurement as a correlate of risk, an association must be observed between these measurements and the clinical endpoint. As discussed in Section 15.3, various statistical approaches such as fitting regression models can be used to fit the data for the clinical endpoint of interest to the immunological measurement (Storsaeter et al 1998; Chan et al 2002; Dunning 2006). Many vaccine studies have shown that antibody titers correlate with risk of infection or disease. In addition to those already mentioned, children with higher immune response to varicella vaccine had lower incidence of chickenpox disease (White et al 1992). In estimating the correlation of the immunological measure with the clinical endpoint, the vaccine status does not necessarily need to be taken into account.

15.4.2 Surrogates of protection

The next two levels of confidence are called surrogates of protection. A surrogate of protection is a correlate of risk that also predicts the level of protective efficacy of the vaccine based on comparison of immunological measurements in the vaccinated and unvaccinated groups. It only makes sense to evaluate an immunological correlate as a potential surrogate of protection if in fact the vaccine is shown to have a protective effect, that is, $\mathrm{VE}_S > 0$. Qin et al (2007) differentiate surrogates of protection that predict vaccine efficacy for the same setting as the source of the data from surrogates of protection predicting efficacy for other settings. The same setting would include a similar population, the same infectious agent, and the same vaccine product. A new setting could be a new population, different strains of the infectious agent, or different vaccine products. Sadoff and Wittes (2007) suggest that the two levels of surrogates of protection be called specific and general surrogates of protection.

The specific surrogates of protection are further classified as statistical surrogates of protection (SoP^S) and principal surrogates of protection (SoP^P). The statistical surrogates of protection are defined in terms of the statistical and observable associations. They satisfy the Prentice (1989) criteria for a surrogate described in Section 15.1.3. The data required to evaluate an immunological marker as a statistical surrogate of protection will be available in most clinical vaccine studies if there is considerable variability of the immunological measurement in the control participants. If there is not much variability in the control group, then it is difficult to evaluate an immunological marker as a statistical surrogate of protection.

The principal surrogates of vaccine protection are based on the principal surrogates proposed by Frangakis and Rubin (2002) using the notation of potential outcomes in causal inference (see Sections 1.4 and 9.3.2). The specific principal surrogates of protection are defined by fixed values of the immune response if assigned vaccine and the immune response if assigned control. The pair of potential immune responses under vaccine and control is assumed fixed before randomization to either vaccine or control, thus the pair is not subject to potential post-randomization selection bias. To begin, consider the simplest case that the potential immune response in the control would be $S(0) = 0$ or some fixed constant c. Let $S(1)$ be the potential response that an unvaccinated subject would have if vaccinated. Let Y be the 0,1 outcome of being infected or not, and Z be the 0,1 assignment to vaccine or control. Assume that the trial is randomized and that there is no interference among the units. For a specific principal surrogate of protection, one needs to estimate

$$\mathrm{VE}(s_1) = 1 - \frac{\Pr[Y = 1|Z = 1, S(1) = s_1]}{\Pr[Y = 1|Z = 0, S(1) = s_1]}. \tag{15.13}$$

Table 15.3 Definitions of three levels of an immunological correlate of protection (adapted from Qin et al 2007 and Gilbert et al 2008)

Term	Definition	Framework for Assessment	Analytic Method
CoR (Correlate of risk)	An immunological measurement S that correlates with the study endpoint Y measuring vaccine efficacy in a defined population	Vaccine trial (efficacy or proof of concept) or observational study	Regression models
Specific SoP (Surrogate of protection for the same setting)	An immunological measurement that is a CoR within a defined population of vaccine recipients and satisfies either:		
SoP^S (Statistical surrogate of protection for the same setting)	Relation between immunological measurement S and endpoint Y is the same in the vaccine and placebo groups	Single large efficacy trial	Statistical surrogate framework
SoP^P (Principal surrogate of protection for the same setting)	The immune response S satisfies two criteria: (1) $\text{VE}_S = 0$ for subjects where vaccine has no effect; (2) $\text{VE}_S > 0$ if vaccine has a sufficiently large effect on S	Single large efficacy trial	Principal surrogate framework
General SoP (Surrogate of protection for new setting)	An immunologic measurement predictive of vaccine efficacy in different settings, such as human populations, viral populations, vaccine lots	Multiple trials and/or post-licensure studies	Meta-analysis

The definition in expression (15.13) implies that the vaccine efficacy at the immune response level s_1 is the relative reduction in the risk for groups of vaccinees with immune response s_1 compared with their risk if they had not been vaccinated. The problem is that in people in the control group for whom $Z = 0$, the value of s_1, the surrogate value under vaccination, is not observed. The main difference between the statistical surrogate of protection and the principal surrogate of protection is that the former is based on what is actually observed in vaccine studies, and the latter is based on information not usually available in any vaccine studies. The problem with statistical surrogates of protection is that what is measured is a mixture of the causal vaccine effects and differences between participants who are infected in the vaccine and unvaccinated groups with values of $S = s$.

To assess whether an immunological measurement is a specific principal surrogate of protection, knowledge about $S(1)$ is needed. That is, one needs to be able to predict the immune response that an unvaccinated participant would have had if vaccinated. Follmann (2006) proposed two approaches to assess what the immune response would have been in the control participants (Section 15.5.5). An immunological measurement is a specific principal surrogate of protection if two conditions are met (Gilbert and Hudgens 2008). First, groups of vaccinees without responses or with the lowest response levels have a risk equal to that had they not been vaccinated. Second, groups of vaccinees with sufficiently high immune response levels have a risk lower than that had they not been vaccinated. This second condition is analogous to assuming there is some threshold measure above which the individuals are protected.

Although it is useful to understand the relation of immune responses to protection against infection and disease within a particular setting, the goal of identifying surrogates of vaccine protection is to replace large scale phase III trials using clinical outcomes with immunological measurements in new settings and for new vaccines. For example, immunological measures of hemagglutination titer are used to approve the new influenza vaccines each year in Europe. To demonstrate that an immunological marker is a general surrogate of protection requires more stringent data requirements than the specific surrogate of protection. It is actually quite difficult without numerous, likely untestable assumptions. To show that an immunological marker is a general surrogate of protection requires that it predict vaccine effects on risk across different populations, for different strains, and different vaccine products. One possible approach would be to use meta-analysis combining information from several studies (Gail et al 1989; Daniels and Hughes 1997).

15.5 Evaluating Principal Surrogate Endpoints

Gilbert and Hudgens (2008) define statistical and principal surrogates of protection formally. Their approach is for specific surrogates of protection and evaluates the immunological marker for the same or similar setting as the trial. They introduce an estimand for evaluating a principal surrogate called a causal effect predictiveness (CEP) surface. The causal effect predictiveness surface quantifies how well vaccine effects on the immunological marker predict causal vaccine effects on the clinical endpoint. The CEP surface can be used to compare the surrogate value of several immunological markers.

15.5.1 Set-up

Consider a randomized, double blind vaccine trial. Assignment is denoted Z, $Z = 1$ for vaccine and $Z = 0$ for control, the discrete or continuous immunological surrogate is S measured at fixed time t_0 after assignment to vaccine or control, and the binary clinical endpoint is Y ($Y = 1$ for disease or infection, 0 otherwise). Gilbert and Hudgens (2008) include an indicator $V = 1$ to denote whether participants are still disease-free at t_0. Later they assume that for any individual, the value of V is the same under vaccine and control. To simplify the presentation, here we assume that everyone is disease-free at t_0, and drop the notation.

Gilbert and Hudgens (2008) consider a two-phase outcome-dependent case-cohort sampling design (Prentice 1986). A case-cohort study is a case-control study in which the source population is a cohort and every person in the cohort has an equal chance of being included in the study as a control, regardless of how much time that individual has contributed to the person-time experience of the cohort (Rothman et al 2008). In phase one of the study, baseline covariates X are measured on everyone, and in phase two, a baseline covariate(s) W is measured for all or most of the cases, participants with $Y = 1$, and for a random sample of those participants who did not develop disease, $Y = 0$. The candidate immunological surrogate S is measured on everyone for whom W is measured. The indicator δ denotes whether W is measured. Of course, W and S could be measured on everyone, but it is not necessary in the case-cohort study. For vaccine trials, S and W can be measured after the trial using stored specimens (Nosten et al 1996, Ballou et al 1995).

15.5.2 *Defining surrogates of protection*

Using this notation, a statistical surrogate of protection defined by Frangakis and Rubin (2002) is evaluated by comparing the risk distributions

$$\text{risk}(s|Z=1) \equiv \Pr(Y=1|Z=1, S=s)$$
$$\text{risk}(s|Z=0) \equiv \Pr(Y=1|Z=0, S=s).$$

If for all values of S, $\text{risk}(s|Z=1) = \text{risk}(s|Z=0)$, then the immunological marker S is a statistical surrogate of protection for the clinical endpoint.

A principal surrogate of protection is defined using potential outcomes of causal inference (see Sections 1.4 and 9.3.2). Denote the potential clinical endpoint by $Y(Z)$ and the potential value of the immunological marker by $S(Z)$ under vaccine assignment Z. The full potential data are iid copies of

$$(Z_i, X_i, \delta_i, \delta_i W_i, S_i(1), S_i(0), Y_i(1), Y_i(0)), \quad i = 1, \ldots, n,$$

assuming no drop-out. The two usual key assumptions of no interference between units (SUTVA) and independence of treatment assignment from the potential outcomes, eg randomization, are made. An immunological marker S is a principal surrogate endpoint if, for all $s_1 = s_0$ the following two risks are equal:

$$\text{risk}_{(1)}(s_1, s_0) \equiv \Pr(Y(1) = 1|S(1) = s_1, S(0) = s_0), \qquad (15.14)$$
$$\text{risk}_{(0)}(s_1, s_0) \equiv \Pr(Y(0) = 1|S(1) = s_1, S(0) = s_0). \qquad (15.15)$$

The contrast of the two risks measures a population-level causal vaccine effect on Y for participants with the potential immunological measures $\{S_i(1) = s_1, S_i(0) = s_0\}$. The statement is equivalent to S being a principal surrogate of protection if in those groups with no causal effect of vaccine on the immunological marker, the vaccine has no causal effect on the clinical outcome of interest (Frangakis and Rubin 2002). Gilbert and Hudgens (2008) propose a second criterion for a principal surrogate of protection, namely that an immunological marker value above a certain level is sufficient to protect against the clinical outcome of interest, a causal analogue of a correlate of protection threshold model(Section 15.2). For example, the difference $s_1 - s_0 > C$, where C is some antibody titer or cell-mediated immune response level, could be sufficient to protect against clinical disease, assuming $s_1 \geq s_0$. Then $\text{risk}_{(1)}(s_1, s_0) < \text{risk}_{(0)}(s_1, s_0)$.

15.5.3 Causal effect predictiveness surface

The causal effect predictiveness surface is defined as a contrast, such as the difference, between the two risks in (15.14) and (15.15)

$$CEP^{risk}(s_1, s_0) \equiv \text{risk}_{(0)}(s_1, s_0) - \text{risk}_{(1)}(s_1, s_0), \tag{15.16}$$

where Gilbert and Hudgens (2008) also consider other contrasts.

The surrogate value of an immunological marker is defined as its capacity reliably to predict the population-level causal effect of vaccination on the clinical endpoint. The surrogate value can be quantified by the nearness of the CEP value to 0 for small differences $s_1 - s_0$, and by how the CEP value, that is, the difference in the risk under vaccine and control, increases as the difference in the two potential immunological measures under vaccine and control, $s_1 - s_0$, increases. Two different immunological markers can have different surrogate values based on differing CEP surfaces.

The marginal CEP curve is defined as a contrast, such as the difference, of the two risks in (15.14) and (15.15) where the risk depends only on the potential immunological marker under vaccine s_1, not also on s_0. When in all participants in the control group, the immunological measure has a 0 or constant value, called the constant biomarker case, such as in equation (15.13), then the CEP surface equals the marginal CEP surface.

As defined by Frangakis and Rubin (2002), an associative measure of a principal surrogate of protection is how large the difference is in the potential outcomes under vaccine and control in people whose potential measures of S are different under vaccine and control. A dissociative measure of a principal surrogate of protection is how large the difference is in the potential outcomes under vaccine and control in people whose potential measures of S are the same under vaccine and control. Intuitively, one would want a principal surrogate of protection to have more of an associative measure than a dissociative measure.

Gilbert and Hudgens (2008) suggest functions of the CEP surface that summarize the surrogate values of an immunological marker. The proportion associative effect, PAE^{ω}, is defined by the ratio of the expected associative effect divided by the sum of the expected associative effect and the expected dissociative measure.

The question is to what extent the expected associative effect is outweighed by the expected dissociative effect. If PAE^{ω} is in the range [0,0.5], then the immunological measure may have no surrogate value. If PAE^{ω} is in the range (0.5,1.0], then it may have some surrogate value.

15.5.4 Estimating the CEP surface

When the immunological marker has 0 or constant value in the control, it is difficult to evaluate it as a statistical surrogate of protection, as described in Section 15.3, although it can be evaluated as a correlate of risk. However, in this special case, an approach can be taken to estimate the CEP surface and marginal CEP curve. The problem in estimating the CEP surface is that we do not observe the immunological responses S under both vaccine and control. So now we include the baseline covariates X and W in the expressions for the two risks in (15.14) and (15.15). Under the assumption of SUTVA and independent assignment mechanism,

$$\text{risk}_{(1)}(s_1, s_0, x, w) = \Pr(Y = 1|Z = 1, S = s_1, S(0) = s_0, X = x, W = w) \,, \tag{15.17}$$

$$\text{risk}_{(0)}(s_1, s_0, x, w) = \Pr(Y = 1|Z = 0, S(1) = s_1, S = s_0, X = x, W = w) \,. \tag{15.18}$$

It would be possible to estimate the two risks if we knew the potential outcomes $S_i(Z)$ of participants if they had been assigned the opposite treatment.

If the response to the immunological marker is 0 or constant in everyone if in the control group, then $\text{risk}_{(1)}(s_1, s_0, x, w)$ can be estimated from the observed data. However, the potential value $S_i(1)$ of the immunological marker if vaccinated in those participants who received control needs to be determined to be able to estimate the CEP surface.

Assume a baseline covariate W predictive of the immunological measure $S(1)$ is measured in both treatment arms (Follmann 2006) (Section 15.5.5). Then a model predicting $S(1)$ from X and W can be fit in the participants in the vaccine group and used to predict the potential value of the immunological measure $S(1)$ for participants in the control group. Details of estimation and inference as well as a test of whether an immunological measure has any surrogate value are in Gilbert and Hudgens (2008). The surrogate marker value of $S(1)$ for people in the control group is treated as missing data. The likelihood contribution for a person in the control group is obtained by integrating the risk over the conditional cumulative distribution function of $S(1)|X, W$ in the vaccinated group.

15.5.5 Augmented designs to assess immune response

Follmann (2006) proposed two augmented vaccine trial designs to help determine whether a particular immune response to a vaccine is actually the causal factor in reducing the infection rate in the vaccinated compared to the unvaccinated group. The first approach involves vaccinating everyone in both the vaccine and control groups before baseline with an irrelevant vaccine. For example, in a pneumococcal vaccine trial, one might vaccinate both the vaccine group and control group with a meningococcal vaccine. Then randomization ensures that the relation between the immune responses to the meningococcal and pneumococcal vaccines observed in the vaccine group is the same as would have been observed in the control group. The potential response to the pneumococcal vaccine in individuals in the control group can be inferred from their response to the meningococcal vaccine and a prediction model based on the relation of the responses to both meningococcal and pneumococcal vaccination in the vaccine group.

In the second approach, all uninfected participants in the control group are vaccinated with the pneumococcal vaccine at the end of the trial and their immune responses are recorded. Then one assumes that the immune response they have at the end of the trial is the response they would have had if vaccinated at the beginning of the trial. By comparing the distribution of immune responses with the full distribution of immune responses in the vaccinated group, because of randomization, one can infer what the distribution of immune responses in the infected participants in the control group would have been. Qin et al (2008) develop details of using case-cohort sampling and a Cox proportional hazards model to assess surrogate endpoint candidates in vaccine trials as developed by Gilbert and Hudgens (2008) using the two different augmented vaccine trial designs.

15.6 Carriage as an Endpoint

Nasopharyngeal carriage is being considered as a target and an endpoint for trials of multivalent pneumococcal congugate vaccines (Käyhty et al 2006). The goal of the PneumoCarr project, an international consortium coordinated in Finland, is to establish reduction of colonization as part of the licensure process of new vaccines. The vaccine efficacy measure is called VE_{col}. Similar to the use of immunological surrogates rather than clinical endpoints, colonization is potentially a much more cost-effective method to evaluate vaccine efficacy than using other clinical endpoints. A second goal of the project is to identify serological correlates of VE_{col}. Information is available at the PneumoCarr website. A new endpoint in pneumococcal vaccine trials is needed. Invasive pneumococcal disease is a rare event that is difficult to study in detail. Its diagnosis is dependent on local medical practices and requires special equipment and training. Acute otitis media as the primary outcome is problematic. Specific diagnosis of pneumococcal bacteria as the infectious agent causing the otitis media needs special procedures to obtain a bacteriological outcome. Otitis media is perceived differently in different parts of the world. Pneumonia as an outcome is problematic because diagnosis and definition of a case are not specific. A lung aspirate is required, which is simply not feasible, so there is no bacteriological endpoint.

Using nasopharyngeal carriage as an endpoint in vaccine trials makes sense for several reasons (Käyhty et al 2006). It is the most important endpoint because preventing carriage will prevent all of the other endpoints directly in the person vaccinated and it will prevent transmission to others, because carriage is the source of infection to others. Nasopharyngeal carriage as a pneumococcal endpoint can teach about other mucosal infections, such as meningococcal carriage. Comparing the relative incidence of the various candidate outcomes, carriage is by far the most frequent. It is also the most accessible endpoint, making it a feasible outcome. Vaccine efficacy for acquisition of carriage, VE_{acq}, based on rate of acquisition been shown to be better than based on prevalence (Rinta-Kokko et al 2009). Nasopharyngeal carriage is abundant both before and after introduction of vaccine. It permits feasible follow-up of dynamics after introduction of vaccines, such as reduction in carriage, and development of antibiotic resistance.

However, the far the known predictors for protection against invasive pneumococcal disease do not predict protection against carriage, spread and mucosal infections. One caveat with nasopharyngeal carriage as an endpoint is the difference in disease potential of different serotypes to various infection sites. Another caveat is the uncertainty in the models used for estimating the acquisition rates and clearance rates to be used in estimating VE_{acq} or VE_{col}. Three types of predictors can be used to measure the effect of vaccination on nasopharyngeal carriage. Prevention of new acquisitions measures direct protection, and can be estimated analogously to $VE_{S,\lambda}$. Prevalence of carriage is a measure of indirect protection. Density of carriage is a measure of direct and indirect protection. Estimation of pneumococcal acquisition and clearance rates based on longitudinal household and school studies is presented in Chapter 11.

Problems

15.1. Estimating predicted efficacy

(a) Show that the estimated model (15.12) for the WHO definition of pertussis gives the predicted attack rates 66.3% and 11.0%.

(b) Another case definition in Storsaeter et al (1998) was whether the study child was laboratory-positive for pertussis and had at least one day cough during the follow-up period. A noncase was a study child who was laboratory negative or laboratory positive but without cough. For this definition, the fitted model was

$$g(x) = 2.003 - 0.146\text{PT} - 1.548\text{FIM} - 1.990\text{PRN} + 1.148(\text{PT} \times \text{FIM}). \tag{15.19}$$

What are the predicted attack rates in the Low and High groups?

15.2. Correlates of risk and surrogates of protection
(a) What are the main differences between a correlate of risk and a surrogate of protection?
(b) What is the difference between a statistical surrogate of protection and a principal surrogate of protection? Under what conditions can either of these be estimated?
(c) What is the difference between a specific surrogate of protection and a general surrogate of protection? Under what conditions could you validate the latter? Which is of more intrinsic interest?

Solutions

Problems of Chapter 2

2.1 (a) level II; (b) $\text{VE}_{S,IR}$, $\text{VE}_{S,\lambda}$, $\text{VE}_{S,PH}$, $\text{VE}_{S,CI}$.

2.2 1.67 .

2.3 (a) 0.91 .

2.4 (a) 0.64; (b) The difference is explained by the assumption of when the soldiers were immunized.

2.5 (a) 0.80, 0.64, 0.93, 0.81; (b) 390, 120.

Problems of Chapter 5

5.6 Prevalence of infection in the women is higher than in men largely because the duration is longer, so there are a greater number of susceptible men than women who are at risk to become new cases, $(1 - P_m) > (1 - P_f)$. The susceptible men make the same number of contacts and have the same transmission probability as the women, but their contact pool, the women, has a higher prevalence of infection, so the incidence rate is higher in the men, $I_m = cpP_f > cpP_m = I_f$. The combined effect in the men of higher incidence rate and greater proportion susceptible results in a higher number of new cases in men than in women.

Problems of Chapter 9

9.3 $\widehat{\text{AVE}}_P = 1 - (10/46)(33/75) = 0.56$ (95% CI 0.10, 0.73).

Problems of Chapter 11

11.1 (a) 0.70; (b) 0.67 .

11.2 (a) SAR: children 0.91; adults 0.91; CPI: children 0.59; adults 0.21; AR: children 0.70; adults 0.47.

Problems of Chapter 12

12.1 (a) Study 1: $\text{SAR}_v = 0.11$, $\text{SAR}_u = 0.43$, $\text{VE}_{S,SAR} = 0.74$ (95% CI 0.29,0.89). Study 2: $\text{SAR}_v = 0.07$, $\text{SAR}_u = 0.43$, $\text{VE}_{S,SAR} = 0.85$ (95% CI 0.39,0.94).

Problems of Chapter 13

13.3 (a)

$$\binom{24}{2}\binom{22}{2}\binom{20}{2}\binom{18}{2}\binom{16}{2}\binom{14}{2}\binom{12}{2}\binom{10}{2}\binom{8}{2}\binom{6}{2}\binom{4}{2}\binom{2}{2} = 1.5 \times 10^{20}.$$

13.4 (a) 80% power, instead of using 0.8416, use $0.8416 \times 1.2 = 1.01$. For type I error of 5%, instead of 1.96, use 2.352. (b) $1.2^2 = 2.44$. (c) Compute the effective sample size by multiplying the person-time y in the sample size calculation by 1.5.

References

1. P Aaby, B Samb, M Anderson, and F Simondon. No long-term excess mortality after measles infection: A community study from Senegal. *Am J Epidemiol*, 143:1035–41, 1996.
2. O Aalen. Heterogeneity in survival analysis. *Stat Med*, 7:1121–1137, 1988.
3. O Aalen. Modelling heterogeneity in survival analysis by the compound Poisson distribution. *Ann Appl Probab*, 2:951–972, 1992.
4. H Abbey. An examination of the Reed-Frost theory of epidemics. *Hum Biol*, 24:201–233, 1952.
5. CL Addy, IM Longini, and MS Haber. A generalized stochastic model for the analysis of infectious disease final size data. *Biometrics*, 47:961–974, 1991.
6. RA Adegbola, O Secka, G Lahai, N Lloyd-Evans, A Njie, S Usen, C Oluwalana, S Obaro, M Weber, T Corrah, K Mulholland, K McAdam, B Greenwood, and PJM Milligan. Elimination of Haemophilus influenzae type b (Hib) disease from The Gambia after the introduction of routine immunisation with a Hib conjugate vaccine: A prospective study. *Lancet*, 366:144–150, 2005.
7. A Agresti. *Categorical Data Analysis*. John Wiley and Sons, New York, 1990.
8. A Agresti and B Coull. Approximate is better than 'exact' for interval estimation of binomial proportions. *Am Stat*, 52:119–126, 1998.
9. JM Albert. Testing for AIDS vaccine efficacy in small sample preclinical studies. *Stat Med*, 15:2371–79, 1996.
10. M Ali, M Emch, M von Seidlein, M Yunus, DA Sack, M Rao, J Holmgren, and JD Clemens. Herd immunity conferred by killed oral cholera vaccines in Bangladesh: A reanalysis. *Lancet*, 366:44–49, 2005.
11. PL Alonso, T Smith, JRM Armstrong Schellenberg, H Masanja, S Mwankusye, et al. Randomised trial of efficacy of SPf66 vaccine against *Plasmodium falciparum* malaria in children in southern Tanzania. *Lancet*, 344:1175–1181, 1994.
12. DG Altman, KF Schulz, D Moher, M Egger, F Davidoff, D Elbourne, PC Gotzsche, and T Lang. The revised CONSORT statement for reporting randomized trials: Explanation and elaboration. *Ann Intern Med*, 134(8):663–694, 2001.
13. R Amador, A Moreno, A Valero, et al. The first field trials of the chemically synthesized malaria vaccine SPf66: Safety, immunogenicity and protectivity. *Vaccine*, 10:179–184, 1992.
14. PK Andersen and RD Gill. Cox's regression model for counting processes: A large sample study. *Ann Statist*, 10:1100–1120, 1982.
15. RM Anderson and RM May, editors. *Population Biology of Infectious Diseases*. Springer-Verlag, Berlin, 1982.
16. RM Anderson and RM May. *Infectious Diseases of Human: Dynamics and Control*. Oxford University Press, Oxford, 1991.
17. H Andersson and T Britton. *Stochastic Epidemic Models and Their Statistical Analysis*. Springer, New York, 2000.

18. N Andrews, R Borrow, and E Miller. Validation of serological correlate of protection for meningococcal C conjugate vaccine by using efficacy estimates from postlicensure surveillance in England. *Clin Diagn Lab Immunol*, 10:780–786, 2003.
19. JJ Angulo. Variola minor in Bragança Paulista County, 1956: Overall description of the epidemic and its study. *Int J Epidemiol*, 5:359–366, 1976.
20. R Antia, JC Koella, and V Perrot. Models of the within-host dynamics of persistent mycobacterial infections. *Proc R Soc Lond B*, 263:257–263, 1996.
21. SS Antia, R Pilyugin and R Ahmed. Models of immune memory: On the role of cross-reacitve stimulation, competition, and homeostasis in maintaining immune memory. *Proc Natl Acad Sci USA*, 95:14926–31, 1998.
22. E Arjas. Survival models and martingale dynamics. *Scand J Stat*, 16:177–225, 1989.
23. JL Aron and RM May. The population dynamics of malaria. In RM Anderson, editor, *Population Dynamics of Infectious Diseases: Theory and Application*, pages 139–179. Chapman and Hall, London, 1982.
24. K Auranen, E Arjas, T Leino, and AK Takala. Transmission of pneumococcal carriage in families: A latent Markov process model for binary longitudinal data. *J Am Stat Assoc*, 95:1044–1053, 2000.
25. K Auranen, J Ranta, AK Takala, and E Arjas. A statistical model of transmission of Hib bacteria in a family. *Stat Med*, 15:2235–2252, 1996.
26. P Baccam, C Beauchemin, CA Macken, FG Hayden, and AS Perelson. Kinetics of influenza A virus infection in humans. *J Virol*, 80(15):7590–9, 2006.
27. NTJ Bailey. *The Mathematical Theory of Epidemics*. Griffin, London, 1957.
28. NTJ Bailey. *The Mathematical Theory of Infectious Diseases and Its Application*. Griffin, London, 2nd edition, 1975.
29. R Bailey. Restricted randomization. *Biometrika*, 70:183–98, 1983.
30. F Ball. A unified approach to the distribution of total size and total area under the trajectory of infectives in epidemic models. *Adv Appl Probab*, 18:289–310, 1986.
31. WR Ballou, J Blood, T Chongsuphajaissidhi, DM Gordon, et al. Field trial of an asexual blood stage malaria vaccine: Studies of the synthetic polymer SPf66 in Thailand and the analytic plan for a phase IIb efficacy study. *Parasitology*, 110:Supp:S25–S36, 1995.
32. P Balmer and R Borrow. Serologic correlates of protection for evaluating the response to meningococcal vaccines. *Expert Rev Vaccines*, 3(1):77–87, 2004.
33. OE Barndorff-Nielson and DR Cox. *Inference and Asymptotics*. Chapman and Hall, New York, 1994.
34. N Basta, ME Halloran, L Matrajt, and IM Longini. Estimating influenza vaccine efficacy from challenge and community-based study data. *Am J Epidemiol*, 168:1343–1352, 2008.
35. NG Becker. Estimation in models for the spread of infectious diseases. In *Proceedings of the XIth International Biometrics Conference*, pages 145–151, 1982.
36. NG Becker. A generalized linear modeling approach to the analysis of a single epidemic. In I Francis, B Manley, and F Lam, editors, *Proceedings Pacific Statistical Congress*, pages 464–467, 1985.
37. NG Becker. *Analysis of Infectious Disease Data*. Chapman and Hall, London, 1989.
38. NG Becker and JJ Angulo. On estimating the contagiousness of a disease transmitted from person to person. *Math Biosci*, 54:137–154, 1981.
39. NG Becker, T Britton, and PD O'Neill. Estimating vaccine effects on transmission of infection from household outbreak data. *Biometrics*, 59:467–475, 2003.
40. NG Becker, T Britton, and PD O'Neill. Estimating vaccine effects from studies of outbreaks in household pairs. *Stat Med*, 25:1079–1093, 2006.
41. NG Becker and R Hall. Immunization levels for preventing epidemics in a community of households made up of individuals of various types. *Math Biosci*, 132(2):205–216, 1996.
42. NG Becker and DN Starczak. The effect of random vaccine response on the vaccination coverage required to prevent epidemics. *Math Biosci*, 154:117–135, 1998.
43. CG Beckett, H Kosasih, I Faisal, et al. Early detection of dengue infections using cluster sampling around index cases. *Am J Trop Med Hyg*, 72(6):777–782, 2005.

44. RB Belshe, KM Edwards, T Vesikari, et al. Live attenuated versus inactivated influenza vaccine in infants and young children. *N Engl J Med*, 356:685–696, 2007.
45. RB Belshe, PM Mendelman, J Treanor, et al. The efficacy of live attenuated, cold-adapted, trivalent, intranasal influenzavirus vaccine in children. *N Engl J Med*, 338:1405–1412, 1998.
46. RB Belshe, WC Gruber, PM Mendelman, et al. Correlates of immune protection induced by live attenuated, cold-adapted, trivalent, intranasal influenza virus vaccine in children. *J Infect Dis*, 181:1133–1137, 2000.
47. S Black, H Shinefeld, B Fireman, and R Hiatt. Safety, immunogenicity and efficacy in infancy of oligosaccharide conjugate *Haemophilus influenzae* type b vaccine in a United States population: Possible implications for optimal use. *J Infect Dis*, 165(Suppl 1):S139–43, 1992.
48. S Black, H Shinefeld, B Fireman, et al. Efficacy, safety and immunogenicity of heptavalent pneumococcal conjugate vaccine in children. Northern California Kaiser Permanente Vaccine Study Center Group. *Pediatr Infect Dis J*, 19:187–195, 2000.
49. MF Boyd, editor. *Malariology*. W.B. Saunders Co., Philadelphia, 1949.
50. P Bremaud. *Point Processes and Queues*. Springer Verlag, New York, 1981.
51. NE Breslow and BE Storer. General relative risk functions for case-control studies. *Am J Epidemiol*, 122:149–162, 1985.
52. KA Brownlee. Statistics of the 1954 polio vaccine trials. *J Am Stat Assoc*, 50:1005–1013, 1955.
53. LJ Bruce-Chwatt. The challenge of malaria vaccine: Trials and tribulations. *Lancet*, i:371–372, 1987.
54. RC Brunet, CJ Struchiner, and ME Halloran. On the distribution of vaccine protection under heterogeneous response. *Math Biosci*, 116:111–125, 1993.
55. W Buchan. *Domestic Medicine: or A Treatise on the Prevention and Cure of Diseases by Regimen and Simple Medicines*. Sleater, Moore, White and Rice, Dublin, 12 edition, 1792.
56. M Burnet and DO White. *Natural History of Infectious Disease*. Cambridge University Press, Cambridge, fourth edition, 1972.
57. T Burzykowski, G Molenberghs, and M Buyse. *The Evaluation of Surrogate Endpoints*. Springer, New York, 2005.
58. BP Carlin and TA Louis. *Bayesian Methods for Data Analysis*. CRC, Boca Raton FL, third edition, 2008.
59. F Carrat, CSahler, M Leuez, et al. Influenza burden of illness: Estimates from a national prospective survey of household contacts in france. *Arch Intern Med*, 162:1842–1848, 2002.
60. S Cauchemez, , PY Boëlle, G Thomas, and AJ Valleron. Estimating in real-time the efficacy of control measures in emerging communicable diseases. *Am J Epidemiol*, 164:591–594, 2006a.
61. S Cauchemez, F Carrat, C Viboud, AJ Valleron, and PY Boëlle. A Bayesian MCMC approach to study transmission of influenza: Application to household longitudinal data. *Stat Med*, 23:3469–87, 2004.
62. S Cauchemez, L Temime, D Guillemot, E Varon, AJ Valleron, G Thomas, and PY Boëlle. Investigating heterogeneity in pneumococcal transmission: A Bayesian MCMC approach applied to a follow-up of schools. *J Am Stat Assoc*, 101:946–958, 2006c.
63. S Cauchemez, L Temime, AJ Valleron, E Varon, G Thomas, D Guillemot, and PY Boëlle. *S. pneumoniae* transmission according to inclusion in conjugate vaccines: Bayesian analysis of a longitudinal follow-up in schools. *BMC Infect Dis*, 6:14, 2006d.
64. S Cauchemez, P-Y Boëlle, CA Donnelly, et al. Real-time estimates in early detection of SARS. *Emerging Infect Dis*, 12:110–113, 2006b.
65. ISF Chan, L Shu, H Matthews, C Chan, R Vessey, et al. Use of statistical models for evaluating antibody response as a correlate of protection against varicella. *Stat Med*, 21:3411–30, 2002.
66. MN Chang, HA Guess, and JF Heyse. Reduction in burden of illness: A new efficacy measure for prevention trials. *Stat Med*, 13:1807–1814, 1994.
67. MA Chaudhary and LH Moulton. A SAS macro for constrained randomization of group-randomized designs. *Comput Methods Programs Biomed*, 83:205–210, 2006.

68. RT Chen, R Weierbach, Z Bisoffi, F Cutts, P Rhodes, S Ramarsosn, C Ntembagara, and F Bizimana. A ‘post-honeymoon period’ measles outbreak in Muyinga Sector, Burundi. *Int J Epidemiol*, 23:185–193, 1994.
69. SE Chick, DE Barth-Jones, and JS Koopman. Bias reduction for risk ratio and vaccine effect estimators. *Stat Med*, 20:1609–1624, 2001.
70. H Chu and ME Halloran. Bayesian estimation of vaccine efficacy. *Clin Trials*, 1:306–314, 2004.
71. H Chu, ME Halloran, and MP Préziosi. Estimating heterogeneous transmission with multiple infectives using MCMC methods. *Stat Med*, 23:35–49, 2004.
72. B Cisse, P Aaby, F Simondon, B Samb, M Soumaré, and H Whittle. Role of schools in the tranmission of measles in rural Senegal: Implications for measles control in developing countries. *Am J Epidemiol*, 149:295–301, 1999.
73. JD Clemens, R Brenner, M Rao, N Tafari, and C Lowe. Evaluating new vaccines for developing countries: Efficacy or effectiveness? *J Am Med Assoc*, 275:390–397, 1996.
74. JD Clemens, DA Sack, J Harris, et al. Field trial of oral cholera vaccines. *Lancet*, 2:124–7, 1986.
75. JD Clemens, DA Sack, J Harris, et al. Field trial of oral cholera vaccines in Bangladesh: Results of one year of follow-up. *J Infect Dis*, 158:60–69, 1988.
76. JD Clemens, DA Sack, JR Harris, et al. Field trial of oral cholera vaccines in Bangladesh: Results from three year follow-up. *Lancet*, 335:270–273, 1990.
77. ML Clements, RF Betts, and BR Murphy. Advantage of live attenuated cold-adapted influenza A virus over inactivated vaccine for A/Washington/80 (H3N2) wild-type virus infection. *Lancet*, 1:705–8, 1984.
78. ML Clements-Mann. Lessons for AIDS vaccine development from non-AIDS vaccines. *AIDS Res Hum Retroviruses*, 14 Suppl 3:S197–203, 1998.
79. ML Clements, MH Snyder, SD Sears, et al. Evaluation of the infectivity, immunogenicity, and efficacy of live cold-adapted influenza B/Ann Arbor/1/86 reassortant virus vaccine in adult volunteers. *J Infect Dis*, 161:869–77, 1990.
80. ML Clements, RF Betts, EL Tierney, et al. Resistance of adults to challenge with influenza A wild-type virus after receiving live or inactivated virus vaccine. *J Clin Microbiol*, 23:73–6, 1986.
81. C Clopper and S Pearson. The use of confidence or fiducial limits illustrated in the case of the binomial. *Biometrika*, 404–413:1934, 26.
82. DR Cox. *Planning of Experiments*. John Wiley and Sons, Inc, New York, 1958.
83. DR Cox. Regression models and life-tables (with discussion). *J R Stat Soc Series B*, 30:284–289, 1972.
84. U D’Alessandro, A Leach, CJ Drakeley, S Bennett, BO Olaleye, GW Fegan, M Jawara, P Langerock, MO George, GAT Targett, and BM Greenwood. Efficacy trial of malaria vaccine SPf66 in Gambian infants. *Lancet*, 346:462–467, 1995.
85. P Damien, J Wakefield, and S Walker. Gibbs sampling for Bayesian non-conjugate and hierarchical models by using auxiliary variables. *J R Stat Soc Series B*, 61:331–344, 1999.
86. MJ Daniels and MD Hughes. Meta-analysis for the evaluation of potential surrogate markers. *Stat Med*, 16:1965–82, 1997.
87. HG Dantes, JS Koopman, CL Addy, ML Zarate, MAV Marin, IM Longini, ES Guttierez, VA Rodriguez, LG Garcia, and ER Mirelles. Dengue epidemics on the Pacific Coast of Mexico. *Int J Epidemiol*, 17:178–186, 1988.
88. S Datta, ME Halloran, and IM Longini. Augmented HIV vaccine trial designs for estimating reduction in infectiousness and protective efficacy. *Stat Med*, 17:185–200, 1998.
89. S Datta, ME Halloran, and IM Longini. Efficiency of estimating vaccine efficacy for susceptibility and infectiousness: Randomization by individual versus household. *Biometrics*, 55:792–798, 1999.
90. M Davidian and DM Giltinan. *Nonlinear Models for Repeated Measurement Data*. Chapman and Hall/ CRC, New York, 1995.
91. B de Finetti. *Theory of Probability*. Wiley, New York, 1974.

92. V DeGruttola, T Fleming, DY Lin, and R Coombs. Perspective: Validating surrogate markers – Are we being naive? *J Infect Dis*, 175:237–46, 1997.
93. O Diekmann and JAP Heesterbeek. *Mathematical Epidemiology of Infectious Diseases: Model Building, Analysis, and Interpretation.* John Wiley, Chichester, 2000.
94. O Diekmann, JAP Heesterbeek, and JAJ Metz. On the definition and the computation of the basic reproduction ratio R_0 in models for infectious diseases in heterogeneous populations. *J Math Biol*, 28:365–382, 1990.
95. K Dietz. The first epidemic model: A historical note on P. D. En'ko. *Austral J Stat*, 30A:56–65, 1988.
96. PJ Diggle, K-Y Liang, and SL Zeger. *Analysis of Longitudinal Data.* Oxford University Press, Oxford, 1994.
97. JH Dingle, GF Badger, and WS Jordan, Jr. *Illness in the Home.* The Press of Western Reserve University, Cleveland, 1964.
98. A Donner. Some aspects of the design and analysis of cluster randomization trials. *Appl Stat*, 47:95–114, 1998.
99. A Donner and N Klar. Cluster randomization trials in epidemiology: Theory and application. *J Stat Plan Inference*, 42:37–56, 1994.
100. AJ Dunning. A model for immunolgoical correlates of protection. *Stat Med*, 25:1485–97, 2006.
101. LK Durham, ME Halloran, IM Longini, and AM Manatunga. Comparison of two smoothing methods for exploring waning vaccine effects. *Appl Stat*, 48:395–407, 1999.
102. LK Durham, IM Longini, ME Halloran, JD Clemens, A Nizam, and M Rao. Estimation of vaccine efficacy in the presence of waning: Application to cholera vaccines. *Am J Epidemiol*, 147:948–959, 1998.
103. B Efron. Forcing a sequential experiment to be balanced. *Biometrika*, 58:403–17, 1971.
104. B Efron. R.A. Fisher in the 21st century. *Stat Sci*, 13:95–122, 1998.
105. B Efron and RJ Tibshirani. *An Introduction to the Bootstrap.* Chapman and Hall, New York, 1993.
106. DRA Ellenberger, A Otten, V Li, et al. HIV-1 DNA/MVA vaccination reduces the per exposure probability of information during repeated mucosal SHIV challenges. *Virology*, 352:216–225, 2006.
107. L Elveback and A Varma. Simulation of mathematical models for public health problems. *Public Health Rep*, 80:1067–76, 1965.
108. LR Elveback, JP Fox, E Ackerman, A Langworthy, M Boyd, and L Gatewood. An influenza simulation model for immunization studies. *Am J Epidemiol*, 103:152–65, 1976.
109. S Eubank, H Guclu, VSA Kumar, MV Marathe, A Srinivasan, Z Toroczkai, and N Wang. Modelling disease outbreaks in realistic urban social networks. *Nature*, 429:180–184, 2004.
110. M Ewell. Comparing methods for calculating confidence intervals for vaccine efficacy. *Stat Med*, 15:2379–2392, 1996.
111. VT Farewell. The use of mixture models for the analysis of survival data with long-term survivors. *Biometrics*, 38:1041–6, 1982.
112. CP Farrington. The measurement and interpretation of age-specific vaccine efficacy. *Int J Epidemiol*, 21:1014–1020, 1992.
113. CP Farrington. Estimation of vaccine effectiveness using the screening method. *Int J Epidemiol*, 22:742–746, 1993.
114. CP Farrington. Relative incidence estimation from case series for vaccine safety evaluations. *Biometrics*, 51:228–235, 1995.
115. CP Farrington. On vaccine efficacy and reproduction numbers. *Math Biosci*, 185:89–109, 2003.
116. MP Fay, ME Halloran, and DA Follmann. Accounting for variability in sample size estimation with applications to nonadherence and estimation of variance and effect size. *Biometrics*, 63:465–474, 2007.
117. F Fenner, DA Henderson, I Arita, et al. *Smallpox and its Eradication.* World Health Organization, Geneva, 1988.

118. NM Ferguson, DAT Cummings, C Fraser, JC Cajka, PC Cooley, and DS Burke. Strategies for mitigating an influenza pandemic. *Nature*, 442:448–252, 2006. doi:10.1038/nature04795.
119. PE Fine and JA Clarkson. The recurrence of whooping cough: possible implications for assessment of vaccine efficacy. *Lancet*, 1:666–69, 1982.
120. PEM Fine. A commentary on the mechanical analogue to the Reed–Frost epidemic model. *Am J Epidemiol*, 106(2):87–100, 1977.
121. PEM Fine. Herd immunity. *Epidemiol Rev*, 15:265–302, 1993.
122. PEM Fine. The interval between successive cases of an infectious disease. *Am J Epidemiol*, 158:1039–1047, 2003.
123. PEM Fine and RT Chen. Confounding in studies of adverse reactions to vaccines. *Am J Epidemiol*, 136:121–135, 1992.
124. PEM Fine and JA Clarkson. Reflections on the efficacy of pertussis vaccines. *Rev Inf Dis*, 9(5):866–883, 1987.
125. PEM Fine, JA Clarkson, and E Miller. The efficacy of pertussis vaccines under conditions of household exposure: Further analysis of the 1978-80 PHLS-ERL study in 21 area health authorities in England. *Int J Epidemiol*, 17(3):635–642, 1988.
126. PEM Fine and K Mulholland. Community immunity. In SA Plotkin, WA Orenstein, and PA Offit, editors, *Vaccines*. Elsevier/Saunders, Philadelphia, 5th edition, 2008.
127. T Fleming and D Harrington. *Counting Processes and Survival Analysis*. Wiley and Sons, New York, 1991.
128. TR Fleming. Intermediate-sized trials for the evaluation of HIV vaccine candidates (abstract). In *Conference on Advances in AIDS Vaccine Development: 8th Annual Cooperative Vaccine Development Groups for AIDS Meeting Program Book.*, page 108, Bethesda, MD, 1996. National Institutes of Health.
129. TR Fleming and DL DeMets. Surrogate endpoints in clinical trials: Are we being misled? *Ann Intern Med*, 125:605–613, 1996.
130. D Follmann. Augmented designs to assess immune response in vaccine trials. *Biometrics*, 62:1161–1169, 2006.
131. D Follmann, MP Fay, and M Proschan. Chop-lump tests for vaccine trials. *Biometrics*, in press:., 2009.
132. BD Forrest, MW Pride, AJ Dunning, et al. Correlation of cellular immune response with protection against culture-confirmed influenza in young children. *Clin Vaccine Immunol*, 15:1042–1053, 2008.
133. J Fox and L Elveback. Herd immunity: Changing concepts. In AL Notkins, editor, *Viral Immunology and Immunopathology*, chapter 16, pages 273–290. Academic Press, New York, 1975.
134. JP Fox, MK Cooney, CE Hall, and HM Foy. Influenzavirus infections in Seattle families, 1975–1979: Pattern of infection in invaded households and the relation of age and prior antibody to occurrensce of infection and related illness. *Am J Epidemiol*, 116:228–242, 1982a.
135. JP Fox, CE Hall, MK Cooney, and HM Foy. Influenzavirus infections in Seattle families, 1975–1979: Study design, methods and the occurrence of infections by time and age. *Am J Epidemiol*, 116:212–227, 1982b.
136. JP Fox, CE Hall, and LR Elveback. *Epidemiology: Man and Disease*. MacMillan, New York, 1970.
137. T Francis, RF Korns, RB Voights, M Boisen, FM Hemphill, JA Napier, and E Tolchinsky. An evaluation of the 1954 poliomyelitis vaccine trials. *Am J Pub Health*, 45:1–63, 1955.
138. DP Francis, SC Hadler, SE Thompson, et al. The prevention of hepatitis B with vaccine: Report of the Centers for Disease Control multi-center efficacy trial among homosexual men. *Ann of Intern Med*, 97:362–366, 1982.
139. CE Frangakis and DB Rubin. Principal stratification in causal inference. *Biometrics*, 58:21–29, 2002.
140. CE Frasch. Regulatory perspectives in vaccine licensure. In RW Ellis and DM Granoff, editors, *Development and Clinical Uses of Haemophilus influenzae Type b Conjugate Vaccines*, pages 435–53. Marcel Dekker, New York, 1994.

141. C Fraser, S Riley, RM Anderson, and NM Ferguson. Factors that make an infectious disease controllable. *Proc Natl Acad Sci USA*, 101:6146–6151, 2004.
142. MJ Gaglani, PA Piedra, GB Herschler, ME Griffith, CA Kozinetz, MW Riggs, C Fewlass, ME Halloran, IM Longini, and P Glezen. Direct effectiveness of the trivalent, cold-adapted, influenza virus vaccine (CAIV-T) against the 2000–2001 influenza A (H1N1) and B epidemic in healthy children. *Arch Pediatr Adolesc Med*, 158:65–73, 2004.
143. MH Gail. Adjusting for covariates that have the same distribution in exposed and unexposed cohorts. In SH Moolgavkar and RL Prentice, editors, *Modern Statistical Methods*, pages 3–18. Wiley, New York, 1986.
144. MH Gail. The effect of pooling across strata in perfectly balanced studies. *Biometrics*, 44:151–162, 1988.
145. MH Gail. A bibliography and comments on the use of statistical models in epidemiology in the 1980s. *Stat Med*, 10:1819–1885, 1991.
146. MH Gail, R Pfeiffer, HC Van Houwelingen, and RJ Carroll. On the meta-analytic assessment of surrogate outcomes. *Biostatistics*, 1:231–46, 1989.
147. MH Gail, WY Tan, and S Piantadosi. The effect of omitting covariates on tests for no treatment effect in randomized clinical trials. *Biometrika*, 75:57–64, 1988.
148. MH Gail, S Wieand, and S Piantadosi. Biased estimates of treatment effect in randomized experiments with non-linear regressions and omitted covariates. *Biometrika*, 71:431–444, 1984.
149. Gambia Hepatitis Study Group. The Gambia Hepatitis Intervention Study. *Cancer Res*, 47:5782–5787, 1987.
150. M Garenne and P Cantrelle. Three decades of research on population and health: the Orstom experience in rural Senegal,1962-1991. In M Das Gupta, P Aaby, M Garenne, and G Pison, editors, *Prospective Community Studies in Developing Countries (International Studies in Demography)*, pages 233–52. Clarendon Press, Oxford, 1998.
151. M Garenne, O Leroy, J-P Beau, and I Sene. Efficacy of measles vaccines after controlling for exposure. *Am J Epidemiol*, 138:182–195, 1993.
152. M Garenne, O Leroy, J-P Beau, et al. Efficacy, safety and immunogenicity of two high-titer measles vaccines: Final report. Technical report, ORSTOM, Dakar, Senegal, 1991.
153. TC Germann, K Kadau, IM Longini, and CA Macken. Mitigation strategies for pandemic influenza in the United States. *Proc Natl Acad Sci USA*, 103:5935–40, 2006.
154. PB Gilbert. Comparison of competing risks failure time methods and time-independent methods for assessing strain variations in vaccine protection. *Stat Med*, 19(22):3065–3086, 2000.
155. PB Gilbert, RJ Bosch, and MG Hudgens. Sensitivity analysis for the assessment of causal vaccine effects on viral load in HIV vaccine trials. *Biometrics*, 59:531–541, 2003a.
156. PB Gilbert, V DeGruttola, MG Hudgens, SG Self, SM Hammer, and L Corey. What constitutes efficacy for a human immunodeficiency virus vaccine that ameliorates viremia: Issues involving surrogate end points in Phase 3 trials trials. *J Infect Dis*, 188:179–193, 2003b.
157. PB Gilbert and MG Hudgens. Evaluating candidate principal surrogate endpoints. *Biometrics*, 64(4):1146–1154, 2008.
158. PB Gilbert, S Lele, and Y Vardi. Maximum likelihood estimation in semiparametric selection bias models with application to AIDS vaccine trials. *Biometrika*, 86:27–43, 1999.
159. PB Gilbert, L Qin, and SG Self. Evaluating a surrogate endpoint at three levels, with application to vaccine development. *Stat Med*, 27:4758–4778, 2008.
160. PB Gilbert, S Self, and M Ashby. Statistical methods for assessing differential vaccine protection against HIV types. *Biometrics*, 54:799–814, 1998.
161. PB Gilbert, S Self, M Rao, A Naficy, and J Clemens. Sieve analysis: Methods for assessing from vaccine trial data how vaccine efficacy varies with genotypic and phenotypic pathogen variation. *J Clin Epidemiol*, 54:68–85, 2001.
162. WR Gilks, CC Wang, B Yvonnet, and P Coursaget. Random-effects models for longitudinal data using Gibbs sampling. *Biometrics*, 49:441–454, 1993.
163. A Gjini, JM Stuart, RC George, T Nichols, and RS Heyderman. Capture-recapture analysis and pneumococcal meningitis estimates in England. *Emerging Infect Dis*, 10:87–93, 2004.

164. I Goldschneider, EC Gotschlich, and MS Artenstein. Human immunity to the meningococcus: I. The role of humoral antibodies. *J Exp Med*, 129:1327–1348, 1969.
165. GT Golm, ME Halloran, and IM Longini. Semiparametric models for mismeasured exposure information in vaccine trials. *Stat Med*, 17:2335–2352, 1998.
166. GT Golm, ME Halloran, and IM Longini. Semiparametric methods for multiple exposure mismeasurement and a bivariate outcome in HIV vaccine trials. *Biometrics*, 55:94–101, 1999.
167. PM Grambsch and TM Therneau. Proportional hazards test and diagnostics based on weighted residuals. *Biometrika*, 81:515–526, 1994.
168. SM Granat, Z Mia, J Ollgren, E Herva, M Das, L Piirainen, K Auranen, and PM Mäkelä. Longitudinal study on pneumococcal carriage during the first year of life in Bangladesh. *Ped Inf Dis J*, 26:319–324, 2007.
169. S Greenland. Interpretation and estimation of summary ratios under heterogeneity. *Stat Med*, 1:217–227, 1982.
170. S Greenland. Interpretation and choice of effect measures in epidemiologic analyses. *Am J Epidemiol*, 125:761–768, 1987.
171. S Greenland. Confounding in epidemiologic studies. *Biometrics*, 45:1309–22, 1989.
172. S Greenland. Absence of confounding does not correspond to collapsibility of the rate ratio or rate difference. *Epidemiology*, 7:498–501, 1996.
173. S Greenland and RR Frerichs. On measures and models for the effectiveness of vaccines and vaccination programs. *Int J Epidemiol*, 17(2):456–463, 1988.
174. S Greenland and JM Robins. Identifiability, exchangeability, and epidemiologic confounding. *Int J Epidemiol*, 15:412–18, 1986.
175. S Greenland and JM Robins. Conceptual problems in the defintion and interpretation of attributable fraction. *Am J Epidemiol*, 128:1185–1197, 1988.
176. S Greenland, JM Robins, and J Pearl. Confounding and collapsibility in causal inference. *Stat Sci*, 14:29–46, 1999.
177. S Greenland and DC Thomas. On the need for the rare disease assumption in case-control studies. *Am J Epidemiol*, 116(3):547–553, 1982.
178. S Greenland, DC Thomas, and H Morgenstern. The rare disease assumption revisited: A critique of "estimators of relative risk for case-control studies". *Am J Epidemiol*, 124(6):869–876, 1986.
179. M Greenwood. On the statistical measure of infectiousness. *J Hyg Camb*, 31:336–351, 1931.
180. M Greenwood and UG Yule. The statistics of anti-typhoid and anti-cholera inoculations, and the interpretation of such statistics in general. *Proc R Soc Med*, 8(part 2):113–194, 1915.
181. H Grosskurth, F Mosha, J Todd, J et al. Impact of improved treatment of sexually transmitted disease on HIV infection in rural Tanzania: Randomised controlled trial. *Lancet*, 346:530–536, 1995.
182. D Guillemot, E Varon, C Bernède, P Weber, L Henriet, S Simon, C Laurent, H Lecoeur, and C Carbon. Reduction of antibiotic use in the community reduces the rate of colonization with penicillin G-nonsusceptible *Streptococcus pneumoniae*. *Clin Infect Dise*, 41:930–938, 2005.
183. L Gustafsson, HO Hallander, P Olin, E Reizenstein, and J Storsaeter. A controlled trial of a two-component acellular, a five component acellular and a whole-cell pertussis vaccine. *N Engl J Med*, 334:349–55, 1996.
184. M Haber, IM Longini, and GA Cotsonis. Models for the statistical analysis of infectious disease data. *Biometrics*, 44:163–173, 1988.
185. ME Halloran. Invited commentary: Challenges of using contact data to understand acute respiratory disease transmission. *Am J Epidemiol*, 164:945–946, 2006, doi:10.1093/aje/kwj317.
186. ME Halloran, S Cochi, T Lieu, M Wharton, and LJ Fehrs. Theoretical epidemiologic and morbidity effects of routine immunization of preschool children with live-virus varicella vaccine in the U.S. *Am J Epidemiol*, 140:81–104, 1994a.
187. ME Halloran, MJ Haber, and IM Longini. Interpretation and estimation of vaccine efficacy under heterogeneity. *Am J Epidemiol*, 136:328–343, 1992.

188. ME Halloran, MJ Haber, IM Longini, and CJ Struchiner. Direct and indirect effects in vaccine field efficacy and effectiveness. *Am J Epidemiol*, 133:323–331, 1991.
189. ME Halloran, FG Hayden, Y Yang, IM Longini, and AS Monto. Antiviral effects on influenza viral transmission and pathogenicity: Observations from household-based trials. *Am J Epidemiol*, 165:212–221, 2007a, doi:10.1093/aje/kwj362.
190. ME Halloran and IM Longini. Using validation sets for outcomes and exposure to infection in vaccine field studies. *Am J Epidemiol*, 154:391–398, 2001.
191. ME Halloran and IM Longini. Community studies for vaccinating schoolchildren against influenza. *Science*, 311:615–616, 2006.
192. ME Halloran, IM Longini, DM Cowart, and A Nizam. Community trials of vaccination and the epidemic prevention potential. *Vaccine*, 20:3254–62, 2002a.
193. ME Halloran, IM Longini, MJ Gaglani, PA Piedra, H Chu, GB Herschler, and WP Glezen. Estimating efficacy of trivalent, cold-adapted, influenza virus vaccine (CAIV-T) against influenza A (H1N1) and B using surveillance cultures. *Am J Epidemiol*, 158:305–311, 2003a.
194. ME Halloran, IM Longini, A Nizam, and Y Yang. Containing bioterrorist smallpox. *Science*, 298:1428–32, 2002b.
195. ME Halloran, IM Longini, and CJ Struchiner. Estimability and interpretation of vaccine efficacy using frailty mixing models. *Am J Epidemiol*, 144:83–97, 1996.
196. ME Halloran, IM Longini, and CJ Struchiner. Design and interpretation of vaccine field studies. *Epidemiol Rev*, 21:73–88, 1999.
197. ME Halloran, IM Longini, CJ Struchiner, MJ Haber, and RC Brunet. Exposure efficacy and change in contact rates in evaluating prophylactic HIV vaccines in the field. *Stat Med*, 13:357–377, 1994b.
198. ME Halloran, PA Piedra, IM Longini, MJ Gaglani, B Schmotzer, C Fewlass, GB Herschler, and WP Glezen. Efficacy of trivalent, cold-adapted, influenza virus vaccine against influenza A (Fujian), a drift variant, during 2003-2004. *Vaccine*, 25:4038–45, 2007b.
199. ME Halloran, M-P Préziosi, and H Chu. Estimating vaccine efficacy from secondary attack rates. *J Am Stat Assoc*, 98:38–46, 2003b.
200. ME Halloran and CJ Struchiner. Study designs for dependent happenings. *Epidemiology*, 2:331–338, 1991.
201. ME Halloran and CJ Struchiner. Causal inference for infectious diseases. *Epidemiology*, 6:142–151, 1995.
202. ME Halloran, CJ Struchiner, and IM Longini. Study designs for different efficacy and effectiveness aspects of vaccination. *Am J Epidemiol*, 146:789–803, 1997.
203. ME Halloran, CJ Struchiner, and A Spielman. Modeling malaria vaccines II: Population effects of stage-specific malaria vaccines dependent on natural boosting. *Math Biosci*, 94:115–149, 1989.
204. ME Halloran, CJ Struchiner, and L Watelet. Epidemiologic effects of vaccines with complex effects in an age-structured population. *Math Biosci*, 121:193–225, 1994c.
205. ME Halloran, NM Ferguson, S Eubank, IM Longini, et al. Modeling targeted layered containment of an influenza pandemic in the United States. *Proc Natl Acad Sci USA*, 105:4639–4644, 2008.
206. WH Hamer. Epidemic disease in England. *Lancet*, 1:733–9, 1906.
207. T Hastie and R Tibshirani. Varying-coefficients models. *J R Stat Soc Series B*, 55:757–796, 1993.
208. CH Hau, TT Hien, NTK Tien, HB Khiem, PK Sac, VT Nhung, RP Larasati, K Laras, MP Putri, R Doss, KC Hyams, and AL Corwin. Prevalence of enteric hepatitis A and E viruses in the Mekong River Delta region of Vietnam. *Am J Trop Med Hyg*, 60:277–280, 1999.
209. FG Hayden, R Belshe, C Villanueva, R Lanno, C Hughes, I Small, R Dutkowski, P Ward, and J Carr. Management of influenza in households: A prospective, randomized comparison of oseltamivir treatment with or without postexposure prophylaxis. *J Infect Dis*, 189:440–9, 2004.
210. FG Hayden, LV Gubareva, AS Monto, et al. Inhaled zanamivir for the prevention of influenza in families. *N Engl J Medicine*, 343:1282–89, 2000.

211. R Hayes, F Mosha, A Nicoll, H Grosskurth, J Newell, J Todd, J Killewo, J Rugemalila, and D Mabey. A community trial of the impact of improved sexually transmitted disease treatment on HIV epidemic in rural Tanzania: 1. Design. *AIDS*, 9:919–926, 1995.
212. RJ Hayes, NDE Alexander, S Bennett, and SN Cousens. Design and analysis issues in cluster-randomized trials of interventions against infectious diseases. *Stat Methods Med Res*, 9:95–116, 2000.
213. RJ Hayes and S Bennett. Simple sample size calculation for cluster-randomized trials. *Int J Epidemiol*, 28:319–326, 1999.
214. RJ Hayes and LH Moulton. *Cluster Randomised Trials: A Practical Approach*. Chapman and Hall/CRC, Boca Raton, FL, 2009.
215. TW Hennessy, RJ Singleton, LR Bulkow, DL Bruden, DA Hurlburt, D Parks, M Moore, AJ Parkinson, A Schuchat, and JC Butler. Impact of heptavalent pneumococcal conjugate vaccine on invasive disease, antimicrobial resistance and colonization in Alaska Natives: Progress towards elimination of a health disparity. *Vaccine*, 23:5464–5473, 2005.
216. HW Hethcote. Qualitative analyses of communicable disease models. *Math Biosci*, 28:335–356, 1976.
217. HW Hethcote and JA Yorke. *Gonorrhea transmission dynamics and control*. Lecture Notes in Mathematics 56. Springer-Verlag, Berlin, 1984.
218. AW Hightower, WA Orenstein, and SM Martin. Recommendations for the use of Taylor series confidence intervals for estimates of vaccine efficacy. *Bull WHO*, 66(1):99–105, 1988.
219. AN Hill and IM Longini. The critical vaccination fraction for heterogeneous epidemic models. *Math Biosci*, 181:85–106, 2002.
220. PW Holland. Statistics and causal inference. *J Am Stat Assoc*, 81:945–960, 1986.
221. RE Hope-Simpson. Infectiousness of communicable diseases in the household. *Lancet*, ii:549–554, 1952.
222. F Hoti, P Erasto, T Leino, and K Auranen. Outbreaks of *Streptococcus pneumoniae* carriage in day care cohorts in Finland – implications for elimination of transmission. *BMC Infect Dis*, 9:102, 2009.
223. MG Hudgens and PB Gilbert. Assessing vaccine effects in repeated low-dose challenge experiments. *Biometrics*, .:in press, 2009.
224. MG Hudgens, PB Gilbert, and SG Self. Endpoints in vaccine trials. *Stat Methods Med Res*, 13:89–114, 2004.
225. MG Hudgens and ME Halloran. Causal vaccine effects on binary postinfection outcomes. *J Am Stat Assoc*, 101:51–64, 2006.
226. MG Hudgens and ME Halloran. Towards causal inference with interference. *J Am Stat Assoc*, 103:832–842, 2008.
227. MG Hudgens, A Hoering, and SG Self. On the analysis of viral load endpoints in HIV vaccine trials. *Stat Med*, 22:2281–2298, 2003.
228. MG Hudgens, IM Longini, ME Halloran, K Choopanya, S Vanichseni, D Kitayaporn, TD Mastro, and PA Mock. Estimating the HIV transmission probability in injecting drug users in Thailand. *Appl Stat*, 50:1–14, 2001.
229. JP Hughes. Using baseline data to design a group randomized trial. *Stat Med*, 24:1983–1994, 2005.
230. JP Hughes. Stepped wedge design. In RB D'Agostino, L Sullivan, and J Massaro, editors, *Wiley Encyclopedia of Clinical Trials*. John Wiley and Sons, Chichester, UK, 2008.
231. JP Hughes, RL Goldenberg, CM Wilfert et al. Design of the HIV Prevention Trials Network (HPTN) Protocol 54: A cluster randomized crossover trial to evaluate combined access to Nevirapine in developing countries. *The Berkeley Electronic Press*, .:http://www.bepress.com/uwbiostat/paper195, 2003.
232. M Hussain, A Melegaro, RG Pebody, et al. A longitudinal household study of *Streptococcus pneumoniae* nasopharyngeal carriage in the UK setting. *Epidemiol Infect*, 133:891–8, 2005.
233. MA Hussey and JP Hughes. Design and analysis of stepped wedge cluster randomized trials. *Contemp Clin Trials*, 28:182–191, 2007.
234. S Jaffar, A Leach, AJ Hall, and et al. Preparation for a pneumococcal trial in The Gambia: Individual or community randomisation. *Vaccine*, 18:633–640, 1999.

235. Y Jemiai, A Rotnitzky, BE Shepherd, and PB Gilbert. Semiparametric estimation of treatment effects given baseline covariates on an outcome measured after a post-randomization event occurs. *J R Stat Soc Series B*, 69:879–901, 2007.
236. D Jenkinson. Duration of effectiveness of pertussis vaccine: Evidence from a 10-year community study. *Br Med J*, 296:612–614, 1988.
237. NP Jewell. On the bias of commonly used measures of association for 2x2 tables. *Biometrics*, 42:351–358, 1986.
238. L Jódar, FM LaForce, C Ceccarini, T Aguado, and DM Granoff. Meningococcal conjugate vaccine for Africa: A model for development of new vaccines for the poorest countries. *Lancet*, 361:1902–1904, 2003.
239. L Jódar, J Butler, G Carlone, R Dagan, et al. Serological criteria for evaluation and licensure of new pneumococcal conjugate vaccine formulations for use in infants. *Vaccine*, 21(23):3265–3272, 2003.
240. S Jones, K Evans, H McElwaine-Johnn et al. DNA vaccination protects against an influenza challenge in a double-blind randomised placebo-controlled phase 1b clinical trial. *Vaccine*, 27:2506–2512, 2009.
241. R Jordan, M Connock, E Albon, A Fry Smith, B Olowokure, J Hawker, and A Burls. Universal vaccination of children against influenza: Are there indirect benefits to the community? A systematic review of the evidence. *Vaccine*, 24:1047–1062, 2006.
242. WS Jordan, FW Denny, GF Badger, S Curtiss, JH Dingle, R Oseasohn, and DA Stevens. A study of illness in a group of Cleveland families. XVII. The occurrence of Asian influenza. *Am J Hyg*, 68:190–212, 1958.
243. JD Kalbfleisch and RL Prentice. *The Statistical Analysis of Failure Time Data*. John Wiley and Sons, New York, 1980.
244. MN Kanaan and CP Farrington. Estimation of waning vaccine efficacy. *J Am Stat Assoc*, 97:389–397, 2002.
245. EL Kaplan and P Meier. Nonparametric estimation from incomplete observations. *J Am Stat Assoc*, 53:457–481, 1958.
246. S Karlin and HM Taylor. *A First Course in Stochastic Processes*. Academic Press, London, 1975.
247. D Katz, J Baptista, SP Azen, and MC Pike. Obtaining confidence intervals for the risk ratio in cohort studies. *Biometrics*, 34:469–74, 1978.
248. H Käyhty, K Auranen, H Nohynek, R Dagan, H Mäkelä, and the Pneumococcal Carriage Group. Nasopharyngeal carriage: A target for pneumococcal vaccination. *Expert Rev Vaccines*, 5:651–667, 2006.
249. MJ Keeling and P Rohani. *Modeling Infectious Diseases in Humans and Animals*. Princeton University Press, Princeton, NJ, 2008.
250. JT Kemper. Error sources in the evaluation of secondary attack rates. *Am J Epidemiol*, 112:457–464, 1980.
251. E Kenah and JM Robins. Second look at the spread of epidemics on networks. *Phys Rev E*, 76:036113, 2007a.
252. E Kenah and JM Robins. Network-based analysis of stochastic SIR epidemic models with random and proportionate mixing. *J Theor Biol*, 249:706–722, 2007b.
253. P Kendrick and G Eldering. A study in active immunization against pertussis. *Am J Hyg, Sect B*, 38:133, 1939.
254. WO Kermack and AG McKendrick. A contribution to the mathematical theory of epidemics. *Proc Roy Soc Lond Ser A*, 115:700–721, 1927.
255. R Kim-Farley, S Bart, H Stetler, et al. Clinical mumps vaccine efficacy. *Am J Epidemiol*, 121:593–597, 1985.
256. JC King, JJ Stoddard, MB Gaglani, KA Moore, L Magder, E McClure, JD Rubin, JA Englund, and K Neuzil. Effectiveness of school-based influenza vaccination. *N Engl J Med*, 355:2523–2532, 2006.
257. N Klar, T Gyorkos, and A Donner. Cluster randomization trials in tropical medicine: A case study. *Trans R Soc Trop Med Hygiene*, 89:454–459, 1995.

258. EG Knox. Strategy for rubella vaccination. *Int J Epidemiol*, 9:13–23, 1980.
259. TD Koepsell, EH Wagner, AC Cheadle, DL Patrick, DC Martin, PH Diehr, EB Perrin, AR Kristal, CH Allan-Andrilla, and LJ Dey. Selected methodological issues in evaluating community-based health promotion and disease prevention programs. *Annu Rev Public Health*, 13:31–57, 1992.
260. RC Kohberger, D Jemiolo, and F Noriega. Prediction of pertussis vaccine efficacy using a correlates of protection model. *Vaccine*, 26:3516–3521, 2008.
261. JS Koopman, SE Chick, CS Riolo, AL Adams, ML Wilson, and MP Becker. Modeling contact networks and infection transmission through networks in geographic and social space using GERMS. *Sex Transm Dis*, 27:617–626, 2000.
262. JS Koopman and RJ Little. Assessing HIV vaccine effects. *Am J Epidemiol*, 142:1113–20, 1995.
263. PAR Koopman. Confidence limits for the ratio of two binomial proportions. *Biometrics*, 40:513–517, 1984.
264. T Leino, F Hoti, R Syrjänen, A Tanskanen, and K Auranen. Clustering of serotypes in a longitudinal study of *Streptococcus pneumoniae* in three day care centers. *BMC Infect Dis*, 8:173, 2008.
265. KY Liang and SL Zeger. Longitudinal data analysis using generalized linear models. *Biometrika*, 73:13–22, 1986.
266. DV Lindley and MR Novick. The role of exchangeability in inference. *Ann Stat*, 9:45–58, 1981.
267. M Lipsitch. Interpreting results from trials of pneumococcal conjugate vaccines: a statistical test for detecting vaccine-induced increases in carriage of non-vaccine serotypes. *Am J Epidemiol*, 154:85–92, 2000.
268. RJA Little and DA Rubin. *Statistical Analysis with Missing Data*. John Wiley, Hoboken, New Jersey, second edition, 2002.
269. IM Longini, S Datta, and ME Halloran. Measuring vaccine efficacy for both susceptibility to infection and reduction in infectiousness for prophylactic HIV-1 vaccines. *J Acq Immun Def Synd*, 13:440–447, 1996.
270. IM Longini and ME Halloran. A frailty mixture model for estimating vaccine efficacy. *Appl Stat*, 45:165–173, 1996.
271. IM Longini, ME Halloran, MJ Haber, and RT Chen. Measuring vaccine efficacy from outbreaks of acute infectious agents. *Stat Med*, 12:249–263, 1993.
272. IM Longini, ME Halloran, A Nizam, M Wolff, PM Mendelman, P Fast, and RB Belshe. Estimation of the efficacy of live, attenuated influenza vaccine from a two-year, multi-center vaccine trial: Implications for influenza epidemic control. *Vaccine*, 18:1902–9, 2000.
273. IM Longini, ME Halloran, A Nizam, and Y Yang. Containing pandemic influenza with antiviral agents. *Am J Epidemiol*, 159:623–633, 2004.
274. IM Longini, ME Halloran, A Nizam, Y Yang, Shufu Xu, DS Burke, DAT Cummings, and JM Epstein. Containing a large bioterrorist smallpox attack: A computer simulation approach. *Int J Infect Dis*, 11:98–108, 2007a.
275. IM Longini, MG Hudgens, ME Halloran, and K Sagatelian. A Markov model for measuring vaccine efficacy for both susceptibility to infection and reduction in infectiousness for prophylactic HIV-1 vaccines. *Stat Med*, 18:53–68, 1999.
276. IM Longini and JS Koopman. Household and community transmission parameters from final distributions of infections in households. *Biometrics*, 38(1):115–126, 1982.
277. IM Longini, JS Koopman, M Haber, and GA Cotsonis. Statistical inference for infectious diseases: Risk-specified household and community transmission parameters. *Am J Epidemiol*, 128:845–859, 1988.
278. IM Longini, A Nizam, S Xu, K Ungchusak, W Hanshaoworakul, DAT Cummings, and ME Halloran. Containing pandemic influenza at the source. *Science*, 309:1083–87, 2005.
279. IM Longini, K Sagatelian, WN Rida, and Halloran ME. Optimal vaccine trials design when estimating vaccine efficacy for susceptibility and infectiousness from multiple populations. *Stat Med*, 17:1121–1136, 1998.

280. IM Longini, A Nizam, M Ali, et al. Controlling endemic cholera with oral vaccines. *PLoS Med*, 4(11):e336. doi:10.1371/journal.pmed.0040336, 2007b.
281. G Macdonald. *The Epidemiology and Control of Malaria*. Oxford University Press, London, 1957.
282. T Madsen. Vaccination against whooping cough. *J Am Med Assoc*, 101:187–188, 1933.
283. L Magder and R Brookmeyer. Analysis of infectious disease data from partners studies with unknown source of infection. *Biometrics*, 49:1110–6, 1993.
284. J de OC Maia. Some mathematical developments on the epidemic theory formulated by Reed and Frost. *Hum Biol*, 24:167–200, 1952.
285. DC Martin, P Diehr, EB Perrin, and TD Koepsell. The effect of matching on the power of randomized community intervention studies. *Stat Med*, 12:329–38, 1993.
286. AR McLean, DJ Nokes, and RM Anderson. Model-based comparison of measles immunization strategies using high dose Edmonston-Zagreb type vaccines. *Int J Epidemiol*, 20:1–11, 1991.
287. WH McNeill. *Plagues and Peoples*. Doubleday, New York, 1976.
288. Medical Research Council. The prevention of whooping-cough by vaccination. *Br Med J*, 1:1463–1471, 1951.
289. DV Mehrotra, X Li, and PB Gilbert. Comparison of eight methods for the dual-endpoint evaluation of efficacy in a proof-of-concept trial. *Biometrics*, 62:893–900, 2006.
290. A Melegaro, Y Choi, R Pebody, and N Gay. Pneumococcal carriage in United Kingdom families: Estimating serotype-specific transmission parameters from longitudinal data. *Am J Epidemiol*, 166:228–235, 2007.
291. A Melegaro, NJ Gay, and GF Medley. Estimating the transmission parameters of pneumococcal carriage in households. *Epidemiol Infect*, 132:433–441, 2004.
292. LA Meyers, ME Newman, and B Pourbohlol. Predicting epidemics on directed contact networks. *J Theor Biol*, 240:400–418, 2006.
293. E Miller and NJ Gay. Epidemiological determinants of pertussis. *Dev Biol Stand*, 89:15–23, 1997.
294. D Moher, KF Schulz, and DG Altman. The CONSORT statement: Revised recommendations for improving the quality of reports of parallel-group randomised trials. *Lancet*, 357:1191–1194, 2001.
295. G Molenberghs, MG Kenward, and E Goetghebeur. Sensitivity analysis for incomplete contingency tables: the Slovenian plebiscite case. *Appl Stat*, 50:15–30, 2001.
296. L Molineaux, RH Morrow, and DA Muir. Epidemiological evaluation of *P. falciparum* vaccines: Suggestions submitted for discussion. *UNDP/World Bank/WHO TDR Working Paper No.14*, 1985.
297. AS Monto, JA Davenport, JA Napier, and TF Francis. Effect of vaccination of a school-age population upon the course of an A2/Hong Kong influenza epidemic. *Bull World Health Organ*, 41:537–542, 1969.
298. AS Monto, JS Koopman, and IM Longini. The Tecumseh study of illness. XII. Influenza infection and disease, 1976-1981. *Am J Epidemiol*, 121:811–822, 1985.
299. AS Monto, ME Pichichero, SJ Blanckenberg, O Ruuskanen, C Cooper, DM Fleming, and C Kerr. Zanamivir prophylaxis: an effective strategy for the prevention of influenza types A and B within households. *J Infect Dis*, 186:1582–8, 2002.
300. M Morris and M Kretzschmar. Concurrent partnerships and the spread of HIV. *AIDS*, 11:641–648, 1997.
301. LH Moulton. Covariate-based constrained randomization of group-randomized trials. *Clin Trials*, 1:297–305, 2004.
302. LH Moulton, JE Golub, B Durovni, SC Cavalcante, AG Pacheco, V Saraceni, B King, and RE Chaisson. Statistical design of THRio: A phased implementation clinic-randomized study of a tuberculosis preventive therapy intervention. *Clin Trials*, 4:190–199, 2007.
303. LH Moulton, KL O'Brien, R Kohberger, I Chang, R Reid, R Weatherholtz, JG Hackell, GR Siber, and M Santosham. Design of a group-randomised *Streptococcus pneumoniae* vaccine trial. *Contr Clin Trials*, 22:438–452, 2001.

304. LH Moulton, KL O'Brien, R Reid, R Weatherholz, M Santosham, and GR Siber. Evaluation of the indirect effects of a pneumococcal vaccine in a community-randomized study. *J Biopharm Stat*, 16:453–462, 2006.
305. KM Murphy, P Travers, and M Walport. *Janeway's Immunobiology*. Garland Science Publishing, New York and London, 7th edition, 2008.
306. TV Murphy, PM Gargiullo, MS Massoudi, et al. Intussusception among infants given an oral rotavirus vaccine. *N Engl J Med*, 344:564–72, 2001.
307. DM Murray. *Design and Analysis of Group-Randomized Trials*. Oxford University Press, New York, 1998.
308. DM Musher. Pneumococcal vaccine: direct and indirect ("herd") effects (editorial). *N Engl J Med*, 354:1522–24, 2006.
309. RE Neustadt and HV Fineberg. *The Swine Flu Affair: Decision-Making on a Slippery Disease*. University Press of the Pacific, Honolulu, 2005.
310. M Newman, A-L Barabási, and DJ Watts. *The Structure and Dynamics of Networks*. Princeton University Press, Princeton, NJ, 2006.
311. KL Nichol, PM Mendelman, KP Mallon, LA Jackson, GJ Gorse, RB Belshe, WP Glezen, and J Wittes. Effectiveness of live, attenuated intranasal influenza virus vaccine in healthy working adults: A randomized controlled trial. *J Am Med Assoc*, 282:137–144, 1999.
312. F Nosten, C Luxemburger, DE Kyle, WR Ballou, et al. Randomised double-blind placebo-controlled trial of SPf66 malaria vaccine in children in northwestern Thailand. *Lancet*, 348:701–07, 1996.
313. O Noya, YG Berti, BA de Noya, et al. A population-based clinical trial with the SPf66 synthetic *Plasmodium falciparum* malaria vaccines in Venezuela. *J Infect Dis*, 170:396–402, 1994.
314. P Olin, F Rasmussen, L Gustafsson, HO Hallander, and H Heijbel. Randomised controlled trial of two-component, three-component, and five component acellular pertussis vaccines compared with whole-cell pertussis vaccine. *Lancet*, 350:1569–77, 1997.
315. PD O'Neill, DJ Balding, NG Becker, M Eerola, and D Mollison. Analyses of infectious disease data from household outbreaks by Markov chain Monte Carlo methods. *Appl Stat*, 49:517–542, 2000.
316. RT O'Neill. On sample sizes to estimate the protective efficacy of a vaccine. *Stat Med*, 7:1279–1288, 1988.
317. WA Orenstein, RH Bernier, TJ Dondero, AR Hinman, JS Marks, KJ Bart, and B Sirotkin. Field evaluation of vaccine efficacy. *Bull World Health Organ*, 63(6):1055–1068, 1985.
318. WA Orenstein, RH Bernier, and AR Hinman. Assessing vaccine efficacy in the field: Further observations. *Epidemiol Rev*, 10:212–241, 1988.
319. DM Oshinsky. *Polio: An American Story*. Oxford University Press, New York, 2005.
320. ME Patarroyo, P Romero, ML Torres, P Clavijo, A Moreno, A Martínez, R Rodríguez, F Guzman, and E Cabezas. Induction of protective immunity against experimental infection with malaria using synthetic peptides. *Nature*, 328:629–632, 1987.
321. ME Patarroyo, R Amador, P Clavijo, et al. A synthetic vaccine protects against challenge with asexual blood stages of *Plasmodium falciparum* malaria. *Nature*, 322:158–161, 1988.
322. K Pearson. Report on certain enteric fever inoculation statistics. *Br Med J*, Nov 5, Nov 19, Dec 3, Dec 17, Dec 31:1243–6,1432,1542,1667–8,1775–6, 1904.
323. MS Pepe, M Reilly, and TR Fleming. Auxiliary outcome data and the mean score method. *J Stat Plan Inference*, 42:137–160, 1994.
324. TR Peters and KA Poehling. Invasive pneumococcal disease: the target is moving. *J Am Med Assoc*, 297(16):1825–6, 2007.
325. R Peto. Experimental survival curves for interval-censored data. *Appl Stat*, 22:86–91, 1973.
326. PHLS Epidemiologic Research Laboratory. Efficacy of pertussis vaccination in England. *Br Med J*, 285:357–9, 1982.
327. PA Piedra, MJ Gaglani, CA Kozinetz, G Herschler, M Riggs, M Griffith, C Fewlass, M Watts, C Hessel, J Cordova, and WP Glezen. Herd immunity in adults against influenza-related illnesses with use of the trivalent-live attenuated influenza vaccine (CAIV-T) in children. *Vaccine*, 23:1540–8, 2005.

328. PA Piedra, MJ Gaglani, CA Kozinetz, GB Herschler, C Fewlass, D Harvey, N Zimmerman, and Glezen WP. Live attenuated intranasal influenza vaccine-trivalent (LAIV-T) administered during the 2003-04 influenza type A (H3N2) outbreak provided immediate, direct and indirect protection in children. *Pediatrics*, 120:e553–e564, 2007.
329. S Pilyugin, J Mittler, and R Antia. Modeling T-cell proliferation: An investigation of the consequences of the Hayflick Limit. *J Theor Biol*, 186:117–129, 1997.
330. SA Plotkin, WA Orenstein, and PA Offit. *Vaccines*. Elsevier/Saunders, Philadelphia, 5th edition, 2008.
331. SL Plotkin and SA Plotkin. A short history of vaccination. In SA Plotkin, WA Orenstein, and PA Offit, editors, *Vaccines*. Elsevier/Saunders, Philadelphia, 5th edition, 2008.
332. RL Prentice. A case-cohort design for epidemiologic cohort studies and disease prevention trials. *Biometrika*, 73:1–11, 1986.
333. RL Prentice. Surrogate endpoints in clinical trials: Definition and operational criteria. *Stat Med*, 8:431–440, 1989.
334. RL Prentice and NE Breslow. Retrospective studies and failure time models. *Biometrika*, 65(1):153–158, 1978.
335. RL Prentice and L Sheppard. Aggregate data studies of disease risk factors. *Biometrika*, 82:113–125, 1995.
336. M-P Préziosi and ME Halloran. Effects of pertussis vaccination on severity: vaccine efficacy for clinical severity. *Clin Infect Dis*, 37:772–779, 2003a.
337. M-P Préziosi and ME Halloran. Effects of pertussis vaccination on transmission: vaccine efficacy for infectiousness. *Vaccine*, 21:1853–1861, 2003b.
338. MP Préziosi, A Yam, M Ndiaye, A Simaga, F Simondon, and SG Wassilak. Practical experiences in obtaining informed consent for a vaccine trial in rural Africa. *N Engl J Med*, 336:370–73, 1997.
339. MP Préziosi, A Yam, SG Wassilak, L Chabirand, A Simaga, M Ndiaye, F Dia, M Dabis, and F Simondon. Epidemiology of whooping cough in a West African community before and after introduction of a widespread vaccination programme. *Am J Epidemiol*, 155:891–6, 2002.
340. L Qin, PB Gilbert, L Corey, MJ McElrath, and SG Self. A framework for assessing immunological correlates of protection in vaccine trials. *J Infect Dis*, 196:1304–12, 2007.
341. L Qin, PB Gilbert, L Corey, MJ McElrath, and SG Self. Assessing surrogate endpoints in vaccine trials with case-cohort sampling and the Cox model. *Ann Appl Stat*, 2:386–407, 2008.
342. AH Rampey, IM Longini, MJ Haber, and AS Monto. A discrete-time model for the statistical analysis of infectious disease incidence data. *Biometrics*, 48:117–128, 1992.
343. ME Ramsay, NJ Andrews, CL Trotter, EB Kaczmarski, and E Miller. Herd immunity from meningococcal serogroup C conjugate vaccination in England: Database analysis. *Br Med J*, 326:365–6, 2003.
344. ME Ramsay, CP Farrington, and E Miller. Age-specific efficacy of pertussis vaccine during epidemic and non-epidemic periods. *Epidemiol Infect*, 111:41–48, 1993.
345. TA Reichert, Sugaya, N, Fedson, DS, et al. The Japanese experience with vaccinating schoolchildren against influenza. *N Engl J Med*, 344:889–896, 2001.
346. PH Rhodes, ME Halloran, and IM Longini. Counting process models for differentiating exposure to infection and susceptibility. Technical Report 94–1, Division of Biostatistics, Emory University School of Public Health, 1994.
347. PH Rhodes, ME Halloran, and IM Longini. Counting process models for differentiating exposure to infection and susceptibility. *J R Stat Soc Series B*, 58:751–762, 1996.
348. WN Rida. Asymptotic properties of some estimators for the infection rate in the general stochastic epidemic model. *J R Stat Soc Series B*, 53:269–283, 1991.
349. WN Rida, PE Fast, R Hoff, and T Fleming. Intermediate-size trials for the evaluation of HIV vaccine candidates: A workshop summary. *J Acquir Immune Defic Syndr Hum Retrovirol*, 16:195–203, 1997.
350. WN Rida and S Sandberg. Modeling the population level effects of an HIV-1 vaccine in an era of highly active antiretroviral therapy. *Bull Math Biol*, 71:648–680, 2009.

351. H Rinta-Kokko, R Dagan, N Givon-Lavi, and K Auranen. Estimation of vaccine efficacy against acquisition of pneumococcal carriage. *Vaccine*, 27:3831–3837, 2009.
352. JM Robins. A new approach to causal inference in mortality studies with sustained exposure period — Application to control of the healthy worker survivor effect. *Math Model*, 7:1393–1512, 1986.
353. JM Robins and S Greenland. Estimability and estimation of excess and etiologic fraction. *Stat Med*, 8:845–859, 1989.
354. JM Robins and S Greenland. Identifiability and exchangeability for direct and indirect effects. *Epidemiology*, 3:143–155, 1992.
355. JM Robins and S Greenland. Adjusting for differential rates of PCP prophylaxis in high-versus low-dose AZT treatment arms in an AIDS randomized trial. *J Am Stat Assoc*, 89:737–749, 1994.
356. JM Robins, MA Hérnan, and BA Brumback. Marginal structural models in causal inference in epidemiology. *Epidemiology*, 11:550–560, 2000a.
357. JM Robins, A Rotnitzky, and DO Scharfstein. Sensitivity analysis for selection bias and unmeasured confounding in missing data and causal inference models. In ME Halloran and Berry DA, editors, *Statistics in Epidemiology, Environment and Clinical Trials*. Springer-Verlag, 2000b.
358. L Rodrigues and P Smith. Case-control approach to vaccine evaluation. *Epidemiol Rev*, 21:56–72, 1999.
359. V Romanus, R Jonsell, and S-O Bergquist. Pertussis in Sweden after the cessation of general immunization in 1979. *Pediatr Infect Dis*, 6:364–71, 1987.
360. P Rosenbaum. *Observational Studies*. Springer-Verlag, Berlin, 1995.
361. PR Rosenbaum. The consequences of adjustment for a concomitant variable that has been affected by the treatment. *J R Stat Soc Series A*, 147:656–666, 1984.
362. R Ross. *The Prevention of Malaria*. John Murray, London, 2nd edition, 1911.
363. R Ross. Some *a priori* pathometric equations. *Brit Med J*, 1:546–7, 1915.
364. R Ross. An application of the theory of probabilities to the study of *a priori* pathometry, Part 1. *Proc R Soc Series A*, 92:204–230, 1916.
365. K Rothman, S Greenland, and TL Lash. *Modern Epidemiology*. Lippincott Williams and Wilkins, Philadelphia, third edition, 2008.
366. A Rotnitzky, JM Robins, and D Scharfstein. Semiparametric regression for repeated outcomes with non-ignorable non-response. *J Am Stat Assoc*, 93:1321–39, 1998.
367. A Rotnitzky, D Scharfstein, T Su, and JM Robins. Methods for conducting sensitivity analysis of trials with potentially non-ignorable competeing casues of censoring. *Biometrics*, 57:103–113, 2001.
368. DB Rubin. Bayesian inference for causal effects: The role of randomization. *Ann Stat*, 7:34–58, 1978.
369. DB Rubin. Discussion of "Randomization analysis of experimental data in the Fisher randomization test" by Basu. *J Am Stat Assoc*, 75:591–593, 1980.
370. DB Rubin. Comment: Neyman (1923) and causal inference in experiments and observational studies. *Stat Sci*, 5:472–480, 1990.
371. DB Rubin. Practical implications of modes of statistical inference for causal effect and the critical role of the assignment mechanism. *Biometrics*, 47:1213–1234, 1991.
372. LG Rudenko, AN Slepushkin, AS Monto, et al. Efficacy of live attenuated and inactivated influenza vaccines in schoolchildren and their unvaccinated contacts in Novgorod, Russia. *J Infect Dis*, 168:881–887, 1993.
373. T Ruuska and T Vesikari. Rotavirus disease in Finnish children: use of numerical scores for clinical severity of diarrhoeal episodes. *Scand J Infect Dis*, 22:259–267, 1990.
374. JC Sadoff and J Wittes. Correlates, surrogates, and vaccines. *J Infect Dis*, 196:1279–81, 2007.
375. M Santosham, M Wolff, R Reid, M Hohenboken, et al. The efficacy in Navajo infants of a conjugate vaccine consisting of *Haemophilus influenzae* type b polysaccharide and Neisseria meningitides outer-membrane protein complex. *New Engl J Med*, 324:1767–72, 1991.

376. LJ Savage. *The Foundations of Statistical Inference*. Methuen, London, 1962.
377. DO Scharfstein, MJ Daniels, and JM Robins. Incorporating prior beliefs about selection bias into the analysis of randomized trials with missing outcomes. *Biostatistics*, 4:495–512, 2003.
378. DO Scharfstein, ME Halloran, H Chu, and MJ Daniels. On estimation of vaccine efficacy using validation samples with selection bias. *Biostatistics*, 7:615–629, 2006.
379. DO Scharfstein, A Rotnitzky, and JM Robins. Adjusting for nonignorable drop-out using semiparametric nonresponse models. *J Am Stat Assoc*, 94:1096–1146, 1999.
380. D Schenzle. An age-structured model of pre- and post-vaccination measles transmission. *IMA J Math Appl Med Biol*, 1:169–191, 1984.
381. HJ Schmitt, H Carl, W von König, et al. Efficacy of acellular pertussis vaccine in early childhood after household exposure. *J Am Med Assoc*, 275:37–41, 1996.
382. D Schoenfeld. Partial residuals for the proportional hazards regression model. *Biometrika*, 69:239–41, 1982.
383. F Sempertegui, B Estrella, J Moscoso, et al. Safety, immunogenicity and protective effect of the SPf66 malaria synthetic vaccine against *Plasmodium falciparum* infection in a randomized double-blinded placebo-controlled trial in an endemic area of Ecuador. *Vaccine*, 12:337–42, 1994.
384. BE Shepherd, PB Gilbert, Y Jemiai, and A Rotnitzky. Sensitivity analyses comparing outcomes only existing in a subset selected post-randomization, conditional on covariates, with application to HIV. *Biometrics*, 62:332–342, 2006a.
385. BE Shepherd, PB Gilbert, and T Lumley. Sensitivity analyses comparing time-to-event outcomes existing only in a subset selected postrandomization. *J Am Stat Assoc*, 102:573–582, 2007.
386. BE Shepherd, PB Gilbert, and DV Mehrotra. Eliciting a counterfactual sensitivity parameter. *Am Stat*, 61:56–63, 2006b.
387. GR Siber. Methods for estimating serological correlates of protection. *Dev Biol Stand*, 89:283–296, 1997.
388. F Simondon, MP Préziosi, A Yam, CT Kane, L Chabirand, I Iteman, G Sanden, S Mboup, A Hoffenbach, K Knudsen, N Guiso, S Wassilak, and M Cadoz. A randomized double-blind trial comparing a two-component acellular to a whole-cell pertussis vaccine in Senegal. *Vaccine*, 15:1606–12, 1997.
389. RJ Singleton, TW Hennessey, LR Bulkow, LL Hammitt, T Zulz, DA Hurlburt, JC Butler, K Rudolph, and A Parkinson. Invasive pneumococcal disease caused by nonvaccine serotypes among Alaska native children with high levels of 7-valent pneumococcal conjugate vaccine coverage. *J Am Med Assoc*, 297(16):1784–92, 2007.
390. PG Smith. Retrospective assessment of the effectiveness of BCG vaccination against tuberculosis using the case-control method. *Tubercle*, 62:23–35, 1982.
391. PG Smith and R Morrow. *Field Trials of Health Interventions in Developing Countries: A Toolbox*. Macmillan, London, 1996.
392. PG Smith, LC Rodrigues, and PEM Fine. Assessment of the protective efficacy of vaccines against common diseases using case-control and cohort studies. *Int J Epidemiol*, 13(1):87–93, 1984.
393. GW Snedecor and WG Cochran. *Statistical Methods*. Iowa State University Press, Ames, sixth edition, 1967.
394. M Sobel. What do randomized studies of housing mobility demonstrate? Causal inference in the face of interference. *J Am Stat Assoc*, 1398–1407:2006, 101.
395. HE Soper. The interpretation of periodicity in disease prevalence. *J R Stat Soc Series A*, 92:34–61, 1929.
396. J Storsaeter, WC Blackwelder, and HO Hallander. Pertussis antibodies, protection, and vaccine efficacy after household exposure. *Am J Dis Child*, 146:167–172, 1992.
397. J Storsaeter, HO Hallander, L Gustafsson, and P Olin. Levels of anti-pertussis antibodies related to protection after household exposureto *Bordetella pertussis*. *Vaccine*, 16:1907–16, 1998.
398. CJ Struchiner and ME Halloran. Randomization and baseline transmission in vaccine field trials. *Epidemiol Infect*, 135:181–194, 2007.

399. CJ Struchiner, ME Halloran, RC Brunet, JMC Ribeiro, and E Massad. Malaria vaccines: Lessons from field trials. *Cadernos do Saúde Pública*, 10(supplement 2):310–326, 1994.
400. CJ Struchiner, ME Halloran, JM Robins, and A Spielman. The behavior of common measures of association used to assess a vaccination program under complex disease transmission patterns – a computer simulation study of malaria vaccines. *Int J Epidemiol*, 19:187–196, 1990.
401. CJ Struchiner, ME Halloran, and A Spielman. Modeling malaria vaccines I: New uses for old ideas. *Math Biosci*, 94:87–113, 1989.
402. H Sugiyama. Some statistical contributions to the health sciences. *Osaka City Med J*, 6:141–158, 1960.
403. Y Sun, PB Gilbert, and IW McKeague. Proportional hazards models with continuous marks. *Ann Stat*, 37:394–426, 2009.
404. Å Svensson. A note on generation times in epidemic models. *Math Biosci*, 208:300–311, 2006.
405. RK Syrjänen, TM Kilpi, TH Kaijalainen, EE Herva, and AK Takala. Nasopharyngeal carriage of *Streptococcus pneumoniae* in Finnish children younger than 2 years old. *J Infect Dis*, 184:451–9, 2001.
406. W Szmuness, CE Stevens, EJ Harley, et al. Hepatitis B vaccine: Demonstration of efficacy in a controlled trial in a high-risk population in the United States. *N Engl J Med*, 303:834–876, 1980.
407. MA Tanner and WH Wong. The calculation of the posterior distributions by data augmentation. *J Am Stat Assoc*, 82:528–540, 1987.
408. B Trollfors and E Rabo. Whooping cough in adults. *Br Med J*, 283:696–697, 1981.
409. B Trollfors, J Taranger, T Lagergard, V Sundh, DA Bryla, R Schneerson, and JB Robbins. Immunization of children with pertussis toxoid decreases spread of pertussis within the family. *Pediatr Infect Dis J*, 17:196–99, 1998.
410. B Trollfors, J Taranger, T Lagergard, et al. A placebo-controlled trial of a pertussis toxoid vaccine. *N Engl J Med*, 333:1045–50, 1995.
411. B Trollfors, J Taranger, T Lagergard, et al. Efficacy of a monocomponent pertussis toxoid vaccine after household exposure to pertussis. *J Pediatr*, 130:532–536, 1997.
412. P Ukkonen and C-H von Bonsdorff. Rubella immunity and morbidity: Effects of vaccination in Finland. *Scand J Infect Dis*, 20:255–259, 1988.
413. M Urdaneta, A Prata, CJ Struchiner, CE Costa, P Tauil, and M Boulos. Evaluation of SPf66 malaria vaccine efficacy in Brazil. *Am J Trop Med Hyg*, 58:378–385, 1998.
414. MV Valero, LR Amador, C Galindo, et al. Vaccination with SPf66, a chemically synthesised vaccine, against *Plasmodium falciparum* malaria in Colombia. *Lancet*, 341:705–710, 1993.
415. F van Loon, JD Clemens, J Chakraborty, MR Rao, BA Kay, DA Sack, M Yunus, M Ali, A Svennerholm, and J Holmgren. Field trial of inactivated oral cholera vaccines in Bangladesh: Results from five years of follow-up. *Vaccine*, 14:162–166, 1996.
416. JW Vaupel, KG Manton, and E Stallard. The impact of heterogeneity in individual frailty on the dynamics of mortality. *Demography*, 16:439–454, 1979.
417. M Vazquez, PS LaRussa, AA Gershon, SP Steinberg, K Freudigman, and ED Shapiro. The effectiveness of the varicella vaccine in clinical practice. *N Engl J Med*, 344:955–960, 2001.
418. T Vesikari, A Karvonen, T Korhonen, et al, and CAIV-T Transmission Study Group. A randomized, double-blind study of the safety, transmissibility and phenotypic and genotypic stability of cold-adapted influenza virus vaccine. *Pediatr Infect Dis J*, 25:590–595, 2006.
419. T Vesikari, T Rautanen, T Varis, GM Beards, and AZ Kapikian. Rhesus *Rotavirus* candidate vaccine. *Am J Dis Child*, 144:285–289, 1990.
420. S Viviani, P Carrieri, E Bah, and AJ Hall et al. 20 years into the Gambia Hepatitis Intervention Study: Assessment of initial hypotheses and prospects for evaluation of protective effectiveness against liver cancer. *Cancer Epidemiol Biomarkers Prev*, 17:3216–3223, 2008.
421. J Wallinga and P Teunis. Different epidemic curves for severe acute respiratory syndrome reveal similar impacts of control measures. *Am J Epidemiol*, 160:509–516, 2004.

422. J Wallinga, P Teunis, and M Kretzschmar. Using social contact data to estimate age-specific transmission parameters for infectious respiratory spread agents. *Am J Epidemiol*, 164:936–944, 2006.
423. DP Webster, S Dunachie, JM Vuola, et al. Enhanced T cell-mediated protection against malaria in human challenges by using the recombinant poxviruses FP9 and modified vaccinia virus Ankara. *Proc Natl Acad Sci*, 102:4836–4841, 2005.
424. R Welliver, Monto AS, Carewicz O, et al. Effectiveness of oseltamivir in preventing influenza in household contacts: A randomized controlled trial. *J Am Med Assoc*, 285:748–754, 2001.
425. CJ White, BJ Kuter, A Ngai, CS Hidelbrand, KL Isganitis, CM Patterson, A Capra, WJ Miller, DL Krah, PJ Provost, RW Ellis, and GB Calandra. Modified cases of chickenpox after varicella vaccination: Correlation of protection with antibody response. *Pediatr Infect Dis J*, 11:19–23, 1992.
426. FM White and M Pagano. A likelihood-based method for real-time estimation of the serial interval and reproductive number of an epidemic. *Stat Med*, 16:2999–3016, 2008.
427. J Whitehead. Fitting Cox's regression model to survival data using GLIM. *Appl Stat*, 29:268–275, 1980.
428. AE Wright. Antityphoid inoculation. *Br Med J*, Nov 12, Nov 26, Dec 10, Dec 24:1343–5,1489–91,1641,1727, 1904.
429. Y Yang, P Gilbert, IM Longini, and ME Halloran. A Bayesian framework for estimating vaccine efficacy per infectious contact. *Ann Appl Stat*, 2(4):1409–1431, 2009a.
430. Y Yang, ME Halloran, and IM Longini. A Bayesian model for evaluating influenza antiviral efficacy in household studies with asymptomatic infections. *Biostatistics*, 10(2):364–373, 2009b.
431. Y Yang, ME Halloran, J Sugimoto, and IM Longini. Detecting human-to-human transmission of Avian A(H5N1) influenza. *Emerging Infect Dis*, 13(9):1348–53, 2007a.
432. Y Yang, IM Longini, and ME Halloran. Design and evaluation of prophylactic interventions using infectious disease incidence data from close contact groups. *Appl Stat*, 55:317–330, 2006.
433. Y Yang, IM Longini, and ME Halloran. A data-augmentation method for infectious disease incidence data from close contact groups. *Comput Stat Data Anal*, 51(12):6582–95, 2007b.
434. Y Yang, IM Longini, and ME Halloran. A resampling-based test to detect person-to-person transmission of an infectious disease. *Ann Appl Stat*, 1:211–228, 2007c.

Index

Printed by Amazon Italia Logistica S.r.l.
Torrazza Piemonte (TO), Italy

51325516R00232